Fitness and Lifestyle Management for Law Enforcement

THIRD EDITION

Nancy Wagner Wisotzki

2008
EMOND MONTGOMERY PUBLICATIONS LIMITED
TORONTO, CANADA

Emond Montgomery Publications Limited
60 Shaftesbury Avenue
Toronto ON M4T 1A3
http://www.emp.ca

Printed in Canada.

We acknowledge the financial support of the Government of Canada through the Book Publishing Industry Development Program (BPIDP) for our publishing activities.

Acquisitions and developmental editor: Tammy Scherer
Marketing director: Dave Stokaluk
Copy editor: Valerie Adams
Supervising editor: Jim Lyons, WordsWorth Communications
Permissions and production editor: Debbie Gervais, WordsWorth Communications
Proofreader: David Handelsman, WordsWorth Communications
Text designer and typesetter: Shani Sohn, WordsWorth Communications
Indexer: Paula Pike, WordsWorth Communications
Cover designer: John Vegter

Library and Archives Canada Cataloguing in Publication

Wagner Wisotzki, Nancy, 1959-
Fitness and lifestyle management for law enforcement / Nancy Wagner Wisotzki. — 3rd ed.

Includes bibliographical references and index.
ISBN 978-1-55239-232-4

1. Police—Health and hygiene. 2. Police—Physical training. I. Title.

HV7936.H4W33 2008 613.02'43632 C2007-903965

To Mom and Dad
(Jean and Carl Wagner)
For the love and guidance and freedom to pursue my path of dreams

To the police officers who have touched my life, especially Larry
Thank you for your inspiration and zest for life
which helps to make health and fitness so important to me

Contents

PREFACE ix
ACKNOWLEDGMENTS xi

PART I Getting Started Toward a Healthy Lifestyle

CHAPTER 1 Wellness and Active Living: A Healthy Lifestyle

Chapter Objectives ... 3
A Wellness Profile ... 3
The Relationship Between Wellness and Fitness ... 4
The Health Benefits of Physical Activity ... 9
The Seven Dimensions of Health ... 10
Requirements for Ontario Police Officers ... 15
Key Terms ... 17
Exercises ... 18
References ... 22

CHAPTER 2 Goal Setting

Chapter Objectives ... 25
The Process of Change ... 25
Factors That Affect Participation in Physical Activity . 29
Understanding Your Goals ... 29
Short- and Long-Term Goals ... 30
Choosing Effective Goals ... 31
Staying On Track ... 31
Rewarding Yourself ... 32
Your Mission Statement ... 33
Examining the Pros and Cons of Change ... 33
Being Fit and Well for Life ... 34
Key Terms ... 34
Exercises ... 35
References ... 38

CHAPTER 3 Time Management

Chapter Objectives ... 39
The Benefits of Time Management ... 40
The Stages of Time Management ... 40
Final Thoughts on Time Management ... 47
Key Terms ... 47
Exercises ... 48
References ... 52

PART II Planning and Maintaining a Fitness Program

CHAPTER 4 Physical Fitness

Chapter Objectives ... 55
What Is Training? ... 56
Health-Related Fitness ... 56
Performance/Skill-Related Fitness ... 58
The Health Benefits of Physical Activity ... 59
The Principles of Physical Training ... 60
Training Methods ... 63
Guidelines for Starting a Fitness Program ... 65
Key Terms ... 66
Exercises ... 67
References ... 72

CHAPTER 5 Cardiorespiratory Fitness

Chapter Objectives ... 73
The Importance of Cardiorespiratory Fitness in Law Enforcement ... 73
The Benefits of Cardiorespiratory Fitness ... 74
Assessing Cardiorespiratory Fitness ... 74
Getting Started on Cardiorespiratory Training ... 76
Creating a Cardiorespiratory Fitness Program ... 79
Key Terms ... 85
Exercises ... 86
References ... 89

CHAPTER 6 Strength and Endurance Training

Chapter Objectives ... 91
The Importance of Strength and Endurance Training 91
The Benefits of Resistance Training ... 92
A Little Bit About Your Body and Muscles ... 93
Types of Muscle Fibre ... 93
The Basics of Strength and Endurance Training ... 94
Guidelines for Strength and Endurance Training ... 97
Example of Different Training Programs ... 99
Variations on Training Routines ... 100
Training Programs ... 108
Key Terms ... 108
Exercises ... 111
References ... 114

CHAPTER 7 Flexibility and Stretching

Chapter Objectives ... 115
Flexibility ... 115
Fast and Slow Muscle Fibres ... 116
The Benefits of Stretching ... 116
How Muscles Cooperate with Each Other ... 117
Types of Muscle Contractions ... 118
Stretching Techniques ... 118
Guidelines for Safe and Effective Stretching ... 119
Upper- and Lower-Body Stretching Exercises ... 120
Key Terms ... 128
Exercises ... 129
References ... 131

PART III *Nutrition and Body Composition*

CHAPTER 8 Nutrition

Chapter Objectives ... 135
Nutritional Concerns in Canada ... 136
Maintaining a Healthy Weight ... 136
Function of Food ... 137
Basic Nutrients ... 137
Canada's Food Guide ... 151
Making Wise Choices with the Four Food Groups ... 153
Understanding Portion Sizes and Labelling ... 153
Understanding the Caloric Value of Nutrients ... 155
Nutrient Content Claims ... 155
How to Read a Food Label ... 155
Understanding the Role of Sodium ... 157
A Quick Overview of Diets ... 158
Drinks That People Use to Enhance Performance ... 160
How to Find the Most Trustworthy Health Information on the Internet ... 163
How Food Companies Are Assisting Canadians with Education and Healthy Eating ... 164
More Nutrition Information ... 166
Key Terms ... 167
Exercises ... 167
References ... 171

CHAPTER 9 Body Composition

Chapter Objectives ... 175
Misguided Views of the Body ... 175
Body Composition ... 177
Metabolism ... 179
Measuring Overweight and Obesity ... 179
Eating Disorders ... 182
Key Terms ... 186
Exercises ... 186
References ... 190

PART IV *Understanding and Managing Potential Health Problems*

CHAPTER 10 Diabetes

Chapter Objectives ... 195
Types of Diabetes ... 196
Children and Diabetes ... 197
Complications Associated with Diabetes ... 197
Risk Factors Associated with Diabetes ... 200
What Happens When You Are Hypoglycemic or Hyperglycemic? ... 201
Symptoms of Diabetes ... 202
Living with Diabetes and Shift Work ... 202
Conclusion ... 203
Appendix: Diabetes Dictionary ... 205
Key Terms ... 207
Exercises ... 207
References ... 211

CHAPTER 11 Cardiovascular Disease

Chapter Objectives ... 213
Cardiovascular Disease: A Canadian Concern ... 214
Anatomy of the Heart ... 218
How the Heart Functions ... 218
Types of Cardiovascular Disease ... 219
Prevention of Cardiovascular Diseases ... 232
Appendix: Cardiovascular Disease Glossary ... 233
Other Points of Interest ... 234
Key Terms ... 234
Exercises ... 235
References ... 240

CHAPTER 12 Back Pain

Chapter Objectives ... 243
The Spine ... 244
Osteoporosis ... 246
The Causes of Back Pain ... 249
Risk Factors ... 250
Preventing Back Pain ... 255
Nutritional Considerations for a Healthier Back ... 259
Treating Back Injuries ... 261
Key Terms ... 261
Exercises ... 262
References ... 267

CHAPTER 13 **Stress**

Chapter Objectives 269
Changing Roles of Law Enforcement and Its Impact on Officers 269
Defining Stress 270
The Types of Stress 270
The Stress Response 270
Stressors 273
Critical Incidents 275
Additional Stress in Your Teens into Adulthood 281
Behaviour Types 282
Coping with Stress 283
Key Terms 290
Exercises 291
References 295

CHAPTER 14 **Shift Work**

Chapter Objectives 297
Shift Schedule 298
Understanding the Importance of Sleep 299
The Effects of Shift Work 299
Coping Strategies 303
More Information 305
Key Terms 306
Exercises 307
References 310

CHAPTER 15 **Common Injuries**

Chapter Objectives 311
General Treatments for Injuries 311
Sorting Out Muscle Soreness 312
Common Sport-Related Injuries 314
Heat-Related Injuries and Illnesses 324
Cold-Related Injuries and Illnesses 326
Exercising in Cold Temperatures 327
Biological and Chemical Hazards in Policing 328
Key Terms 330
Exercises 331
References 334

PART V *Preparing to Meet Law Enforcement Fitness Standards*

CHAPTER 16 **Preparing to Meet Law Enforcement Fitness Standards**

Chapter Objectives 337
Physical Readiness Evaluation for Police (PREP) Test 338
Physical Abilities Requirement Evaluation (PARE) Test 341
Ontario Police Fitness Award (OPFA) Standards 348
Peel Regional Police Service Fitness Standards 353
Physical Fitness Log 356
References 358

APPENDIX

ASSIGNMENTS

ASSIGNMENT 1.1
Wellness 361

ASSIGNMENT 1.2
Informed Consent for Training and BFOR Testing 369

ASSIGNMENT 2.1
Assessing Your Values 371

ASSIGNMENT 2.2
Determining What Success Means to You 373

ASSIGNMENT 2.3
Developing Your Short-Term Goals to Achieve Long-Term goals 377

ASSIGNMENT 2.4
Summary of Goal-Setting Results—Successes, Barriers, and Strategies to Overcome Challenges 381

ASSIGNMENT 2.5
Mission Statement 383

ASSIGNMENT 3.1
Where Does All Your Time Go? 385

ASSIGNMENT 3.2
Tracking Your Time 387

ASSIGNMENT 3.3
Your To-do List for This Week 391

ASSIGNMENT 3.4
Assessing Your Level of Procrastination 393

ASSIGNMENT 4.1
Health Benefits of Physical Activity 395

ASSIGNMENT 4.2
Physical and Psychological Benefits of Physical Activity 397

ASSIGNMENT 4.3
Reviewing your fitness training goals 399

ASSIGNMENT 5.1
Assessing Your Cardiorespiratory Fitness Level 401

ASSIGNMENT 5.2
Determining Your Resting Heart Rate and Target Heart Rate 403

ASSIGNMENT 5.3
Setting Up Your Cardiorespiratory Fitness Program 405

ASSIGNMENT 6.1
Determining Your One-Repetition Maximum (1RM) for Bench Press 409

ASSIGNMENT 6.2
Designing Your Strength and Endurance Training Program 411

ASSIGNMENT 7.1
Designing a Stretching Program 415

ASSIGNMENT 8.1
Portion Distortion 419

ASSIGNMENT 8.2
Nutritional Labelling 421

ASSIGNMENT 9.1
Determining Your Body Mass Index (BMI) 423

ASSIGNMENT 9.2
Determining Your Waist Circumference (WC) 425

ASSIGNMENT 9.3
Determining Your Waist-to-Hip Ratio (WHR) 427

ASSIGNMENT 10.1
Are You at Risk for Diabetes? 429

ASSIGNMENT 11.1
First Aid for Heart Attack and Stroke Victims 431

ASSIGNMENT 11.2
Are You at Risk for Heart Disease? 433

ASSIGNMENT 12.1
Healthy Back Assessment 435

ASSIGNMENT 13.1
The Life Experience Survey 437

ASSIGNMENT 13.2
What Is Your Behaviour Type? 443

ASSIGNMENT 14.1
Understanding Shift Work Based on Sleeping Patterns 445

ASSIGNMENT 14.2
How Will You Cope with Shift Work? 447

ASSIGNMENT 16.1
Physical Fitness Log 449

GLOSSARY OF TERMS 455

INDEX 461

Preface

Law enforcement is a physically demanding profession. It requires officers to acquire important skills and physical abilities related to optimal health and a high level of personal fitness. Entrance requirements have evolved over the years to reflect the physical demands of the job, particularly in the adoption of Bona Fide Occupational Requirements (BFORs) testing, which assesses the minimum physical requirements for police officers. However, we are seeing a nation of young people with a lower level of general fitness. Although they are still able to pass the entrance test, many cannot meet the standards after a short period of time on the job. This may not be problematic early in a career; however, over time, health issues, combined with lower fitness levels, may put individuals at risk for injury and disability both on the job and at home.

Officers have to continually adapt to diverse situations. Whether it is school violence, gang warfare, the impact of the Internet (for example, identity theft, Internet child luring), road rage, SARS, or terrorism, police must respond quickly and appropriately and with the correct use of force, sometimes risking their lives to do their jobs. Officers must also deal with stress from a variety of sources. Financial, political, mental, and physical stressors all challenge officers in the performance of their duties. Yet, it is amazing how committed and resilient individuals can be, even when faced with some of the horrific aspects of the job.

In the physically demanding profession of policing, health means not only the absence of disease but the ability to do the job over the length of a career while maintaining one's quality of life. This means that the onus falls on the individual to maintain a healthy fitness level in order to ensure a balance for the demands of both career and home life.

Most officers are aware of the importance of being fit in order to meet the physical demands of the job. They are also concerned with reducing on- and off-duty injuries due to overexertion and preventing diseases such as coronary heart disease. Officers also understand the importance of emotional well-being, slowing the aging process, maintaining the mental capacity to do the job, and maintaining a healthy weight. While individuals are at school or enrolled in entrance training, such as recruit training at the Ontario Police College, they are motivated to participate in physical training. Once that mandatory commitment (external motivation) is removed, many drop off the fitness radar. Some explain to me that life gets in the way. Between long shifts, duties, and court and family commitments, fitness takes a back seat. But it is imperative to fit physical activity into your life, both in terms of personal time and family involvement, so that your quality of health will improve and your physical fitness level will be maintained.

This workbook has been prepared with these goals in mind. Just as your instructors will tell you that learning is lifelong commitment, physical activity must be thought of as equally important. This workbook will introduce you to issues and concepts of crucial importance to law enforcement personnel, including wellness and physical fitness, time management, nutrition, hypokinetic diseases (such as obesity, diabetes, and cardiovascular disease), back pain, stress, shift work, and common injuries. It is not enough to meet the minimum requirements of the job to get hired; police work requires a lifetime commitment to yourself and your family to ensure that you find a balance and ensure quality of life both on the job and off.

This workbook is designed to give you some basic information and tools to assist you in making appropriate choices. Although there is a plethora of information out there regarding fitness and health issues, this workbook specifically addresses issues relating to law enforcement. Having the knowledge and coping skills to deal with the demands of the job and daily life will be key to your success in policing. Quality of life—both on the job and off—through awareness, positive choices, and physical fitness will be your choice to make.

This new edition includes expanded coverage of nutrition (including discussion of the new *Canada's Food Guide*), a new chapter on diabetes, new end-of-chapter questions, updated references, and illustrations to help explain some of the topics. Photographs and techniques to illustrate weight training exercises are available at www.emp.ca/fitness for those who are new to training.

For each chapter in this workbook, there are numerous textbooks written on the specific topics covered. I encourage you to continue researching these topics and expand your knowledge in order to assist in your personal growth. I hope that you develop a passion for the policing profession and find its rewards as meaningful as I have in working with students and police officers in this field. Good luck.

Acknowledgments

I was always amazed by the support and encouragement that I received from individuals in the police fitness field as I pursued the update of this workbook. To members of the Police Fitness Personnel of Ontario—especially Gary Goguen, Shelley Howes, Joanne Pendrak, Marion Reeves, Robert Séguin, Claire Shaw, and Peter Shipley—I want to thank you for your encouragement, input, and suggestions. Your commitment to police officers' fitness and well-being in Ontario is reflected in your devotion not only to your individual services but to all officers in the province. At Georgian College, I would like to thank Ruth Vesterback, Janice Pepe, and Linda Lee Couse for their editing comments. I would like to thank Tammy Scherer, Valerie Adams, and Jim Lyons, who has provided me with encouragement, editorial guidance, and positive input throughout this process. I would especially like to thank students Jadie Stainthorp and Neil Hubley for their photographic endeavours and comic relief when things were not going as planned. Special thanks to the students in the Law and Security Administration, Police Foundations, and Applied Degree for Police Studies programs at Georgian College (as well as my firefighting students), who continue to aspire to great things in their professional and personal lives and who share those accomplishments with me so that I am continually inspired to love what I do. Finally, I would like to thank my family—Larry, Alexandra, and Christine—for their love and patience during the writing of this third edition.

PART I

Getting Started Toward a Healthy Lifestyle

CHAPTER 1

Wellness and Active Living: A Healthy Lifestyle

CHAPTER OBJECTIVES

After completing this chapter, you should be able to:

- Explain the concepts of fitness, active living, vitality, health, and wellness.
- Describe the health benefits of physical activity.
- Describe some of the steps you can take to achieve a healthy lifestyle.
- Evaluate the physical competencies you need to meet the requirements of a law enforcement career.

Wellness has grown to mean different things to different people. For some people, wellness equates to a certain level of fitness, while others perceive wellness as freedom from illness. This chapter discusses the concepts of fitness, active living, vitality, health, and wellness. As you prepare for a career in law enforcement, you will be required to scrutinize your health and physical fitness level to determine your readiness to meet the occupational demands expected as part of the job. The goal of this chapter is to enable you to assess your wellness and commitment to lifelong fitness and make some decisions on how you may achieve that level.

A WELLNESS PROFILE

Wellness can be defined as a way of life where you make decisions and choices to enjoy the highest level of health and well-being possible. Wellness includes the idea that life is a journey that must be enjoyed and continually fine-tuned in order to benefit as much as possible from all aspects of your life. This means taking the appropriate steps to prevent illness and to lead a richer, more balanced, and satisfying life.

Here is a list of behaviours and habits necessary for wellness:

- taking responsibility for your own health (including research on health issues, regular checkups, and asking questions) and taking an active role in the decisions you make about your life
- learning to manage stress effectively
- maintaining high self-esteem and being able to interact successfully with others
- understanding your sexuality and having satisfying intimate relationships
- avoiding tobacco and other drugs; using alcohol wisely, if at all
- eating well, exercising, and maintaining a normal weight
- understanding the Ontario health care system and what health benefits your employment entitles you to
- knowing the facts about cardiovascular (heart and blood vessel) disease, diabetes, cancer, sexually transmitted diseases and other infections, and injuries, and using your knowledge to protect yourself against them
- understanding how the environment affects your health and taking appropriate action to protect yourself against hazards in the environment
- having a sense of satisfaction with life and appreciating the different stages of life
- achieving a balance in all dimensions of health

THE RELATIONSHIP BETWEEN WELLNESS AND FITNESS

Physical Activity

physical activity
all leisure and non-leisure body movement that results in an expenditure of energy

Physical activity is all leisure and non-leisure body movement that reduces the risk for many diseases, helps control weight, and strengthens muscles, bones, and joints. For older adults, it can also reduce the risk for falls. This bodily movement produced by skeletal muscles results in an expenditure of energy. We know that people's health and well-being improves with daily moderate levels of activity. Moderate activities can include walking briskly, mowing the lawn, dancing, swimming, or bicycling. Occupational physical activity can include walking, hauling, lifting, pushing, carpentry, shovelling, and packing boxes.

Exercise

exercise
a form of leisure-time physical activity that is planned, structured, and repetitive; its main objective is to improve or maintain physical fitness

Exercise is a form of leisure-time physical activity that is planned, structured, and repetitive. Its main objective is to improve or maintain physical fitness. The benefits of exercise are improved health, resistance to diseases caused by inactivity, and the capacity to perform daily activities with vigour. People who make exercise a part of their everyday activities will likely be fitter than those who do not exercise, and will, therefore, enjoy better health and more energy to perform daily tasks more effectively and skillfully.

For those who suffer from arthritis or osteoporosis, exercise increases the range of motion and improves bone density. This improves the quality of daily living, and allows simple tasks to be done without risk of injury or pain. This becomes even more important in law enforcement, with its physical demands, whether it is wearing your belt weighing 5–10 kg or being involved in an altercation.

Physical Fitness

Physical fitness has to do with a person's health and performance, specifically in the areas of cardiorespiratory fitness, body composition, muscular strength and endurance, and flexibility. A physically fit person can perform moderate to vigorous levels of physical activity without undue fatigue.

- **Health-related fitness** involves aspects of fitness that are linked to a person's health. For example, people who perform weight-bearing exercises in their middle years are less likely to be afflicted with decreasing bone density in their later years. In law enforcement, this may help in a situation where you must physically respond to the demands of an altercation.
- **Performance/skill-related fitness** is the degree of fitness required to perform a particular job or sport. A person who exercises regularly will likely develop better motor skills (including coordination, agility, speed, and reaction time) and the endurance, muscular strength, and cardiorespiratory power and capacity necessary for peak performance. Law enforcement officers must respond to emergency situations all the time. Impaired speed and reaction time can cost them their lives or the lives of others who depend on them.

physical fitness
a person's health and performance, specifically in the areas of cardiorespiratory fitness, body composition, muscular strength and endurance, and flexibility

health-related fitness
the aspects of fitness that are linked to a person's health

performance/skill-related fitness
the degree of fitness required to perform a particular job or sport

Regular physical activity should include activity most days of the week, preferably each day. Five or more days of the week should include at least 30 minutes (which can be done in 10-minute increments) of moderate-intensity activities, and three days of the week should include 20–60 minutes of vigorous-intensity activities (US Department of Health, 1996).

PERSONAL PERSPECTIVE

About five years ago, I had the privilege to meet a grad whom I had not seen since the late 1980s. He had returned to Barrie to work, and connected with me through a student that he had hired. The student confided that this grad was avoiding coming to see me not because he did not want to come and talk, but because he was embarrassed by his physical condition. As I thought about this justification, I realized that I had represented an extrinsic motivation for his being successful in class (passing the course and being physically fit). It taught me that I had missed the boat in terms of helping students with the intrinsic motivational skills needed to help them maintain or return to fitness after graduation. Hopefully, as you read chapter 2, you will discover both the intrinsic and extrinsic motivational skills needed to be successful throughout the career that you have chosen. I ultimately reconnected with that grad, and over the years have supported him in realizing those intrinsic reasons to be physically active again.

Active Living

active living
a way of life in which individuals make meaningful and satisfying physical activities an integral part of daily living

Throughout the 1990s and early 2000s, research revealed that most Canadians were not active enough to receive health benefits from regular physical activity. This level of physical inactivity has reached epidemic proportions. According to Fitness Canada (1991), **active living** is a way of life in which people make meaningful and satisfying physical activities an integral part of daily living.

The percentage of Canadians who are overweight or obese has risen dramatically in recent years, mirroring a worldwide phenomenon (Katzmarzyk, 2002; Tremblay et al., 2002). According to the 2004 Canadian Community Health Survey: Nutrition (Garriguet, 2004), from 1978 to 2004, the percentage of Canadian adults who were obese rose from 14 percent to 23 percent (Tjepkema, 2006). This increase is associated with an increased risk of type II diabetes, cardiovascular diseases, psychosocial difficulties, osteoarthritis, some cancers, gallbladder disease, and premature mortality (National Institutes of Health, 1998).

We know that poor nutrition and lack of physical activity are primary contributors to weight gain. Although Health Canada has done intensive promotion of healthy eating and physical activity, obesity continues to increase.

According to Garriguet (2004), 23.1 percent of Canadians aged 18 or older—an estimated 5.5 million adults—have a body mass index (BMI) of 30 or more, indicating that they are obese, and 8.6 million or 36.1 percent of adults were overweight. From the 1978–79 survey, the most striking increase is in young people under 35 years old, whose obesity levels have risen from 8.5 percent to 20.5 percent in 2004. From the survey, we know that poor nutrition, lack of or little physical activity, and social-economical differences may play more of a role in obesity rates for women than for men. What is of even greater concern is that 26 percent of Canadian children and adolescents aged 2 to 17 were overweight or obese (a figure that has doubled since 1978–79), and 8 percent were obese (triple that of 1978–79). Lack of fruits and vegetables in the diet, as well as inactivity due to watching TV, playing video games, or using a computer, contribute to the increase in weight (Garriguet, 2004). It is estimated that physical inactivity costs at least $2.1 billion annually in direct health care costs and an estimated annual economic burden of $5.3 billion (Katzmarzyk, 2004). It is estimated that the total cost in Canada of illness, disability, and death attributed to chronic diseases amounts to over $80 billion annually (FPTAC, 2002; Health Canada, 2002a).

An interesting note regarding causes of mortality. Although cardiovascular disease has been the main cause of death in Canada in the last 25 years, it is on the decline (from 47 percent in 1979 to 32 percent in 2004). The second main cause of death has been cancer and its share has been growing (from 23 percent in 1979 to 30 percent in 2004). Scientists are predicting that cancer will eventually surpass cardiovascular disease as the leading cause of death in Canada (see figure 1.1) (Statistics Canada, 2004).

Active living is essential to improved health, well-being, and quality of life. There are three types of activities you need to keep your body healthy: endurance activities, flexibility activities, and strength activities (PHAC, 2004). These topics will be covered in other chapters of this book. An active lifestyle helps increase bone density, energy levels, physical fitness, and muscular strength; improves endurance,

FIGURE 1.1
Percentage Share of Deaths due to Cardiovascular Diseases, Cancer, and Both Causes, Canada, 1979 to 2004

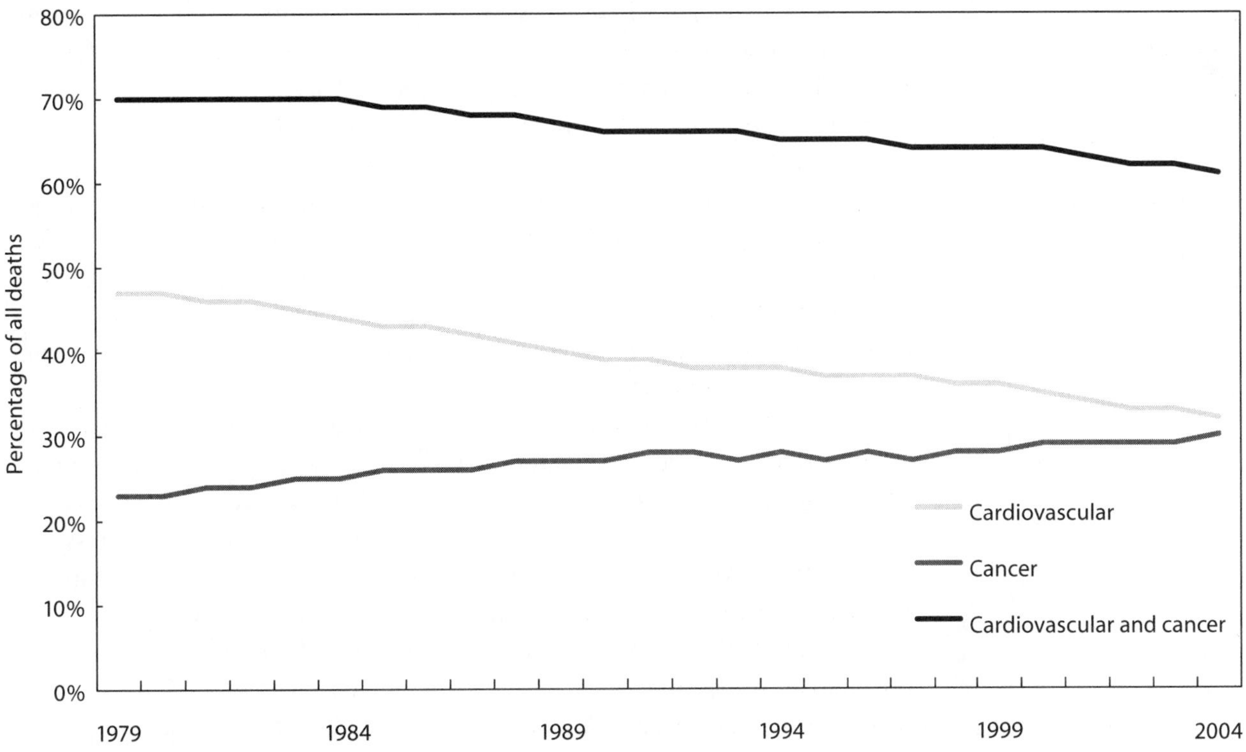

Source: Statistics Canada, *Mortality, summary list of causes* (2004). Released April 27, 2007. Catalogue 84F0209XIE, p. 10.

flexibility, motor coordination, and general health; prevents disease; and reduces body fat.

Active living is also about finding opportunities to become physically active at home, school, work, and in the community. Getting involved in charity walkathons or joining the workplace baseball team can, for example, be an important part of active living. All activities of this kind provide physical, social, emotional, and spiritual benefits that lead to an improved quality of life. As a result, the Public Health Agency of Canada (PHAC, 2004) has taken the federal role of encouraging and assisting Canadians to be physically active through awareness and programs that may facilitate the integration of physical activity within communities throughout Canada.

So how do these facts affect potential employees in the field of law enforcement? How does the field promote the importance of physical fitness as it relates to the demands of the job? Is the onus solely on potential employees to ensure that they can meet the demands of the job? How do law enforcers maintain a proper level of fitness? Should employers ensure that their employees maintain a healthy level of fitness by providing facilities or opportunities to participate in various forms of physical fitness? Ultimately, who is responsible for fitness? The box on the next page provides a perspective on these issues.

PERSONAL PERSPECTIVE

In the early 1980s, when I first started teaching in the Law and Security Administration (LASA) program at Georgian College in Barrie, Ontario, fitness was a mandatory course. The police and firefighting services were the only two employers in Ontario to enforce fitness standards at that time. All students in the LASA program had to meet police fitness standards, even if policing was not their career choice.

During the mid- and late 1990s, we again addressed the program's fitness requirements. In the first-year curriculum, fitness instruction took on a wellness and active living approach. It became the students' responsibility to meet set fitness criteria that would enable them to continue into a second-year fitness class. If a student could not meet these criteria or decided not to continue fitness classes, he or she chose other course options.

One of the positive outcomes of this new approach was the stronger lifelong commitment to fitness. The negative side of an optional second-year fitness course was the number of students who quickly lost interest in maintaining a healthy weight and lifestyle. Again, it became an issue of extrinsic motivation (surviving first-year fitness) rather than an intrinsic commitment to themselves (keeping active throughout their lives).

With the introduction of the Police Foundations Program in 1997, students face a heavier onus than ever before to meet the fitness requirements of the career they have chosen. Standards now exist for police, corrections workers, and court security officers. With a dual responsibility to achieve Bona Fide Occupational Requirements (BFOR, discussed as part of the Physical Abilities Requirement Evaluation [PARE] test in chapter 16), there is a greater onus on students to maintain their fitness at a level that allows them to successfully meet the physical job requirements of law enforcement. Note that being fit is not necessarily the same as meeting the minimum requirements of the various police, RCMP, and correctional services standards. Students who are fit, however, are easily meeting the required standards when they apply for a career in law enforcement.

In the fall of 2001, the Ontario Police Service's Physical Readiness Evaluation for Police (PREP) reduced graduation requirement in the shuttle run from level 7.5 to the applicant standard of level 6.5. As a result of this change, we are seeing new concerns from a fitness perspective. Are applicants as fit as they should be for the physical demands and lifestyle they face in law enforcement? Many can barely pass level 6.5 when they graduate from the Ontario Police College. What happens in six months, two years, five years, and ten years from now? Will this reduction of the exit requirement result in health issues and real costs, in terms of sick days and higher rates of injury, down the road to police agencies that may not have as fit a workforce? These questions are still of major concern to the Police Fitness Personnel of Ontario, who are the fitness promotion body for Ontario police officers.

Vitality

Vitality is an integrated approach to healthy living that shifts the focus away from rigid ideals, dieting, and overly prescriptive exercise toward acceptance of a range of body shapes and sizes and an emphasis on healthy eating, active living, and a positive self-image and body image (Active Living, 1998).

vitality
an integrated approach to healthy living that shifts the focus away from rigid ideals, dieting, and overly prescriptive exercise toward acceptance of a range of body shapes and sizes and an emphasis on healthy eating, active living, and a positive self-image and body image

In the 1990 report The Well-Being of Canadians: Highlights of the 1988 Campbell's Survey (Health Canada, 1990; Fitness Canada, 1991), it was shown that weight-related problems were a possible health risk for nearly 50 percent of Canadians. The report also found that an increasing number of Canadians were overweight, and that even people within a healthy weight range were preoccupied with weight loss.

In 1991, Health Canada and Fitness Canada responded to the report by launching the Vitality program to promote overall personal well-being, enhanced quality of life, and maintenance of a healthy weight. The program's philosophy was that Canadians should be empowered to make positive choices in the areas of healthy eating, active living, and positive self-image and body image (Fitness Canada, 1991). This philosophy has been promoted in the ParticipACTION commercials featuring Joanne McLeod and Hal Johnson. We also see more organizations sponsoring walking, swimming, and cycling activities to encourage Canadians to get involved in fitness and stay healthy. For example, the Ontario Police College sponsors a Torch Fun Run, with proceeds going to various organizations, including the Canadian Cancer Society.

The Vitality program's aim is to enhance Canadians' physical, psychological, and social well-being. The focus is on creating environments that support healthy choices within the home, school, workplaces and communities involving eating, being active, and feeling good about oneself (Health Canada, 2002b).

Health

Health and wellness are related concepts. Good **health** means being able to function independently in a constantly changing environment. **Wellness** is the ability to function at your best. Wellness is a holistic approach to life, and those who may not have ideal health can still have quality of life.

health
the ability of an individual to function independently in a constantly changing environment

wellness
the ability of an individual to optimally function at his or her best

THE HEALTH BENEFITS OF PHYSICAL ACTIVITY

Health experts who want to convince people to follow a more active lifestyle and make healthier choices must convince those people that physical activity is an integral part of a healthier life. The following are some of the health benefits of a lifestyle that includes physical activity (Pitts, 1996; Bouchard & Shephard, 1991; Klonoff, 1994):

- a reduced risk of coronary heart disease, non–insulin-dependent diabetes, obesity, osteoporosis (a reduction in bone mass), reproductive and colon cancer, hypertension (high blood pressure), and stroke
- help with maintaining a healthy body weight and more desirable body image
- increased strength, energy, and stamina
- improved cardiorespiratory function
- improved functioning of the lungs

- improved functioning of the digestive and excretory organs
- improved agility, speed, and coordination
- increased range of motion in joints
- improved general posture
- increased resistance to mental fatigue
- greater ability to cope with the intellectual demands of college and full-time or part-time jobs
- better stress management
- reduced anxiety and depression
- improved sleep
- higher self-esteem and perceived quality of life

In 2002, the federal government developed an integrated pan-Canadian Healthy Living Strategy (PHAC, 2005). Under the Public Health Agency of Canada, goals were set to improve health and reduce health disparities in Canada. The aim was to focus on children and youth to address physical inactivity and unhealthy eating. The Healthy Living Network was set up in 2003 for communication and health information to provide support for communities and educators in improving health quality in Canada. Healthy living incorporates appropriate choices with healthy eating, refraining from smoking, having a support system in place, and staying physically active whether at home, school, or work. There is an emphasis on the reduction of diseases and prevention of injuries.

Turn to **assignment 1.1**, "Wellness" (in the appendix). Complete the questionnaires to determine how ready you are to make healthier choices concerning habits, nutrition, stress management, and physical activity.

THE SEVEN DIMENSIONS OF HEALTH

Originally, health was defined as the absence of disease. In the late 1970s and 1980s, many exercise physiologists, kinesiologists, and health educators concluded that this definition was too restrictive. They decided that good health should be defined as wellness and equated with "healthy living." According to the Physical Activity, Fitness, and Health Consensus Statement (Quinney, Gauvine, & Wall, 1994), health has physical, social, and psychological dimensions, each of which lies along a continuum. Positive health is associated with a capacity to enjoy life and to withstand challenges; it is not merely the absence of disease.

There are seven dimensions in all to good health. All of the individual dimensions must work together to create good health. One weak dimension can affect all the others. The dimensions are as follows:

1. *Physical* Physical health involves looking after your body as best you can. This means eating properly, exercising, avoiding unhealthy behaviours and substances, making responsible decisions about sex, being aware of the symptoms of disease, having regular checkups, and taking steps to prevent injuries.

2. *Emotional and psychological* Emotional and psychological health involves maintaining a positive self-concept; dealing constructively with feelings; developing such qualities as optimism, trust, and self-confidence; and being able to cope with the challenges of daily stressors. It also involves self-acceptance, controlling your emotions, and knowing when to seek support.
3. *Intellectual* Intellectual health involves valuing lifelong learning and challenging yourself while searching for answers and solutions. It also involves being able to analyze and evaluate a situation and proposing alternatives or solutions. As well, intellectual health includes self-awareness and learning from life experiences.
4. *Spiritual* Spiritual health involves searching for meaning and purpose in your life. It also involves coming to terms with what is right and wrong, whether through religion, meditation, art, or some other practice. Spiritual health may involve developing faith in a being or power beyond yourself, as well as the capacity for compassion, altruism, joy, and forgiveness. Research has found that "intrinsic religiosity" plays a role in speedier recovery from depression, anxiety, and illness, and can contribute to a longer life expectancy (Hummer et al., 1999).
5. *Social and interpersonal* Social and interpersonal health involves being able to develop meaningful relationships, cultivating a network of supportive friends and family members, and contributing to the community. It also includes valuing diversity—accepting people for who they are. Statistics show that people who are socially isolated are at higher risk of developing illness and even dying (Cacioppo, 2002).
6. *Environmental* Environmental health involves respecting and protecting the environment at the local level and beyond, protecting yourself from environmental hazards, and minimizing the negative impact of your behaviour on the environment.
7. *Occupational* Occupational health involves deriving satisfaction from the accomplishments and challenges of your job while maintaining a balance between work and the rest of your life.

There are so many demands on law enforcement officers, who deal with the physical demands of altercations, the emotional demands of domestic calls, the intellectual demands of having to make sound decisions (sometimes almost instantly), the spiritual demands of coming to terms with deaths and other tragic events they witness, the interpersonal demands of dealing with the public, the environmental demands of working in all weather and other conditions, and the occupational demands of encountering society at its best and worst. It is important to be healthy in all of these areas in order to do your job effectively and safely.

Today, with advances in health care that help to cure or reduce the spread of infectious diseases, we have seen the **mortality** (death) rate decline. People live well into their 70s and 80s, and more people will reach 100 years old in the 21st century than ever before. **Morbidity** (illness) rates show us that people are becoming ill less from common infectious diseases than in past generations.

mortality
number of deaths in a population, usually expressed as an annual rate

morbidity
number of ill people in a population, usually expressed as an annual rate

However, just because we are living longer doesn't mean that we are healthier. Less than 15 percent of the older population is participating in regular fitness activities. It is estimated that more than 67 percent of our youth are inactive and 50 percent are not active enough to receive the health benefits associated with exercise (de St. Auboin, 1997). This inactivity, combined with less walking and more driving, watching TV more, spending more time on computers and video games, and a poor diet of fatty fast foods, has led to a generation that is less active than 30 years ago (Anderson, 2000). With the academic changes in high school curriculum in Ontario, there are fewer physical fitness classes and an apparent devaluing of the importance of physical activity in young people's lives.

This is why the federal government has pushed for education programs like Active Living, Physical Activity Guide, and Healthy Living, which are aimed at addressing health and wellness. By informing people about the seven dimensions that work together for good health, we may improve the quality of Canadians' lives.

Wellness

Wellness applies to all ages, socio-economic groups, and levels of ability or disability. Wellness relies on personal empowerment—people taking charge of their lives. Many disabled people, for example, find ways to live healthy, physically active lives. As Donald Ardel (1987, p. 131) points out, "Wellness is not a goal to be attained but a process to be maintained." It runs along a continuum (see figure 1.2).

At each phase of your life, physical fitness, active living, and wellness take on different degrees of importance. For those entering the field of law enforcement, physical skills and abilities are becoming a prerequisite for employment. During the middle and later phases of a law enforcement career, active living and health-related issues come to the fore. Physical activity also becomes an employer's issue when it is associated with sick days and Workplace Safety and Insurance Board claims.

Twenty years ago, fitness in the law enforcement context was treated exclusively as a hiring issue, but today it is viewed more broadly. We now see campaigns to address fitness throughout a person's law enforcement career. For example, Ontario Police College fitness staff and the Police Fitness Personnel of Ontario (PFPO; see the box on the next page) have implemented a yearly fitness lapel pin initiative to encourage ongoing fitness for all officers. Since 1988, the PFPO has rewarded officers who meet the criteria with the pin to recognize their commitment to fitness. Over 25,000 fitness tests have been performed over the years since the program's inception, an average of 3,000 to 5,000 pins annually.

FIGURE 1.2 Wellness/Illness Continuum

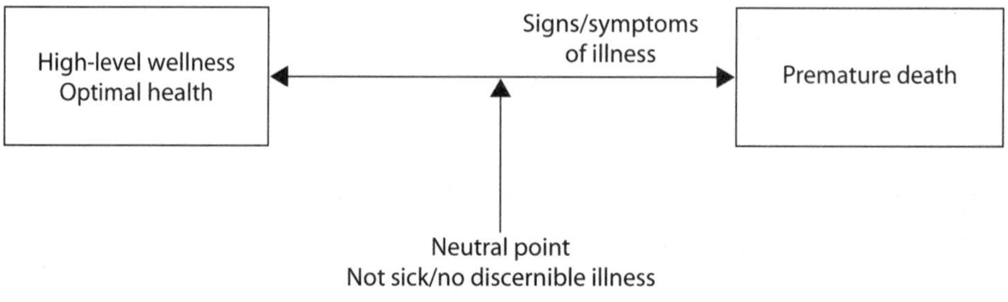

Source: Adapted from R.V. Hockey, *Physical fitness: The pathway to healthful living* (7th ed.) (Boston: Mosby-Year Book, 1993), p. 18. Reproduced with permission of The McGraw-Hill Companies.

POLICE FITNESS PERSONNEL OF ONTARIO

The PFPO, an organization sanctioned by the Ontario Association of Chiefs of Police, has a mandate to promote fitness and health awareness within the policing community. In addition to its yearly fitness pin awards, the PFPO offers awareness programs on topics such as maintaining a healthy back, nutrition, fitness and shift work, and cardiovascular disease.

During the mid- and late 1980s, we had to rethink our standards for two reasons. First, fewer students were entering policing and other fields with less stringent standards. Second, students were arriving at college less fit than their predecessors, because fitness programs were no longer mandatory throughout the high school years. As a result, the program lowered its fitness standards, although through the academic advisory process we continued to encourage students to meet police standards.

Since the 1980s, the physical and occupational skills of various public employees have been tested by the Ontario Police Service's Physical Readiness Evaluation for Policing (PREP) test, the RCMP's Physical Abilities Requirement Evaluation (PARE) test. The Ontario Correctional Service is in the process of developing a Bona Fide Occupational Requirements (BFOR) standard called FIT-CO—Fitness Test (for Ontario) Correctional Officer Applicants.

Ontario's PREP test has been made challenging with the introduction of the push–pull machine, which simulates the motions of pushing and pulling during an altercation, and the arm-restraint device, which simulates the motion of holding onto a person while bringing her or his arms together for handcuffing. Upper-body strength and cardiorespiratory (heart and respiratory system) endurance are also tested.

When the PREP was introduced, there were concerns about the number of women who are not meeting the PREP test's minimum standards (Ruttan, 1998). In 1998, for example, 656 of the 739 males who were tested by the Toronto force passed, but only 73 of the 148 females tested were successful. With proper training, in 2001, 94 percent of the women in the second year of the Police Foundations Program at Georgian College met the graduation standards for both the PREP and the PARE. There is a definite learning curve for these machines, but upper-body strength and aerobic conditioning are also important. However, if people are physically motivated as well as educated about the requirements, they should have no difficulty passing by the time they graduate from their law enforcement programs. The keys to success lie in familiarity with the equipment and a commitment to a personal fitness program designed to meet the standards, including a strong aerobic and strength-training program. Most are able to get through the pursuit and restraint component; however, there is a greater percentage of individuals who find it aerobically challenging to get to level 6.5 on the shuttle run and to continue to maintain and/or improve above that level.

How can law enforcement officers be convinced to integrate physical fitness into their lives? Simply telling people that physical activity is good for them is not sufficient motivation. There must be some intrinsic or extrinsic motivation for becoming and remaining fit (see the box on the next page). A commitment to lifelong wellness and fitness is an intricate part of achieving your career goals. This workbook provides information that will allow you to make positive health and lifestyle changes, but ultimately, it is up to you to make the choice regarding your health and fitness level.

IT'S NEVER TOO LATE

At 37 my father had his first angina attack. It happened when he started to feel crushing chest pains while we were visiting Expo 67. I remember how exciting it was for me as a child to travel through the crowds in an ambulance and receive VIP treatment while my father lay very still. Eventually, his chest pains subsided, and we continued our tour the next day. In 1970, when he was 40, he suffered a massive heart attack caused by a blockage of the left coronary artery.

When I got older and started learning about heart disease, I realized that my father had been a time bomb waiting to go off. He led a sedentary life and was a meat-and-potatoes man who worked six days a week, walked only a few short steps to work, and smoked two and a half packs of cigarettes a day.

After the heart attack my father spent six weeks in a hospital. Today, heart attack patients are out of the hospital in days, but in 1970 the medical staff did not know what to do with him, because heart research did not begin to make great strides until the mid-1970s. By the time my father was finally released from the hospital, he had given up smoking and begun daily one-hour walks in which he covered up to 6 km; he has stuck to this walking program religiously ever since.

In 1983, two days before my mid-term on the physiology of heart disease, my father suffered another heart attack. Although he had had a stress test a week earlier, there had been no sign of an impending heart attack (a stress test uses exercise to evaluate whether the heart and blood vessels are working properly). I remember how he denied that he was having another heart attack. Mental stress—not problems with eating or exercise—caused this attack. Afterward, my father made further changes to his lifestyle and outlook on health.

In December 2003, my father suffered his third heart attack and had quadruple bypass surgery. It truly is amazing that after three heart attacks, an aortic aneurysm, and kidney problems, technology has advanced so far as to enable my family to continue to have him present.

Sometimes we get caught up in the career we have chosen and forget about our health. Law enforcement officers, for example, tend to eat on the run and fail to maintain a balanced diet. As a result of shift work, court appearances, and overtime, many become rundown from lack of sleep. Fitness seems to be the first thing that is left out of an officer's daily routine. The most common excuse that I hear from officers is that they don't have time for fitness. As a result, I see many who are overweight, who have back problems, and who are suffering from stress-related issues that should not be present at such young ages. I hope that reading this book will lead you to a greater appreciation of the importance of fitness. Taking care of your health is an important part of leading a long, productive, and rewarding life. We work to enjoy the rewards of retirement. Make sure that you are healthy enough to enjoy those rewards.

REQUIREMENTS FOR ONTARIO POLICE OFFICERS

The following pages provide an overview of some of the standards for a police officer in the province of Ontario (OPP, 2002). See if you have these skills and abilities, and look very carefully at the medical requirements to see whether you can pass them.

In 1996, the Ontario Association of Chiefs of Police (OACP) developed a standardized police applicant process. From this process, they developed one set of standards police services could use to look for applicants through a centralized system. They stated that

> [a] career in policing is primarily about one thing: working with people to ensure public safety through crime prevention and law enforcement. ... Police work is demanding. A police constable must work shifts, including evenings, nights, and weekends, at all times of the year. It affects an individual's health, perspective on life, and family life. This is not a job that everyone will like or can do well. Many cannot work shifts.

In Ontario, you must meet certain minimum requirements as outlined in Ontario's *Police Services Act*. One of these requires you to "be physically and mentally able to perform the duties of the position, having regard to your own safety and the safety of members of the public."

Competencies

In addition to the minimum requirements set out in the *Police Services Act*, you must possess specific competencies, which are skills, abilities, behaviours, and attitudes that are essential to law enforcement work. The two categories specified for the job of policing are essential competencies and developmental competencies (OPP, 2002).

Essential competencies must be demonstrated before you can become a police officer (OPP, 2002):

1. Analytical Thinking: The ability to analyze situations and events in a logical way, and to organize the parts of a problem in a systematic way.
2. Self Confidence: A belief in your own abilities and judgment, and a recognition of personal limitations and development needs.
3. Communication: The ability to demonstrate effective listening, verbal and written communication skills.
4. Flexibility/Valuing Diversity: The ability to adapt your approach in a variety of situations, and to work effectively with a wide cross section of the community representing diverse backgrounds, cultures and socioeconomic circumstances.
5. Self Control: The ability to keep your own emotions under control and to restrain negative actions when provoked or when working under stressful conditions.
6. Relationship Building: The ability to develop and maintain a network of contacts, both inside and outside the police service.
7. Achievement Orientation: The desire for continuous improvement in service or accomplishments.

8. Medical/Physical Skills and Abilities: Job-related medical/physical skills and abilities, including vision, hearing, motor skills, cardiovascular endurance and upper-body strength.

Developmental competencies can be acquired through training after you have been hired as a police officer. However, some police services may require these competencies in new applicants, thus making these conditions for hiring. The following 11 competencies have been identified as developmental:

1. Information Seeking: The ability to seek out information from various sources before making decisions.
2. Concern for Safety: The ability to exercise caution in hazardous situations in order to ensure safety to self and others.
3. Assertiveness: The ability to use authority confidently and to set and enforce rules appropriately.
4. Initiative: Demonstrated ability to be self-motivated and self-directed in identifying and addressing important issues.
5. Cooperation: The ability to collaborate with others by seeking their input, encouraging their participation and sharing information.
6. Negotiation/Facilitation: The ability to influence or persuade others by anticipating and addressing their interests and perspectives.
7. Work Organization: The ability to develop and maintain systems for organizing information and activities.
8. Community-Service Orientation: Proven commitment to helping or serving others.
9. Commitment to Learning: Demonstrated pattern of activities which contribute to personal and professional growth.
10. Organizational Awareness: Understanding of the dynamics of organizations, including the formal and informal cultures and decision making processes.
11. Developing Others: Commitment to helping others improve their skills.

When you apply to become a police officer in Ontario, you will also have to go through a medical/physical skills and abilities test (OPP, 2002). These abilities are equally important to determine prior to applying to the service. It is prudent to do these tests while you are still in school to ensure that you have the ability to apply and meet these standards. This test measures

- *Vision* Uncorrected (no eyeglasses or contact lenses) visual acuity must be at least 20/40 (6/12) with both eyes open. Corrected visual acuity must be at least 20/20 (6/6) with both eyes open. There are also minimum requirements for farsightedness, colour vision, depth perception, peripheral vision, and other vision-related areas.

  Don't wait until you apply to find out whether you meet these standards. Too many students who have not done their own research have found out after two years of college that they will never be able to meet the standards, especially for colour vision. Statistically, more males are colourblind than females.
- *Hearing* You must have normal hearing at frequencies of 500 to 4000 Hz, as measured by an audiometer.

- *Physical fitness* This part of the test assesses whether you have the physical skills and abilities to pass the PREP in 162 seconds or less, with a shuttle run to a level of stage 6.5 (this is explained in more detail in chapter 16). This test does *not* assess your fitness level.

  This is the one test over which you have total control. For some people, it will take only one or two times to acquaint themselves with the equipment and successfully meet the standard. For others, it may take the entire two years of training at college to gain the required physical strength and aerobic endurance. Ultimately, you are the only one who can ensure your success.

Informed Consent for Fitness Testing

Part of the requirement prior to testing for police services is to ensure that you are medically safe to do the testing. Expectations are that with a PAR-Q you are assuring the assessor that you are physically able to do the testing without limitations. The informed consent takes that one step further to address due diligence to ensure that you know about the test protocols and are aware of the stress that they may put you under. The informed consent also ensures that you have followed appropriate guidelines to ensure that you are able to perform the tasks safely. Turn to **assignment 1.2**, carefully read the informed consent form, sign it, and return a copy to your instructor. If you require further clarification, make sure to ask your instructor.

Local Needs of Police Services

Apart from the competencies listed above, police services may require certain special skills and abilities in order to address urgent issues pertaining to the specific service or community. A local need may be a second language, a special type or level of computer skills, prior experience in working with abused women and troubled youth, the ability to relocate, and so on.

As you go through the chapters of this book, remember to think about some of these competencies. When you set your goals in chapter 2, you may have to include some competencies to work on so you can demonstrate those skills to the agency you apply to. Ultimately, you will have to determine whether you have chosen the right career.

KEY TERMS

physical activity

exercise

physical fitness

health-related fitness

performance/skill-related fitness

active living

vitality

health

wellness

mortality

morbidity

EXERCISES

Review

1. Healthy living can be defined as

2. The seven dimensions of good health are

3. Why is it important to put equal emphasis on each dimension of good health?

4. How does wellness apply to law enforcement?

5. What does physical fitness mean to you?

6. What is the difference between health-related and performance-related fitness?

7. Describe the difference between active living and vitality.

8. List some of the ways you can improve your health based on the information in this chapter.

9. Which of the 8 essential and 11 developmental competencies required of Ontario police do you possess? Which ones do you need to work on?

10. What are some of the concerns that police have when dealing with issues around being overweight or obese?

11. What are some of the benefits of reducing weight?

Multiple Choice

1. The wellness concept emphasizes which of the following?
   a. reliance on the health care system
   b. personal responsibility for well-being
   c. a complete absence of disease
   d. adequate medical insurance coverage
   e. exercising to maximum heart rate every day

2. Which of the following is one of the dimensions of wellness?
   a. health
   b. sexual health
   c. environmental health
   d. cardiovascular health
   e. nuclear health

3. Which of these statements is true about a wellness lifestyle?
   a. the rewards of wellness are delayed
   b. living to an old age is a benefit to living a wellness lifestyle
   c. college is a time to think about wellness
   d. wellness involves gaining control of your life
   e. all of these choices are true

4. The wellness/illness continuum identifies a neutral point. This neutral point is where
   a. premature death occurs
   b. no discernible illness exists
   c. medical intervention is important
   d. a person is physically fit
   e. a high level of wellness is enjoyed

5. The practice of leaving work at work is an example of which dimension of wellness?
   a. social
   b. spiritual
   c. occupational
   d. emotional
   e. intellectual

6. Dealing effectively with a stressful situation is an example of which dimension of wellness?
   a. social
   b. spiritual
   c. occupational
   d. emotional
   e. intellectual

7. Taking time to read up on a subject that interests you is an example of which dimension of wellness?
   a. social
   b. spiritual
   c. occupational
   d. emotional
   e. intellectual

8. Developing a good network of friends both within and outside your career is an example of which dimension of wellness?
   a. social
   b. spiritual
   c. occupational
   d. emotional
   e. intellectual

9. Finding a rewarding career in law enforcement is an example of which dimension of wellness?
   a. social
   b. spiritual
   c. occupational
   d. emotional
   e. intellectual

10. Which of the following is a benefit of regular physical activity?
    a. greater resistance to mental fatigue
    b. reduced risk of heart disease
    c. better stress management
    d. improved agility
    e. all of these

REFERENCES

Active Living. (1998). Available at http://www.activeliving.ca/activeliving/alc/faq.html.

Anderson, R.E. (2000). The spread of the childhood obesity epidemic. *Canadian Medical Association Journal, 163*(11), 1461-1462. Available at http://www.cmaj.ca/content/vol163/issue11/.

Ardel, D. (1987). The health benefits of exercise (part 1): A round table. *The Physician and Sports Medicine, 15,* 131ff.

Bouchard, C., & Shephard, R. (1991). *Physical activity, fitness and health: A model and key concepts.* Consensus Doc-017, August 22, document prepared for the International Consensus Symposium on Physical Activity, Fitness and Health.

Bouchard, C., & Shephard, R.J. (1994). Physical activity, fitness and health: The model and key concepts (pp. 77-88). In C. Bouchard, R.J. Shephard, & T. Stephens (Eds.), *Physical activity, fitness and health.* Champaign, IL: Human Kinetics.

Cacioppo, J.T., et al. (2002). Loneliness and health: Potential mechanisms. *Psychosomatic Medicine, 64,* 407-417.

de St. Auboin, B. (1997). *Get serious! Promote physical activity.* Ontario Physical and Health Education Association (Winter), 24-25.

Federal/Provincial/Territorial Advisory Committee on Population Health (FPTAC). (2002). Advancing integrated prevention strategies in Canada: *An approach to reducing the burden of chronic diseases.* Ottawa: Health Canada.

Fitness Canada. (1991). *Active living: A conceptual overview.* Ottawa: Government of Canada.

Garriguet, D. (2004). *Nutrition: Findings from the Canadian Community Health Survey.* Statistics Canada. Catalogue no. 82-620-MIE. Ottawa: Minister of Industry.

Health Canada. (1990). *The well-being of Canadians: Highlights of the 1988 Campbell's survey.* Ottawa: Supply and Services Canada.

Health Canada. (2002a). *Economic burden of illness in Canada.* Catalogue no. H21-136/1998. Ottawa: Health Canada.

Health Canada. (2002b). *Vitality: A positive approach to healthy living.* Available at http://www.hc-sc.gc.ca/fn-an/nutrition/weights-poids/positive_approach-approche_sain_e.html#1.

Hockey, R.V. (1993). *Physical fitness: The pathway to healthful living* (7th ed.) Boston: Mosby-Year Book.

Hummer, R.A., et al. (1999). Religious participation and U.S. adult mortality. *Demography, 30*(2), 273-285.

Katzmarzyk, P.T., & Janssen, I. (2004). The economic costs of physical inactivity and obesity in Canada: An update. *Canadian Journal of Applied Physiology, 29*(1), 90-115.

Klonoff, Elizabeth A. (1994). Predicting exercise adherence in women: The role of psychological and physiological factors. *Preventive Medicine, 23,* 257-262.

National Institutes of Health. 1998. Clinical guidelines on the identification, evaluation, and treatment of overweight and obesity in adults—The evidence report. *Obesity Research, 6*(Supp. 2), 51S-209S.

Ontario *Police Services Act,* RSO 1990, c. P.15, as amended.

Ontario Provincial Police (OPP). (2002). To be a constable. Available at http://www.opp.ca.

Pitts, E.H. (1996). The surgeon general's call to action. *Fitness Management, 12*(9), 36-38.

Public Health Agency of Canada. (2005). *Healthy living strategy.* Ottawa: Supply and Services Canada. Available at http://www.phac-aspc.gc.ca/hl-vs-strat/index.html.

Public Health Agency of Canada. (2004). *Healthy living unit.* Ottawa: Supply and Services Canada.

Quinney, H.A., Gauvine, L., and Wall, A.E.T. (Eds.) (1994). *Toward active living: Proceedings of the International Conference on Physical Activity, Fitness and Health.* Champaign, IL: Human Kinetics.

Ruttan, S. (1998, June 25). Toronto Police Service Fitness Coordinator. Telephone conversation.

Statistics Canada, Health Statistics Division. (2004). *Mortality, summary list of causes.* Catalogue no. 84F0209XIE. Available at http://www.statcan.ca/english/freepub/84F0209XIE/84F0209XIE2004000.htm.

Tjepkema, M. (2006). Adult obesity in Canada: Measured height and weight. In *Nutrition: Findings from the Canadian Community Health Survey.* Statistics Canada. Catalogue no. 82-620-MWE2005001. Ottawa: Minister of Industry. Available at http://www.statcan.ca/english/research/82-620-MIE/2005001/pdf/aobesity.pdf.

Tremblay, M.S., Katzmarzyk, P.T., & Willms, J.D. (2002). Temporal trends in overweight and obesity in Canada, 1981–1996. *International Journal of Obesity, 26,* 538-543.

US Department of Health and Human Services. (1996). *Physical activity and health: A report of the Surgeon General.* Atlanta: US Department of Health and Human Services, Centers for Disease Control and Prevention National Center for Chronic Disease Prevention and Health Promotion.

CHAPTER 2

Goal Setting

CHAPTER OBJECTIVES

After completing this chapter, you should be able to:

- Understand how self-esteem, attitude, and intentions play a role in participation in physical activity.
- Understand the process of setting short- and long-term goals.
- Assess your values and formulate goals that reflect those values.
- Create a mission statement that will give direction to the decisions you make throughout the course of your life.

As a law enforcement student, you are working toward various goals. Your first goal was achieved when you were admitted into your law enforcement program. To achieve your other goals, you must set up pathways to success. In this chapter, you will assess your values, set short- and long-term goals for yourself, and create a mission statement. By setting goals and creating a mission statement, you will begin to see more meaning and direction in your life.

Remember that you are in charge of your law enforcement career. Managing it will be a lifelong process. You will have to find a balance that is right for you and the people around you.

THE PROCESS OF CHANGE

As the demands of law enforcement change, employers are looking for people with both academic training and practical experience gained through paid or volunteer work. Law enforcement agencies want independent decision makers and self-directed learners who have a positive attitude toward work. Candidates need a well-rounded education (including math and computer literacy), communication skills (including a good command of vocabulary and grammar), interpersonal and time-management skills, flexibility, dependability, and a lifelong commitment to physical activity. To be successful, people in law enforcement must be able to adapt to the changing demands of their field and set their goals accordingly.

Behavioural psychologists have undertaken a great deal of research to understand why people find it difficult to follow through on major lifestyle changes or goals. Lifestyle behaviours can have a negative effect on people's ability to stay healthy and free from disease or disability. Unfortunately, many people succumb to behaviours that lead to illness, including alcohol and drug abuse, smoking, inappropriate dieting, and insufficient physical fitness.

After studying people who committed themselves to health-related behavioural changes, Prochaska, Norcross, and DiClemente (1994) discovered that people pass through five distinct stages of change: pre-contemplation, contemplation, preparation, action, and maintenance. Some people pass through all five stages in sequence, whereas others bounce back and forth between stages or get stuck at one stage. Some people, therefore, never achieve their goals. Table 2.1 lays out the five stages of change.

extrinsic motivation motivation to perform a task or goal based on external rewards

Extrinsic motivation does not keep people participating in exercise programs for long. Extrinsic motivation emphasizes doing a certain behaviour for a reward or outcome. In other words, the motivation is external to the individual. People with extrinsic motivation focus on such rewards as losing weight, quitting smoking, being physically fit, and being less prone to disease.

People can become so focused on the outcomes that they ignore the process (why they are exercising). Many individuals ignore developing positive, intrinsic experience from exercise—that is, exercise for exercise's sake. This is why most will lose interest in participating in regular physical activity or sticking to a smoking

TABLE 2.1 The Five Stages of Change

Stage	Description	Examples
1. Pre-contemplation	The individual does not believe that a problem exists and resists changing his or her behaviour.	• "Why should I quit smoking? Winston Churchill drank and smoked into his nineties." • "Why should I exercise? My weight is the same as it was 10 years ago."
2. Contemplation	The individual understands and appreciates the importance of changing his or her behaviour, but is unable to take that step.	• "I know that I should stop smoking, but right now I'm too stressed out to try." • "I know that if I exercised I would have more energy, but I don't have the time for an exercise program."
3. Preparation	The individual intends to act on his or her goals.	• "I've marked a weight-control session on my calendar." • "I've set aside three hours next week to work out."
4. Action	The individual commits time and energy to seeing his or her goals realized.	• "I worked out four times this week." • "I'm doing upper-body exercises, including chin-ups and push-ups, so that I will be able to complete the push component of the PREP test without any difficulty."
5. Maintenance	The individual has realized his or her goals and is now working to safeguard his or her accomplishments.	• "I've been able to stay at my target weight for the last six months and I'm going to continue my weight-control program because I feel better than I've ever felt." • "I look at that two-year-old pack of cigarettes in the cupboard and realize that cigarettes don't control my life anymore."

Source: Prochaska, J.O., Norcross, J.C., & DiClemente, C.C. (1994). The five stages of change. In *Changing for good* (pp. 36-50). New York: William Morrow. Reprinted by permission of HarperCollins Publishers.

cessation program within the first six months of trying—they quickly lose their motivation when they are not realizing their goals. Those who are **intrinsically motivated** to exercise regularly or lose weight are motivated by the activity itself. Those who adopt attitudes and behaviours for a healthy lifestyle usually have a positive attitude toward themselves and others as well as a zest for life. They are individuals who include physical activity as part of their daily routine.

intrinsic motivation
motivation to perform a task or goal based on enjoyment of doing the task itself

PERSONAL PERSPECTIVE

A few years ago I had an opportunity to talk to a grad who was doing background checks for her police service. After our interview, she shared with me something that I have been acutely aware of in my students for years. She told me that she had hated fitness classes when I had made her run (remember that you are the one who chooses to come into a program with set courses, which you should research before entering). She said that she really enjoyed running now and could see why I had tried to make fitness part of her everyday life. Her motivation for telling me this was that she had just completed her first half marathon, and wanted me to know what a difference doing fitness for personal reasons had made in her life.

I realized two things. The first was that, at times, students believe that it is someone else's responsibility to make them successful (or not). The second was that at times I motivate students extrinsically through marks rather than helping them to see the intrinsic rewards of fitness. This can apply to just about anything, from success in fitness to academics to goals in everyday life. We need to find those values that are important to us and shift from extrinsic motivation (outcomes) to intrinsic motivation (process for its own sake) if achieving those goals is going to be part of our everyday life. So where does your motivation come from?

Prochaska, DiClemente, and Norcross (1992) identify nine processes of change that affect one's ability to progress through the five stages (see table 2.2). These processes of change include both obvious and non-obvious activities, events, and experiences that affect individuals attempting to change their behaviour. This means that you have to be doing the right things at the right time and in the right stage in order to see positive change. Unless you are ready to embrace the changes necessary for success, the change will not happen. Are you ready to see your efforts through to completion?

We know that lifestyle behaviours are affected by thoughts and feeling of the individual and the impact of those around that individual. **Self-esteem** (how one feels about oneself and one's characteristics) is at the centre of one's success. If an individual has negative feelings including depression, helplessness, and loneliness, he or she is likely not able to develop positive lifestyle behaviours. We know that those who are successful in developing and maintaining healthy lifestyle behaviours have high self-esteem. They are actively involved in physical activities and have good dietary practices.

self-esteem
how one feels about oneself and one's characteristics

There are several dimensions involved in determining the level of a person's self-esteem. Intellectual, social, emotional, and physical dimensions combine to affect behaviour, and our perception of this behaviour will influence a healthy lifestyle. If individuals have a positive perception of themselves (that is, a higher level of self-esteem), even if they are not in great shape, they will still have positive outcomes from what they do in terms of physical activity. However, if they possess a negative perception (that is, a poor self-image due to unrealistic cultural, media, and peer pressure), unrealistic expectations and unhealthy lifestyle choices usually result.

self-efficacy one's ability to take action and perform a specific behaviour

This confidence in your ability to take action and perform a specific behaviour is known as **self-efficacy**. Those who are successful have the confidence to believe

TABLE 2.2 The Nine Processes of Change

Processes	Description	Examples
Consciousness raising (belongs to stages 1 and 2)	The individual seeks out information that will assist him or her in reaching his or her goal.	• Learning to use the push–pull machine • Understanding that one will not be physically fit unless one works out three or more times a week
Social liberation (belongs to stages 1, 2, 3, and 4)	The individual implements alternatives for ensuring success.	• Encouraging group participation in running • Identifying alternative fitness activities on campus that will help one to become fit
Emotional arousal (belongs to stages 2 and 3)	The individual draws on emotional experiences to instigate changes in behaviour.	• Watching a family member go through a similar situation that does not result in a positive outcome • Analyzing the information provided for the college's alcohol awareness week
Self-evaluation (belongs to stages 2 and 3)	The individual weighs the benefits against the drawbacks.	• Telling oneself, "If I give up smoking I will be able to run without relying on my puffer." • Asking oneself, "What will happen if I accept a ride from this person, who I know has been drinking?"
Commitment (belongs to stages 3, 4, and 5)	The individual now believes in himself or herself and assumes responsibility for changing his or her behaviour.	• Creating an action plan and following through on it • Setting specific time limits for achieving one's goals
Reward (belongs to stages 3, 4, and 5)	The individual rewards himself or herself for changing his or her behaviour.	• Feeling good about oneself and encouraging oneself to succeed • Putting incentives in place to encourage oneself to move forward along the road to success
Countering (belongs to stages 3, 4, and 5)	The individual is prepared to initiate further behavioural changes if the original changes do not work.	• Using a treadmill as an alternative to exercising outside when it is raining • Encouraging another person to help one complete a task that cannot be completed alone
Environmental control (belongs to stages 3, 4, and 5)	The individual alters his or her environment to avoid being tempted by problem behaviours.	• Waking up half an hour early to have time for a workout • Writing a note to oneself about not forgetting one's workout
Helping relationships (belongs to stages 3, 4, and 5)	The individual solicits support from family and friends to change problem behaviours.	• Enlisting a friend as a workout partner • Entering into a written workout "contract" with a friend

Source: Adapted from Prochaska, J.O., DiClemente, C.C., & Norcross, J.C. (1992, September). In search of how people change. *American Psychologist*, *47*, 1102-1114.

that they have internal control over their behaviour. They believe in themselves and do not allow external influences to sabotage their efforts for change. They have the ability to visualize the success they will achieve, and reinforce that success with positive self-talk (such as "I am a strong person who is committed to seeing these changes in myself"). Those who have strong self-efficacy also surround themselves with individuals who support these changes, encourage their attempts, and revel in their successes.

FACTORS THAT AFFECT PARTICIPATION IN PHYSICAL ACTIVITY

Ultimately, there are three main reasons why people participate in physical activity. They include health benefits (for example, preventing a heart attack), enjoyment, and self-image (for example, losing weight).

Health benefits are easy to recognize—"I want to get in shape," "I want to be able to see my child graduate," "I want to feel better." Many individuals are looking for improved strength and stamina, stress reduction, or reduced risk of certain diseases. Often this motivation comes when someone experiences a serious illness or health problem.

health benefits
improvements to physical, mental, and psychological health

Belief that physical activity will lead to this success is key. Through personal experience, observation, and education, those that commit to physical activity have determined expected outcomes and believe they will be successful (self-efficacy).

belief
acceptance of an idea on the basis of knowledge and conviction

Having the right **attitude** (value added to one's belief) when stepping into a fitness program is also a key to success. Going into any activity with a positive attitude will help the success of the outcome.

attitude
value added to one's beliefs

The right **intentions** are important in the success of a fitness program. Those who have made informed decisions, designed a plan of action, and made a commitment are more likely to be successful at staying on a fitness program. For these intentions to work, the plan must be realistic. Individuals need to be aware of the obstacles they may face (for example, shift work, which does not allow them to work out the same time each day) and should determine success markers, sources of support, and rewards for their successes. Individuals must enjoy the physical activity they are doing—very few people who hate running, for example, will ever complete a marathon.

intentions
a determination to achieve an aim

UNDERSTANDING YOUR GOALS

Once you are able to make positive changes in your behaviour, you will have a greater chance of achieving your goals. To achieve your goals, you must understand what they are and why they are important to you. Take, for example, your long-term goal of a career in law enforcement. One possible reason you are attracted to this field is that you like the physical challenges it presents. You know you can meet these challenges because you value physical fitness and have made it a part of your life. Therefore, what you value is reflected in your goal. **Values** are the things that matter most to us and guide our daily behaviour, activities, and decisions. **Assignments 2.1**, **2.2**, and **2.3** are designed to help you set your goals (see the appendix).

values
the things that matter most to us and guide our daily behaviour, activities, and decisions

Assignment 2.1 begins the process by asking you to assess your values. Turn to **assignment 2.1** now.

SHORT- AND LONG-TERM GOALS

In setting your goals, you need to look at short-term goals (for example, goals for the next semester, the next year, or the next two years) and long-term goals (goals for 5 and 10 years down the road). Short-term goals are as simple as passing the test on Thursday, meeting fitness requirements for the semester, or earning a 3.4 grade point average for the year. Short-term goals are smaller and more manageable than long-term goals and exist within limited time frames. Long-term goals can last a lifetime and are a better reflection of who you are as a person and where your interests lie. Long-term goals may have to be adjusted due to changing circumstances in one's life (for example, adjusting when you will take time off to travel due to a job opportunity).

Five kinds of goals (both short- and long-term) drive your life:

personal goals
goals that reflect our personality—who we are, how we think, and how we look

- *Personal goals* **Personal goals** reflect your personality—who you are, how you think, and how you look. Are you prepared to make fitness a lifelong commitment? Do you value your health? Do you have short- or long-term goals that include overcoming personal obstacles?
- *Family and relationship goals* Have you thought about relationships? What kind of lifestyle are you interested in? Will it involve a significant other or children? Do you get on well with your family? What does "family" mean to you? Are your goals the same as those of your significant other (if you have one)?

professional goals
goals that reflect your career aspirations

- *Professional goals* **Professional goals** reflect your career aspirations. What career would you like to pursue? Do you have the academic background and basic skills that law enforcement is looking for? Are you prepared to do what is required by your course of study to achieve your career goals? Do you have the basic skills to successfully pass the police selection process in Ontario, Corrections Canada aptitude testing, or private security screening? Do you have the medical clearance that agencies require (that is, have you had a full medical examination, had your eyes tested for vision and colour blindness, etc.)?
- *Financial goals* Are you choosing a career that will financially support the lifestyle you want? Can you handle loans, credit cards, and other financial obligations? Have you demonstrated a good credit rating?
- *Lifestyle goals* Do you want to travel before getting a full-time job? Where do you want to live? Are you prepared to move anywhere in the province or country to have the career of your choice? Will you commit some of your leisure time to volunteer work with the Girl Guides, the Scouts, sports teams, Neighbourhood Watch, a crisis-intervention team, or similar groups?

Go to **assignment 2.2** (in the appendix) and begin to determine which goals are important to you and what it means to you to be successful.

CHOOSING EFFECTIVE GOALS

Understanding values makes us aware of why we choose certain goals and prepares us to make more effective decisions about our lives. According to the Canadian Society for Exercise Physiology (2003), goals should be meaningful, realistic, specific, and progressive if they are to be attainable.

- *Meaningful goals* are freely chosen goals. A goal cannot be imposed on someone else. Over the years, former law enforcement students have told me how much they disliked running as part of their program. They would run when I instructed them to, but not outside class. It was only after they graduated and realized that maintaining their health and fitness was an important part of their work that they started running for themselves. The moral is that even if someone else opens the door to future wellness, ultimately only you can choose to walk through it.
- *Realistic goals* take individual abilities and constraints into account. Improvements in health and physical performance happen slowly. For example, weight loss does not happen overnight. One needs to establish behavioural and performance goals that are measured out in small increments. For example, if you are sedentary, beginning an exercise program in which you engage in physical activity just three times a week may be a realistic choice for you and allow you to see results. If you set your goals too high, you are more likely to become disappointed and give up.
- *Specific goals* are goals that are clearly formulated. If your goals are not specific, you will not have a sense of direction or purpose.
- *Progressive goals* are goals that build toward a larger purpose. Short-term goals are necessary for producing the results that motivate people to pursue larger, long-term goals. Thus, where fitness is concerned, people need to see short-term results to remain committed to lifelong fitness goals.

Now that you know something about choosing effective goals, go to **assignment 2.3** (in the appendix) to see whether your prioritized goals meet the criteria of effectiveness. The first time through goals setting, most people do not have all of their goals listed. Some people have more difficulty thinking past the next semester. Take a break and go back at it again if you are having some difficulty setting goals. This is an important process you need to have established.

Fifty percent of people who start a fitness program are no longer participating in it six months later (Gledhill, 2001). How can you ensure that you don't become one of those statistics?

STAYING ON TRACK

We inevitably put up obstacles and resistance when we are trying to change. Here are some suggestions to help you deal with some of these problems.

- When your desire to continue a negative behaviour is stronger than the motivation and commitment to change, remember that change does not always happen overnight and the behaviour may have to become more annoying or a greater health risk before you are able to change. Smokers, for example, usually make three or four attempts to break their habit. Don't be too hard on yourself.

social involvement the support of other people to assist you in achieving your goals

- **Social involvement** is a key issue in obtaining goals. Many people, especially young people, pursue activities that are governed more by whom they do those activities with rather than what they do. In this case, the buddy system keeps people involved in the activity. If you have the support of family and friends in the early stages of an activity, you will more likely have a successful behavioural change and continued commitment to that activity. Find the support you need. If your family or close friends can't offer you support, find a support group that will. Monetary commitment to an aerobics class, for example, keeps many people going until they can exercise for other reasons.
- If an activity just isn't for you, try something else. People who have been turned off aerobics classes, for example, can get the same benefits from a program that incorporates martial arts into the moves.
- Although some activities can reduce stress, you may have to take time out from one if you feel that is adding stress to your life. Try something new, or take a small break and then reapproach the activity from a different angle.
- Focus on the real problem. Some people blame others for their inability to change, making excuses and putting things off. Accepting responsibility for your actions and refocusing on the goal may help you succeed.

In addition, the five Cs make activities enjoyable and achievable (Canadian Society for Exercise Physiology, 1996):

1. *Competence* People are more likely to engage and maintain participation in a program that they feel competent doing while being able to learn new skills.
2. *Challenge* The skill needs to match the ability of the individual. If the challenges are too hard, an individual will give up quickly. Conversely, to keep motivation up, the skill must constantly become more challenging.
3. *Control* A sense of personal control leads to higher motivation. This goes back to intrinsic motivation (e.g., improving one's time in the mile-and-a-half run) rather than extrinsic motivation (e.g., passing the requirements of the course).
4. *Choice* By choosing a variety of activities to achieve a goal, people have a greater chance of obtaining their goal.
5. *Commitment* People who have sufficient competence and are involved in a challenging situation that they choose are more likely to stay motivated and committed to the activity.

REWARDING YOURSELF

Behaviours that are rewarded tend to be repeated. Building in different types of rewards to reinforce your efforts will increase your chances of success. Rewards can include treats, breaks from other tasks, monetary rewards (such as a new outfit), and special activities (such as a movie). Remember that everyone has setbacks. Learn from each experience, and try to avoid negative thoughts and comments. Focus on the positive, and move on from there.

Turn to **assignment 2.3**, "Developing Your Short-Term Goals to Achieve Long-Term Goals" (in the appendix). Use the chart "Smart Goal Setting & Action Planner" to develop your action plan. You will determine what steps to take to work toward your goals and what indicators will show you that you are successful. Also determine some rewards to keep yourself motivated. Two to three weeks before the end of the semester, look at **assignment 2.4**, "Summary of Goal Setting Results," and determine how things went.

YOUR MISSION STATEMENT

Having assessed your values, priorities, and long-term goals, you are ready to begin creating your **mission statement**. Your mission statement will reflect your values and goals and be a road map that guides you through life for the next five years.

mission statement
a concise statement of one's major values and goals, meant to give direction to the decisions one will make throughout the course of one's life

It may take a few attempts to create a mission statement that accurately reflects your values and goals. A mission statement is a very personal document about what you want out of life and are striving to achieve. Make sure that your mission statement is dynamic—that is, flexible enough to respond to changes in your life. As your life progresses, so will your goals and mission statement. Remember to think in terms of both professional and personal priorities.

The following is an example of a mission statement:

> My mission is to devote my talents and abilities to continue teaching in the law enforcement field and to encourage and help people (regardless of their age, nationality, and economic background) achieve a safe environment that will promote a positive attitude toward behavioural changes in terms of fitness and knowledge in the area of law enforcement, which is free from discrimination and prejudice. I will strive to balance work with family time, physical activity, and independent growth, while remembering that my family and friends are my first priority.

Remember that your mission statement is exclusively yours. It empowers you to have control over the decisions you must make. The mission statement must truly reflect your goals and guide your everyday decisions.

Turn to **assignment 2.5** (in the appendix) to create your mission statement.

EXAMINING THE PROS AND CONS OF CHANGE

We know that behavioural change has both short-term and long-term benefits and costs. For example, time commitment to activities must change in order for you to participate in physical activity at least 30 minutes each day. Sometimes just getting to where you are working out may take away from social activities, and participation in physical activities becomes a balancing act. In the case of long-term benefits, the decreased risk of cardiovascular diseases, cancers, and premature death may be motivated by a family death.

As you work on your goals, focus on the effects that are most meaningful to you. Remember that in order for these goals to be successful, they must be tied to your values of success.

BEING FIT AND WELL FOR LIFE

Your first attempts at behavioural change may take a bumpy road. For some people, staying at the maintenance stage will be difficult the first time through. To stay fit and be ready for a career in law enforcement takes a great deal of effort. When you are able to maintain this healthy behavioural change, you will realize that this empowerment will lead you to try to achieve new goals. It takes effort, and will constantly change as new information affects your choices. Although you do not have total control over every aspect of your life, especially your health, you do have the ability to create a lifestyle that minimizes your health risks while maximizing your well-being and enjoyment through life. Good luck.

KEY TERMS

extrinsic motivation

intrinsic motivation

self-esteem

self-efficacy

health benefits

belief

attitude

intentions

values

personal goals

professional goals

social involvement

mission statement

EXERCISES

Review

1. What are values?

2. What five kinds of goals drive our lives?

3. Describe the five stages of change using an example from your life.

4. How can the nine processes of change help you achieve your goals?

5. Why is it important to understand values when choosing goals?

6. Describe the four characteristics that make goals attainable.

7. Define self-efficacy, and describe how you would boost your own.

8. What is a mission statement? How can you apply a mission statement to a career in law enforcement?

Multiple Choice

1. Prochaska et al.'s five stages of change include precontemplation, contemplation, preparation, ________________, and ________________.
   a. goal setting, behavioural change
   b. consciousness raising, social liberation
   c. commitment, behavioural change
   d. motivation, support
   e. action, maintenance

2. The stage of change where people acknowledge that they have a problem and are considering doing something about it is the ________________ stage.
   a. precontemplation
   b. contemplation
   c. preparation
   d. action
   e. there is no such stage

3. Which of the following are *processes* in the Prochaska et al. change model?
   a. emotional arousal, contemplation, social liberation
   b. countering, commitment, consciousness raising
   c. maintenance, action, precontemplation
   d. helping motivate, reward, precontemplation
   e. preparation, action, commitment

4. The key to effective behaviour change is
   a. writing a goal statement and posting it in a prominent place
   b. enlisting the help of those around you
   c. identifying the stage of change you are in and using the correct techniques for that stage
   d. setting up a reward system for each process
   e. having a lot of desire and willpower

5. The stage of change in which a person is actively participating in a fitness program for two years is an example of the ________________ stage.
   a. precontemplation
   b. contemplation
   c. preparation
   d. action
   e. there is no such stage

6. People who deny that they need to practise for law enforcement evaluation tests or stop smoking to make the tests easier are in the ________________ stage.
   a. precontemplation
   b. contemplation
   c. preparation
   d. action
   e. there is no such stage

7. In the nine processes of change, social liberation involves
   a. researching information regarding your goal
   b. implementing alternatives to ensure success
   c. drawing on emotional experiences to change your behaviour
   d. weighing the benefits of the change against the consequences
   e. believing in yourself and assuming responsibility for changing your behaviours

8. Countering is a process that involves
   a. rewarding yourself for making changes in your life
   b. weighing the benefits of the change against the consequences
   c. researching information regarding your goal
   d. being prepared to initiate further behavioural changes if the original changes do not work
   e. altering your environment to avoid being tempted by problem behaviours

9. Self-esteem
   a. is dependent on what people think about you
   b. is dependent on social behaviours and physical attributes
   c. is how one looks at one's emotional status
   d. is how one feels about oneself and one's characteristics
   e. is not taken into consideration when someone tries to help motivate someone else into participating in fitness.

10. The three major reasons why people participate in a fitness program are
   a. health benefits, self-image, and enjoyment
   b. health benefits, self-efficacy, and learning a new skill
   c. self-image, self-efficacy, and self-esteem
   d. self-image, learning a new skill, and determination
   e. to learn a new skill, to master that skill, and to meet people

11. Having the right intentions to participate in a fitness program includes
   a. having extrinsic motivation to keep you going
   b. making an informed decision, designing a program, and making a commitment
   c. designing a program, looking for extrinsic motivation, and setting goals for yourself.
   d. having someone design a program that is based on extrinsic motivation with high-expectation goals.
   e designing a program that is based on extrinsic motivation with low-expectation goals.

12. When it comes to values around physical activity, they are based on
   a. daily behaviours, attitude, and goal setting
   b. daily behaviours, fitness programs available, and physical prowess
   c. daily behaviours, individual decisions, and facilities available
   d. daily behaviour, activities available, and individual decisions
   e. daily behaviour, attitude, and physical prowess.

REFERENCES

Canadian Society for Exercise Physiology. (2003). *The Canadian physical activity, fitness and lifestyle approach: CSEP—health and fitness program's health-related appraisal and counselling strategy.* Ottawa: Author.

Gledhill, N. (2001, October 26). *The latest research.* Paper presented at the OASES 13th Annual Professional Development Day and Internet Conference, Toronto, Ontario.

Prochaska, J.O., DiClemente, C.C., & Norcross, J.C. (1992, September). In search of how people change. *American Psychologist, 47,* 1102-1114.

Prochaska, J.O., Norcross, J.C., & DiClemente, C.C. (1994). The five stages of change. In *Changing for good* (pp. 36-50). New York: William Morrow.

CHAPTER 3

Time Management

CHAPTER OBJECTIVES

After completing this chapter, you should be able to:

- Understand the importance of time management.
- Evaluate your time-management skills.
- Manage your time more effectively.

Are you back at school after a number of years? Do you have one or more part-time jobs? Do you have time-consuming family or volunteer commitments? Are you on your own for the first time? If you answered yes to any of these questions, then as a student you need to be aware of your time. Students who fall behind in their work face the stress of trying to keep up. If you can keep up, not only will you be able to follow along with more confidence in class, but you will also experience less stress. If you can develop a balance between school, work, and social life, you will be successful in your endeavours.

In the previous chapter, you learned about setting short- and long-term goals. In this chapter, you will start to see how your goals can be achieved by managing your time well. Time management is essential for successful people in any line of work. In law enforcement, officers are expected to capably manage the time demands of shift work, court appearances, family life, and personal life. Many people who do shift work struggle to maintain a normal routine in their personal life. Those who work 12-hour shifts soon realize that their four-day workweek seems to be consumed by work, travelling back and forth between home and work, and sleep. If court time is added to workdays or days off, it becomes a struggle to organize all their activities. Paper workloads have increased exponentially. There is now a requirement to produce more detailed reports, answer emails, and be more accountable for your time. In high school, many of you had four courses per semester, but now have six to eight courses per semester. At times you can feel overwhelmed by twice the workload.

Setting goals, organizing your time, and adhering to a schedule are critical to a less stressful lifestyle. There is no excuse for officers who cannot carry out a job such as responding quickly to a call because they have mismanaged their time. As in any profession, failure to complete a task can have adverse career repercussions. To be effective, officers must be skilled at juggling different duties. Therefore, as someone pursuing a career in law enforcement, you must make a conscientious effort to manage your time effectively.

THE BENEFITS OF TIME MANAGEMENT

Time management is a way of taking short-term goals and dividing them into manageable daily, weekly, and monthly increments, which in turn makes your long-term goals more achievable. Here are some other benefits of time management:

- It gives meaning to daily activities by increasing one's productivity, accountability, and commitment to the tasks at hand.
- It gives you a sense of order, progress, and success.
- It gives you a sense of control over your life.
- It distinguishes between priorities and non-priorities.
- It helps you deal with mundane tasks in a more effective manner.
- It helps you deal with the boredom of the task.
- It helps to improve your relationships both on and off the job.
- It allows you to do the things that have to be done while having time to do the things you want to do.
- It reduces stress and provides more enjoyment of everyday life.

At the heart of time management is an important shift in focus: you concentrate on results instead of on being busy. Many people spend their days in a frenzy of activity but achieve very little because they are not concentrating on the right things. Studies show that every interruption uses up to 5 minutes in addition to the actual time spent dealing with the interruption, because it takes this amount of time to get back to the task at hand (Georgian College Corporate Training and Consulting, 2001). In **assignment 3.2** you will determine how much time you spend effectively during a one-week period. Some people convert wasted time into a dollar amount (number of hours wasted times hourly salary) to see how much they lost. Money lost can speak volumes, and usually helps to motivate people to rethink how they use their day. Often a lack of time leaves us angry and hostile, unable to focus and maintain our productivity.

What remains unseen is the toll on people and organizations in terms of stress and even illness. Ultimately, those who have good time-management skills are those who enjoy their job.

THE STAGES OF TIME MANAGEMENT

According to Seaward (2004), time management should be broken down into three stages: prioritizing, scheduling, and implementing.

As was discussed in chapter 2, you have to know what your goals are and why, and then prioritize them. The next step is to use a daily appointment book to schedule your activities. Scheduling adds clarity to your day. You must, of course, follow through on (implement) your scheduled activities, or your prioritizing and scheduling become pointless.

The remainder of this chapter will help you evaluate how well you manage your time and get you started on developing your time-management skills. Start by turning to **assignment 3.1** (in the appendix) and determining whether you know where your time is spent. Then go to **assignment 3.2** and actually monitor where you are spending your time. This assignment will help those who need to make better use of their time. Every last detail should be written down, including the time it takes to shower, dress, commute, attend meetings, make phone calls, clean the house, cook dinner, pick up the children from school, take them to after-school activities, and eat meals. Also include time for entertainment or exercise, such as driving to the gym, going for a walk, watching television, surfing the Internet, and answering emails and text messages.

It is important that the first step in efficient time management is organizing the workspace or home. Even if one's schedule is well ordered, if the office and filing system are a disaster, time will be wasted trying to work efficiently in a disorderly place.

Prioritizing Your Activities

To get on track in your use of time, you need to devise an *action plan* or *to-do list* that arranges the things that need to get done under the headings "Essential Activities," "Regular Activities," and "Optional Activities." Some people use calendars or meeting makers to schedule their time more effectively. If you have things written down, you are less likely to forget an assignment, a meeting, or an activity.

- *Essential activities* These are activities you must take care of no matter what, such as attending class, going to work, keeping a medical appointment, putting gas in your car, and paying bills.
- *Regular activities* These are activities that you normally carry out daily or a few days each week. Examples include preparing meals, working out, and doing homework. Regular activities are important but, in terms of scheduling, they offer more flexibility than essential activities offer.
- *Optional activities* This category includes activities you would like to do but can reschedule without much sacrifice, such as a trip to the mall, a social telephone call, and attending a sports event.

See if you can categorize the activities you have ahead of you this week.

Scheduling Your Activities

In addition to including an action plan or to-do list, your daily appointment book should record the following:

- Due dates for papers, projects, presentations, and tests.
- Birthdays, anniversaries, and other special occasions.
- Benchmarks for steps toward a goal, such as due dates for sections of a project, a deadline for losing 2 kg, or a date on which you need to contact someone.
- Important meetings, medical appointments, and due dates for bill payments.
- Your employment schedule (paid and volunteer work).
- Your travel time to get to and from activities.
- Your workout schedule.
- Commitments of a personal nature.

Turn to **assignment 3.3** (in the appendix) and determine your to-do list for this week. Figure out, based on importance, what needs to, should, or could be done this week, and then try mapping out the list on the activity chart. Here are some hints to ensure that your scheduling is effective:

- *Take time to think about time.* Spending 10–15 minutes on time-management planning at the beginning of your day can save time later. Often when individuals write down every last activity, they find that there is very little time left for sleeping. The end result is that many activities must be pared down, eliminated, consolidated, or delegated. It is important to prioritize your activities.
- *Refer to your schedule.* Make sure your daily appointment book and to-do list are easily accessible. Keeping a log may help you identify time-robbers. Word-processing programs contain calendars that can be easily accessed and put to effective use.
- *Develop a game plan.* Allow for at least two evenings to study for a major test. Major research papers require more time. Set time aside to type up papers, and make sure you have an extra cartridge for your printer before you start—you don't want to run out of ink a few hours before a paper is due.
- *Recognize the limits on your time.* There are only 168 hours in a week. Don't set yourself up for failure by asking too much of yourself. Remember that self-discipline is very important if you want to be successful.
- *Categorize a week's worth of hours.* By estimating how many hours your regular activities will take this week, you'll be able to determine how much time you have for other activities. Remember to leave some blocks of time open in case an activity takes longer than expected.
- *Make the most of class.* Read the assignment or chapter before class rather than reading just before a test. You will understand lectures better and be able to take better notes. Read your notes at the end of the day or at least at the end of each week.
- *Schedule downtime.* Everyone needs time to relax and refresh. Make sure your downtime schedule includes activities you enjoy. Remember to enjoy life.
- *Keep your workspace in order.* Piles of paper can be distracting, and you can spend a lot of time looking for misplaced notes or articles. Handle a paper or bill only once—do not become a paper shuffler. Spending 10 minutes at the end of the day to get things in order can save valuable time and give you a fresh start on tomorrow.
- *Remember that practice makes perfect.* Time management, like any new skill, takes time to perfect. Don't forget to review your overall approach to scheduling once in a while to see whether you need to make any changes.
- *Reward yourself.* Plan rewards for yourself for attempting to keep to a schedule and reducing wasted time.

Implementing Your Activities

After you have scheduled your activities, you must follow through on them. Otherwise, you will find yourself falling behind as new tasks arise.

You can also run into implementation problems when you fail to prioritize your activities or set an unreasonable schedule for yourself. You need to avoid procrastination and other time traps (see Keyes, 1991; Rice, 1992; Schafer, 1996).

PROCRASTINATION AND OTHER TIME TRAPS

Many people fail to achieve their goals because they procrastinate over immediate tasks. **Procrastination** is postponing unpleasant or burdensome tasks. Procrastination is often deliberate, especially when you are facing a frightening prospect, such as having to get a major task done in very little time. Turn to **assignment 3.4** (in the appendix) to determine your level of procrastination. If you find yourself with no time left to revise and proofread a paper, feel a rush of adrenalin when you finish a paper ten minutes before it is due, and often pull all-nighters, you may have procrastination issues. Some of the reasons people procrastinate include fear of failure, fear of success (work too hard and lose perspective around you), fear of losing autonomy (wanting control over when and how you have to do something instead of following instructions), and fear of being alone (having to do a solitary activity without someone helping or being around). These fears can paralyze us and keep us from taking action, until discomfort and anxiety overwhelms us and forces us to get the task done or give up (Burka, 2004).

procrastination
the postponement of unpleasant or burdensome tasks

Here are some strategies for fighting procrastination. Remember, there are no quick fixes. You aren't going to wake up tomorrow and never procrastinate again. However, you might figure out how to do one or two simple tasks that will help you finish a draft a little earlier or reduce your level of stress.

- Weigh the benefits of completing the task against the drawbacks of procrastinating. If you have two assignments that are due the next day, you may not be able to spend the time that you should on each, and will have to determine which one may be worth more or which one is more beneficial (in terms of marks) to complete with more details.
- Reward yourself for completing a task. Punishing yourself every time you put something off won't help you change. Try to be a little less critical of yourself.
- Ask for help with school, work, and domestic tasks. Learn to delegate (but don't dump all the work on someone else).
- Don't expect to be perfect—just do your best.
- Set goals that can realistically be accomplished in the time you have. Connect daily activities to your work and life goals.
- Adopt a positive attitude.
- Get started—the worst thing you can do is make excuses or perform other tasks simply to avoid the task you don't want to face.
- Analyze a task and break it down into manageable parts.
- Make time for exercise and relaxation so that you can rejuvenate and develop a fresh perspective.
- Screen out the telephone, text messages, Internet, email, the television, and junk mail. If you are already overloaded, do not let these take the place of the task at hand.

Here are some strategies to help prepare for tests:

- Identify the best time to study, whether it is morning, afternoon, or early evening. If your classes don't start until the afternoon, use your free time in the morning to get studying out of the way.
- Review your notes after your class. If they don't make sense, the information is still fresh in your head to correct them or to make a note to ask your teacher to clarify the information.
- Study the more challenging components first, when you are less fatigued. When you become tired, it's easier to cover the material you enjoy more.
- Study in the same place each time—you'll be able to focus on the task more quickly. Stay off the bed; 10-minute naps can easily turn into two-hour naps.
- If you are falling asleep, take a 10-minute nap. Put the alarm on loud enough to hear it immediately, and come back to the material more refreshed.
- Use waiting time (public transportation, the hour between classes) to learn something small or write things out on cue cards that you can go over in order to help you memorize facts.
- Treat school as a full-time job. Remember that for every hour you are in class, you probably will be expected to do one to two hours of work outside the classroom. It takes time to read texts, read the blackboard, and study for tests. If you have to work, know your limits and try to stick to set hours that you can handle.

Here are some time-management tips that may help to prevent becoming overwhelmed in the first place:

- *Don't say yes when you really don't have the time.* Learn to say no graciously. Although this is one of the hardest skills to learn, you will experience less stress and be able to enjoy some time to yourself when you learn to say no to people.
- *Avoid studying during those times of the day when you are the least productive.* If you are a morning person, try to do your homework in the morning. Even if you have only a short time for homework in the morning, use that time effectively.
- *Think ahead.* By thinking ahead you won't forget things or waste time. Don't be the student who tries to convince the teacher that it was the computer's fault for crashing 10 minutes before your assignment was due.
- *Limit your social time.* Socializing is important, but going out five nights a week is not going to bring you success in school. Limit your phone conversations. Most importantly, don't give in to peer pressure.
- *Delegate.* Some things you must do for yourself, but there are times when you can ask for a favour (just be sure you do one in return). Be reasonable about how many tasks you really can do. Don't get to the point where you are overwhelmed; cut the task down or ask for help even if you are part of the way through it.
- *Don't try to do too much.* Many people do too much and become stressed or suffer chronic time urgency. **Chronic time urgency** is not just the result

chronic time urgency
a constant state of stress due to putting pressure on yourself to do too much in too little time

of external pressure, but occurs when people put pressure on themselves to perform an unreasonable number of tasks. They think that they must always be productive and complete their tasks in the shortest possible time with no help. People who experience chronic time urgency become agitated because they always feel that they are in a hurry and will let others down if they cannot complete everything they set out to do. Leave some time open for unplanned events that are beyond your control.

- *Learn to limit the number of times you use chat lines, text messaging, email, or the phone.* Specifically set aside a certain time frame for these activities, and stick to it even if you are not finished (that is, first thing in the morning, just before lunch, and an hour before shutting down your computer). Sometimes it's better to leave a detailed message explaining specifically what information you require rather than responding to two or three additional messages.
- *Do not multitask when on the phone or having face-to-face conversations with another person.* This will reduce the conversation time as well as making sure that key information is conveyed.
- *Ask for help.* There are a multitude of individuals at your college who are there to assist you, including faculty, counsellors, learning strategists, and librarians. Learn what other resources your college has to offer. Many colleges have writing centres, math labs, and career centres. Some offer e-learning programs, such as SkillSoft eLearning, that are designed to help with basic computer skills, word processing, and Web design.

  Try to realize that you must work at a pace that is conducive to health, and set only realistic goals. Step back now and then and ensure that your priorities are reasonable. Stop hurrying when there is no need to hurry.

ORGANIZING ASSIGNMENTS

Here are some helpful tips for when you are working on an assignment with a deadline:

- There is no "right" way to break up the work and start—it depends on your personality.
- You can begin in the middle of the assignment and work out, start with the most difficult part, the most important part, or the most profitable part (the part that has the most marks attached to it).
- Nibble at the corners, ease into a tough assignment by doing the simple, routine, or the more pleasant parts of it.
- Consider the deadline. Some people work best "under the gun," while others suffer shell shock. Regardless, make sure you at least understand the task so that if you need information or equipment it will be there when the deadline looms. There is no excuse for running out of paper or printer ink.
- Some people work in bursts and intersperse other activities, such as a workout, before returning to a project. Others need to stay focused and work continuously to get it done. Schedule your time according to your strengths.

GROUP WORK AND DELEGATION

One of the skills that a law enforcement employer is looking for is an ability to work effectively in groups. So much time can be wasted if you don't have the right group or have assigned the wrong person to a task. It can be very frustrating to be assigned by your boss or teacher to a group that you know has weaker individuals who have difficulty contributing. Here are some tips to help with group work:

- If you are allowed to choose your group, choose people who complement your work ethics (not necessarily work the same way you do) and work well in team settings.
- Decide what needs to be delegated. Determine what can and cannot be delegated, ensuring that both popular and unpopular components, and important and less important components, are delegated.
- Choose the right person for the job. Ensure that the workload is evenly distributed and that individuals are given authority over their work.
- Set goals for different tasks. Start with small projects to ensure that the group is on the right track. Define from the outset how well the group wants each task accomplished—what will be considered a "good" job? That will save frustration and time later. Agree on deadlines.
- As a group, agree who is in charge of overseeing the project. Plan periodic reviews and schedule them when you first start the assignment. Make sure everyone knows his or her role from the start. Then stand back and allow individuals to do their jobs.
- At the periodic reviews and when the final product is brought together, make sure to review the project before handing it in. Hold people accountable for their contribution.

RUNNING AN EFFECTIVE MEETING

A well-run meeting proceeds without wasted motion from beginning to end. If it is well planned, has a defined purpose, follows an agenda, and proceeds crisply, it will be an effective meeting. Unfortunately, many meetings do not go well—they may be too long, deal too much with extraneous issues, include people who arrive late and disrupt the flow, and so on. Here are some tips for having an effective meeting:

- Give people ample notice so that they can prepare based on the agenda sent out, be able to notify you whether they can attend, and arrive on time.
- Start at the appointed time, whether everyone is there or not. Ignore late arrivals—keep the agenda rolling and keep to the time limit you have set for the meeting.
- Have a purpose that all participants know and understand (e.g., analyze or solve a problem, achieve a training objective, or reconcile a conflict).
- Have an agenda that is organized to achieve the purpose and that ensures that everyone is on the same page.
- Include as participants only those who will contribute to or gain something from the meeting. Do not allow small groups to start up separate conversations.

- Stick to the agenda, with no wasted time or motions. Restate the relevant points of the agenda when the discussion veers from the objectives.
- Ask open-ended questions to obtain different points of view and to make sure that everyone's point of view is being heard.
- Allow participants to understand their role, come prepared, and make contributions. Prevent individuals from dominating the discussion by asking them to allow others to speak.
- Make sure that one person chairs the meeting. The chair should summarize what has been accomplished so everyone has the same understanding.
- Have a post-meeting follow-up where necessary. Include off-target subjects to be discussed at a later meeting.

FINAL THOUGHTS ON TIME MANAGEMENT

Remember that the more you use your time-management skills, the closer you will be to achieving your long-term goals. It is very important to follow a schedule. If you fail to keep to your schedule, ask yourself why and attempt to change the behaviours that caused the problem. If you need help, ask. Every college campus has counselling services to help you make your academic career a success. A faculty member can point you in the right direction if you are unsure where to turn.

Remember that you have to find a balance between work and play. As Schafer (1996, p. 493) advises, "Learn to live with unfinished tasks—only a corpse is completely finished."

KEY TERMS

procrastination

chronic time urgency

EXERCISES

Review

1. Why is it important to organize your time?

2. How does time management relate to goal setting?

3. Briefly describe the three headings under which activities can be prioritized.

4. What are some effective methods to assist you with your schedule?

5. What is procrastination? How can it be overcome?

6. What are some of the signs that may indicate that you are procrastinating?

7. What are some other time traps? How can they be overcome?

8. What can you do to prevent multimedia and electronic devices from monopolizing your time?

9. What can you do to make studying time more effective?

10. How can you organize yourself to ensure that all your assignments are completed and handed in on time?

Multiple Choice

1. Which of the following is a health-related consequence of an unrealistic schedule?
   a. creating stress
   b. being late for classes
   c. missing your bus or car pool
   d. failing to return calls
   e. forgetting your textbooks in the cafeteria

2. Travel to and from school and work, household chores, and child care are examples of
   a. free time
   b. work time
   c. committed time
   d. lost time
   e. valued time

3. What is the first step to managing time effectively?
   a. analyzing your current time use
   b. establishing priorities
   c. making a schedule
   d. monitoring your current time use
   e. creating a calendar of your monthly events

4. Writing down your goals will help you to
   a. organize them
   b. evaluate them
   c. remember them
   d. publish them
   e. share them with others

5. Managing your time by organizing and scheduling activities will
   a. not make a difference
   b. give you more control over daily stress
   c. give you no more time for other activities
   d. just be a paper exercise
   e. let others see how busy you are

6. The three stages of good time management are
   a. prioritizing, scheduling, and involving
   b. scheduling, implementing, and assessing
   c. scheduling, organizing, and implementing
   d. prioritizing, organizing, and implementing
   e. prioritizing, scheduling, and implementing

7. In recent years, the amount of time the average person spent at work has
   a. decreased
   b. increased
   c. remained the same
   d. fluctuated up and down
   e. depended on each person's needs

8. Which is most likely to suffer due to a lack of time?
   a. work
   b. chores
   c. sleep
   d. relationships
   e. travel time

9. "Killing two birds with one stone" in time management means
   a. rescheduling recreation regularly
   b. arranging recreation during work
   c. combining recreation with other leisure activities
   d. planning recreation at least two or three weeks early
   e. avoiding recreation to get work done

10. Chronic time urgency refers to
    a. teachers assigning you too much homework
    b. putting too much pressure on yourself to perform a number of tasks
    c. having your family expect you to help clean around home before doing your homework
    d. organizing a number of tasks to get them done in time
    e. setting realistic goals for yourself

REFERENCES

Burka, J.B., & Yuen, L.M. (2004). *Procrastination: Why you do it, what to do about it.* New York, NY: Da Capo Press.

Georgian College Corporate Training and Consulting. (2001). *Time management training.* Barrie, ON: Author.

Georgian College (2007). Current student web page. Available at http://www.georgianc.on.ca/current/.

Keyes, R. (1991). *Timelock: How life got so hectic and what you can do about it.* New York: Ballantine Books.

Rice, P.L. (1992). *Stress and health.* Pacific Grove, CA: Brooks/Coles.

Schafer, W. (1996). *Stress management for wellness* (3rd ed.). Orlando, FL: Holt, Rinehart and Winston.

Seaward, B.L. (2004). *Managing stress: Principles and strategies for health and wellbeing* (4th ed.). Boston: Jones and Bartlett.

PART II

Planning and Maintaining a Fitness Program

CHAPTER 4

Physical Fitness

CHAPTER OBJECTIVES

After completing this chapter, you should be able to:

- Explain how health-related and performance/skill-related fitness are important in law enforcement.
- Describe the benefits of exercise, both physical and psychological.
- Understand the principles of physical training and how to apply them in your fitness program.
- Describe the proper way to start a fitness program.

In this chapter, you will learn about the components of physical fitness and the benefits of physical activity. As you begin your studies toward a career in law enforcement, you must also begin a fitness program that trains you to endure the physical challenges of policing. This chapter will help you understand why physical fitness is important in policing.

As was pointed out in chapter 1, physical activity is all leisure and non-leisure body movement that results in an expenditure of energy. Physical fitness, however, measures a person's health and performance using a set of attributes that are either health-related or performance/skill-related, as well as key concepts in training principles. This chapter will look at these attributes.

Physical activity is so important. We know that Canadians are now more active in their leisure time than they were two decades ago, but the majority are still not active enough overall for long-term health and well-being (Coalition for Active Living, 2004). Overweight children experience physical and psychological health problems during childhood. They are at increased risk of developing chronic diseases later in life, because they are more likely to become overweight adults (Perez, 2003). Four out of five Canadian adolescents do not participate in the recommended volume of physical activity suggested by Canada's *Physical Activity Guide.* Slightly more primary school than secondary school youth are physically active on a daily basis (19 percent versus 17 percent (Canadian Adolescents at Risk Research Network, 2004). The most profound concern is that there has been a progressive increase in the body mass index (BMI) of Canadian youth (aged 7 to 13) from 1981 to 1996, with the prevalence of obesity in this age group more than doubling over this period. Vigorous physical activity defined as at least three bouts of 20 minutes per week) among youth has decreased, and smoking among secondary school students continues to be common (Plotnikoff, 2004). The implications of health-related diseases associated with physical inactivity can be reversed if individuals are willing to take ownership of their physical well-being. As you research the components of physical training, remember the goals you set in chapter 2. They will assist you in determining which goals may be more important.

WHAT IS TRAINING?

In the simplest terms, training refers to making your body more efficient. If you can train your body through general fitness activities (for example, running or weight training), you will be able to do parts of your job more efficiently (for example, chasing potential criminals, enduring a physical altercation, or being able to function at 4 a.m. when asked to search for a lost person).

This process and the changes that take place are dependent on the individual who is training and the goals that he or she has set. It may be to gain more muscle, to reduce body fat, to have the best time on the 1.5 mile run at the fitness pin test, or to reduce stress.

Training is an individual process. It depends on the objectives of the workout and the attributes of the individual involved. There are a number of ways in which to modify your body's attributes, and each person must understand that there may be a variety of options available to achieve those changes. Finding out which way works best for you will take time and effort. Human performance results cannot be completely standardized. In other words, no one program works the same for each person. It is impossible to expect that a fitness instructor would be able to give your entire class the same program and have the same results by the end of the course. Ultimately, you will have to do a great deal of training to find out which program you are most successful at.

HEALTH-RELATED FITNESS

The Police Fitness Personnel of Ontario (PFPO) has advocated the importance of health-related fitness in policing for over 20 years. It has promoted a fitness pin award that looks at components to support the fact that officers that are fit will be able to do their jobs more effectively and safely.

The five components of health-related fitness are cardiorespiratory endurance, muscular strength, muscular endurance, flexibility, and a healthy body composition. Regular physical activity leads to improvements in all five areas.

Cardiorespiratory Endurance

cardiorespiratory endurance
heart and respiratory system endurance; the ability to perform prolonged large-muscle activities at moderate to high intensity

Cardiorespiratory endurance (heart and respiratory system endurance) is the ability of the heart to pump blood throughout the body efficiently. This means your body can perform prolonged large-muscle activities, such as swimming or jogging, at moderate to high intensity. It is probably the most important component of fitness. When you regularly engage in activities that improve cardiorespiratory endurance, you enhance your body's ability to regulate blood flow and use oxygen and other fuels. As a result, you lower your resting heart rate and blood pressure, and your ability to dissipate heat increases. Having the stamina for a foot chase is one example of how cardiorespiratory endurance is important in law enforcement.

Muscular Strength

Muscular strength is the amount of force a muscle can produce with a single maximum effort. Strong muscles are important for daily activities such as climbing stairs, vacuuming, and carrying groceries. Strong muscles provide good structural support for the back and help prevent back and leg pain. Muscular strength is also important in recreational activities. It helps us, for example, jump higher in volleyball, hit a tennis ball harder, and kick a soccer ball farther.

muscular strength
the amount of force a muscle can produce with a single maximum effort

Abundant muscle tissue is important for overall health. A greater muscle mass increases the body's metabolism rate (the rate at which the body breaks down food, producing energy). It also gives you more strength to perform daily activities such as lifting and pulling heavy objects. Strength training is vital to prevent diseases such as osteoporosis. Muscular strength can be developed by training with weights or by doing calisthenic exercises, such as push-ups, that do not require special equipment.

Muscular Endurance

Muscular endurance is the ability of a muscle to sustain a prolonged contraction or to contract over and over again. Muscular endurance is important for injury prevention and proper posture. Without strong back and abdominal muscles, one's spine is subjected to stress that can result in lower-back pain. For law enforcement officers, who must carry an equipment belt weighing 7 to 9 kg, abdominal strength is important. Muscular endurance exercises involve applying a force to the muscle that is greater than what the muscle is used to. Muscular endurance can be achieved by exercising with weight-training equipment. In these exercises, light weights are combined with a high number of repetitions.

muscular endurance
the ability of a muscle to sustain a prolonged contraction or to contract over and over again

Flexibility

Flexibility is the ability to move the joints freely through their full range of motion. As one ages, lack of flexibility can create poor posture and be debilitating. Stiff joints and a restricted range of motion can lead to lower-back problems, an issue that we will look at in chapter 11. Without flexibility, it is easier to get hurt when reaching or twisting inappropriately. Flexibility leads to muscles that are more supple and less prone to injury. Flexibility can be maintained by following a regular fitness program.

flexibility
the ability to move the joints freely through their full range of motion

Body Composition

Body composition (discussed in greater detail in chapter 9) refers to the proportion of lean tissue (muscle and bone) to fat in the body. A healthy body composition requires a large proportion of lean tissue and a small proportion of fat. Fat is important for organ protection, for control of heat production and heat loss, and as a source of energy that the body can use. However, people with excessive fat risk joint problems, back pain, heart disease, high blood pressure, stroke, gallbladder disease,

body composition
the proportion of lean tissue to fat in the body

cancer, and other illnesses. The healthiest way to lose fat is to exercise and to adhere to a sensible diet recommended by your doctor. Weight training is the best way to increase lean tissue mass.

PERFORMANCE/SKILL-RELATED FITNESS

The six components of performance/skill-related fitness are speed, coordination, reaction time, agility, balance, and power. These are greatly enhanced when you exercise regularly. Although not considered essential for a healthy life, the six components are especially important in law enforcement—for example, if you are involved in a foot chase, a physical altercation, or a rescue. All of these situations require you to be in top physical condition and able to respond to trouble quickly and appropriately. Both health-related and performance/skill-related fitness are evaluated by the Physical Readiness Evaluation for Policing (PREP) test, the Physical Ability Requirement Evaluation (PARE) test, and the Police Officer Physical Abilities Test (POPAT). (The POPAT was developed for police in British Columbia and has been modified to create a PARE test based on the analysis of specific demands for RCMP and Corrections Canada jobs.) These tests will be discussed in detail in chapter 15.

Speed

Speed is the ability to move quickly. During a foot chase, for example, a law enforcement officer requires leg and foot speed.

Coordination

Coordination involves the mind and body working together to perform motor tasks smoothly and accurately. Good coordination is needed, for example, to jump over obstacles, kick a soccer ball, and hit a golf ball. Using firearms also requires good coordination. Without it, hitting a target is almost impossible.

Reaction Time

Reaction time is the time that elapses between stimulation and the beginning of one's reaction to the stimulus. For a law enforcement officer, being able to react quickly to a volatile situation can mean the difference between success and failure and even between staying alive and getting killed.

Agility

Agility is the ability to rapidly and accurately change the body's direction of movement. Skiing, mountain biking, and self-defence are examples of activities that require agility.

Balance

Balance refers to the body's ability to maintain equilibrium while stationary or moving. Walking across a support beam, performing on a balance beam, and self-defence are activities that require good balance.

Power

Power is the ability to transform energy into force at a rapid rate. Power is necessary in sports such as discus throwing and the shot put. In law enforcement, power is necessary to move a person out of the way, scale a wall, or jump a railing.

Before reading any further, go to **assignment 4.1** (in the appendix) and see if you can list some of the health benefits of physical activity.

THE HEALTH BENEFITS OF PHYSICAL ACTIVITY

Regular physical activity produces long-term improvements in body function. These benefits are both physical and psychological.

Physical Benefits

The health of Canadians has been a huge issue with researchers. Many papers and research grants have addressed this issue in hopes of providing a business case for the government to do something about our health status. These studies have pointed out that there are key benefits of physical activity, including:

- increased nervous system and sensory adaptation, allowing muscles to react in a shorter time (Bouchard et al., 1990)
- increased ability of muscle tissue to sustain long bouts of endurance activities without undue fatigue (Bouchard et al., 1990; Shephard, 1997)
- prevention of cardiovascular decline, which has been shown to decline by as much as one-half in inactive adults between the ages of 30 and 70 (Wagner, 1992)
- improved strength, increased lean muscle, and decreased body fat (Bouchard et al., 1990; Pitts, 1996)
- increased responsiveness of the sympathetic nervous system (the part of the autonomic nervous system that regulates your reaction to stress—that is, speeds up the heart rate, narrows blood vessels, and raises blood pressure), making the body's energy system more efficient (one result of this is the ability to burn fat during endurance activities) (Bouchard et al., 1990)
- stronger cardiorespiratory system, which reduces the risk of cardiovascular diseases by reducing resting heart rate and increasing stroke volume (the amount of blood the heart can pump out with each beat) (Bouchard et al., 1990; Klonoff, 1994)
- control of joint swelling and pain (Bouchard et al., 1990)
- decreased risk of non-insulin-dependent diabetes (Bouchard et al., 1990; Pitts, 1996)
- stronger immune system (however, if you overtrain, you can weaken your immune system) (Bouchard et al., 1990)
- increased bone density, thereby reducing the risk of osteoporosis or broken bones (Bouchard et al., 1990; Klonoff, 1994)

Psychological Benefits

A regular fitness program offers not only physical but also psychological benefits. Some of the psychological benefits are as follows:

- decreased symptoms of stress (McAuley & Wall, 1994)
- an improved appearance, which in turn contributes to a more positive self-image, greater confidence, and better interaction with others (McAuley & Wall, 1994)
- more energy (McAuley & Wall, 1994)
- improved moods and greater resistance to mental depression (Shephard, 1997; Anspaugh, 1996)
- better sleep (McAuley & Wall, 1994)
- better eating habits and better care of personal health (McAuley & Wall, 1994)
- better job satisfaction with better morale, increased productivity, and reduced absenteeism (Elias & Murphy, 1986)
- improved ability to live independently as you age (McAuley & Wall, 1994)

Physical inactivity costs the Canadian health care system at least $2.1 billion annually (Katzmarzyk, 2000) in direct health care costs, and the estimated total annual economic burden is approximately $53 billion (Katzmarzyk, 2004). The Canadian government has undertaken the development of a healthy living strategy with an emphasis on physical activity, where areas such as healthy weights, mental health, and injury prevention will be identified (Ministry of Health, 2005).

Turn to **assignment 4.2** (in the appendix) and list the physical and psychological benefits of physical activity that are most important to you.

THE PRINCIPLES OF PHYSICAL TRAINING

The goal of physical training is to bring about some of the physical and psychological benefits discussed above and to improve the body's functioning. Although there is inevitably a limit to the level of fitness and performance you can attain—a limit that varies from person to person—physical training gives everyone the chance to experience at least some of the physical and psychological benefits of physical activity.

Particular fitness outcomes require particular exercises. For example, to conform to the aerobic component of the Bona Fide Occupational Requirement (BFOR) (discussed as part of the PARE test in chapter 16), you have to be willing to devote some time to running. Léger (1982; Léger & Lambert, 1985) equates level 6.5 in the shuttle run component of the PREP to running 1.5 miles in approximately 11 minutes and 30 seconds. The level at which one completes the shuttle run does not necessarily correlate to the time that it takes the person to run 1.5 miles; although results do indicate that those who can successfully run 1.5 miles in the specified time have no difficulties in completing level 6.5 in the shuttle run.

The basic principles of physical training are specificity, progressive overload, reversibility, individuality, and recovery (Canadian Society for Exercise Physiology, 1996).

The Principle of Specificity

The **principle of specificity** refers to the ability of the body to adapt to a particular type and amount of stress placed on it. To develop a particular fitness skill, one must choose exercises tailored to that skill. Over the past 15 years, the primary reason many law enforcement students have failed the 1.5-mile run or shuttle run has been their lack of commitment to aerobic training—specifically running. Although weight training and cycling provide some cross-training effects, nothing can take the place of running. Similarly, the demands of the push–pull machine and the arm-restraint device are best met by an upper-body strength training program. A commitment to law enforcement requires a well-rounded fitness program with training components tailored to cardiorespiratory endurance, strength, and flexibility.

principle of specificity refers to the ability of the body to adapt to a particular type and amount of stress placed on it

The specificity principle is sometimes referred to as the SAID (specific adaptation to imposed demand) principle. Muscle adaptation will occur when you place a specific demand for improvement on a specific skill. It is important, then, to train to a high aerobic level to be successful in aerobic training. It is also important to train anaerobically to manoeuvre easily up and down the stairs on the PREP and PARE BFORs. It is also imperative that you have leg strength to easily use the push–pull machine.

Progressive Overload

Progressive overload refers to providing a greater stress or load on the body than it is used to. The body needs to be subjected to increasing gradual demands in order to produce continual improvements. If the body is not worked hard enough or, on the other hand, is worked too hard, physical training will not produce benefits. Excessive exercise may in fact cause detraining and injuries.

The **principle of overload** takes into account that both the skeletal and cardiac muscles adapt to the overloading. This means that the body becomes more efficient and able to handle greater loads. For example, in order to easily complete a 1.5-mile run, your training has to go from a jog to a run, from running for 20 minutes to 40 minutes, and increasing your pace from about 9 to 12 km/h. If you decrease your levels of exercise, the gains that you achieved will start to disappear.

principle of overload refers to training and overloading our muscles that help us to adapt to more and more stress

Progressive overload is accomplished by gradually increasing these criteria, which together are known as the FITT principle:

- *Frequency* Most objectives require a training level of three to five times a week. People whose fitness level is low should begin with three times a week, and then gradually build up to five. Once your goals are reached, physical activity two or three times a week is needed to maintain your fitness level.
- *Intensity* To benefit from an exercise, you need to gradually increase the intensity of the exercise over the course of your training program—for example, slowly increasing the weight pushed or pulled for strength training, by gradually raising jogging speed to increase cardiorespiratory intensity, or by stretching muscles more and more with each workout to increase flexibility. But increasing the intensity of a workout must be done in small steps to avoid injuries. Also, for beginners, intensity is less important than frequency and duration.

- *Time* (duration) Exercise produces benefits only if your exercise sessions last for extended periods of time. And as you progress, you should increase the duration of the sessions. A runner who wants to increase cardiorespiratory endurance, for example, may begin with 20-minute sessions and slowly move up to 60-minute sessions (20–60 minutes is normal for endurance training).
- *Type of exercise* The exercises relate to the specific program you are involved with. In aerobic training, they include activities that work large-muscle groups and that can be done in a rhythmic fashion, such as brisk walking, cycling, swimming, and running. In weight training, they include activities that focus on the muscles that you want to strengthen or increase.

The Principle of Progression

With training and overloading, our muscles are able to adapt to more and more stress. In order to continue to see improvements, individuals must continue to increase the stress placed on their muscles. This means that over time, if the number of repetitions or sets of exercises are not adjusted, the muscles will begin to adapt and not gain in strength or size.

The Principle of Individuality

Each body's response to exercise is different. Several factors come into play, including physical and psychological makeup, age, gender, the ability to recover after a workout, and susceptibility to injury. These all play a part in designing a program. For example, in weight training, individuals must either change the number of reps or sets they are performing, or for a few weeks change their entire program, in order to confuse the muscles into having to work in a different way and cause changes at the cellular level.

The Principle of Reversibility

principle of reversibility refers to all the benefits of exercise that are lost if you stop training

According to the **principle of reversibility**, all of the benefits of exercise are lost if you stop training. Atrophy occurs when muscles undergo periods of complete or near-complete inactivity. In fact, up to 20 percent of exercise benefits can be lost in the first two weeks of not training, and as much as 50 percent can be lost in less than two months. Not only do muscles lose strength with disuse, but they also decrease in size. Detraining is the term used to describe the time period in which someone who has undergone a significant amount of training either stops completely or to a large extent. This happens for a number of reasons, including the inability to train because of an injury, the lack of an available open gym when an individual is off-shift, a lack of motivation, or the need for family time. One way to prevent much of this loss is to maintain the intensity of your workouts, even if you cannot maintain the frequency and duration.

The Principle of Diminishing Returns

The principle of diminishing returns is based on the fact that a person's training gains will reflect that person's prior level of training. People who have had little training make significant gains both in terms of strength and aerobic capacity.

Those that are highly trained make relatively small gains. For example, those that start running at the beginning of a course for the first time are able to see significant decreases in their times (sometimes by as much as 3–4 minutes), while those that are runners usually only see gains (their time for their run decreases by less than one-half of a minute). It becomes very important to try new training methods or different equipment in order to see more gains.

Devising an exercise program that is most suited to you depends on your goals, the requirements of the law enforcement community, and your fitness level. Depending on your size, you may be spending substantially more time in a program to meet the demands of the BFOR standards and preparing for the demands of the job.

The Principle of Recovery

The **principle of recovery** is tied to the recuperation time or amount of rest required after a workout. It is important to realize that torn muscle tissue needs time to repair. In cardiorespiratory training, beginners should exercise three times a week and leave at least a day between each session. Similarly, in weight training, beginners should allow a day's rest between each day of training. In strength training, beginners may need 48 hours or more between workouts. Also, be aware that more demanding exercise programs typically require more rest between training sessions.

principle of recovery refers to the recuperation time or amount of rest required after a workout

People who do not feel a small increase in strength after each workout, or experience pain with each workout, may need to change how often they work out.

Turn to **assignment 4.3** (in the appendix) and review your fitness training goals.

TRAINING METHODS

When training for the BFOR tests, it becomes necessary to focus on increasing your speed, endurance, strength, agility, and flexibility. To achieve these goals, a number of training methods have been devised to provide variety and challenge, including periodization, concurrent training, interval training, Fartlek training, resistance training, and plyometric training.

Periodization

Periodization refers to the overall training plan where an individual maximizes performances at peak times. This reduces the risk of injury and mental burnout. In sports, training periods are separated into off-season, pre-season, and in-season. There is a distinct period where athletes learn necessary skills and motor development, and then gradually improve in skill, strength, and endurance while competing in their sport. Some of you may want to consider this as a method for reaching your goals. In order to successfully pass fitness standards, individuals need to set up programs. These should include a small period in order to become familiar with the BFOR equipment. The preparation period that follows should include a high-volume, low-intensity training program in order to learn the routine. This should be followed by a strength phase, where strength is built up to be able to do a task with ease, and a power phase to address the fact that training intensity increases while volume may be decreasing. The competitive or in-season stage usually combines shorter periods of training specific skills at more intense levels with tapering

periodization overall training plan where an individual maximizes performances at peak times

or complete rest just prior to a competition. In terms of meeting BFOR standards, this means that individuals need to train generally for increasing their level of fitness. Then they are required to train on the equipment needed to practise the push–pull, arm-restraint, the shuttle run, and victim relocation, as well as jumping over objects and interval training on stairs. The final stage would be to ensure that the individual could easily get to level 6.5 on the shuttle, do the equipment movements with ease, and be able to complete the circuit in the required time frame prior to testing.

Concurrent Training

concurrent training
training for either strength or power at the same time you train for endurance

Concurrent training refers to the principle that you train for either strength or power at the same time you train for endurance. Those who train more generally have leaner muscle mass and lower body fat composition, which makes the tasks of the job easier to do.

Interval Training

interval training
training that is based on the concept that the body's energy systems can make both aerobic and anaerobic gains by training with relatively intense exercises followed by period of recovery

Interval training is based on the concept that the body's energy systems can make both aerobic and anaerobic gains by training with relatively intense exercises followed by a period of recovery. Intensity and recovery times depend on the individual's level of fitness. For example, runners will do intervals of 400 metres to train for 1.5-mile (2.41 km) runs. By attempting to increase the number of repetitions and varying the speed, many runners are able to reduce their time on the run.

Fartlek Training

fartlek training
interval training of distances at intense levels followed by recovery periods at predetermined intervals

Fartlek training (derived from the Swedish term for "speed play") refers to interval training of distances at intense levels followed by recovery periods at predetermined intervals. Fartlek provides an excellent endurance and strength session and also helps to improve speed and race awareness. It is known to stress both the aerobic and anaerobic energy pathways. The theory behind it is to run at a set pace, take a break, and begin again. This becomes a very structured interval training program (for example, run 200 m, walk 100 m, and repeat). Fartlek has grown into a popular method of training used by runners to provide an enjoyable and constructive alternative to simply pounding the streets with no purpose and plan. It is more free form, and done over a variety of terrains (for example, hills, sand beaches).

Resistance Training

resistance training
the most common form of weight training which incorporates exercises that result in gains to muscle mass and strength as well as the potential for improved flexibility and range of motion

The most common form of weight training is **resistance training**. There are gains to muscle mass and strength, as well as potential for improved flexibility and range of motion. This form of training is usually associated with a reduced number of injuries. Resistance training benefits are dependent on the number of repetitions and sets, the rest periods between exercises, and the intensity and volume of workouts.

Plyometric Training

plyometric training
a form of resistance training that works on developing strength and power

Plyometric training is a form of resistance training that works on developing strength and power. Through a series of drills, usually using your own body weight or with medicine balls, exercise bands, stability balls, or weighted vests, individuals develop programs that include exercises that have explosive movements through countermovements to build muscular energy and power. Examples include squat-jumps, box drills, hopping, and ballistic medicine ball drills. Individuals have to be highly motivated to do this kind of training.

GUIDELINES FOR STARTING A FITNESS PROGRAM

To ensure that you enjoy exercising and do it safely, here are some guidelines for starting a fitness program:

- *Start slowly.* When you begin your program, remember that duration and frequency should take precedence over intensity. If you are experiencing muscle soreness 48 hours after your workout, or are experiencing a lack of energy or decreased physical performance, you are probably suffering from overtraining and are at risk of injury. Remember that you are making a lifelong commitment to fitness, so it is not important to get in shape as fast as possible. Instead, gradually build up to your desired fitness level, and then work on maintaining that level.
- *Train specifically to meet the job demands of law enforcement.* Your body will adapt to the demands that you place on it. You need to focus on upper-body strength, cardiorespiratory endurance, and flexibility training to stay as healthy as you can throughout your career.
- *A proper warm-up and cool-down are absolutely necessary.* The former should gradually warm up the muscles, including the heart, so that they can respond to the demands of your physical activity. A warm-up should include exercises that increase your heart rate as well as stretch all muscle groups, and include low-intensity movements similar to the exercises you will be doing. A cool-down should bring the body back to normal by using slow and gradual movements to prevent pooling of blood.
- *Think about the order in which you do your exercises.* Start with the large muscle groups and work your way down to the smaller ones. Training large muscle groups (such as thighs, chest, and back) will take a majority of your energy; therefore, you need to do them when you are at your strongest. Smaller muscles (such as biceps, triceps, and forearms) should be trained after larger muscles because they don't require as much energy to train.
- *Get enough fluids into your system.* Two hours before a workout you should have at least 0.5 L of a cool drink. During a workout, you should have 150–225 mL of fluid every 15 minutes. After a workout, you should drink about 1 L for every kilogram of body weight lost. You can determine how much body weight you lose during a workout by weighing yourself before and after the workout. Drinking water is a good way to replenish your fluids. Sports drinks are also acceptable, although many people find them too hard on their digestive systems and need to dilute them.
- *Train regularly.* Remember that you need a regular workout routine. Three to five times a week is necessary to see results from endurance training and to maintain those results. People who exceed the recommended number of workouts, however, risk injury.

- *Train with a partner.* The motivation and encouragement that you get from a fitness partner will help you through the hard times when your fitness routine does not seem to be producing results. A partner is also invaluable in weight training as a spotter and generally to ensure that you are adhering to the proper techniques.
- *Remember that everyone has a unique physical makeup.* Everyone progresses at a different rate or experiences different improvements. Fitness is a very personal thing. If you compare yourself to others, you may set yourself up for failure, especially if the others are already at a higher fitness level.

KEY TERMS

cardiorespiratory endurance
muscular strength
muscular endurance
flexibility
body composition
principle of specificity
principle of overload
principle of reversibility
principle of recovery
periodization
concurrent training
interval training
fartlek training
resistance training
plyometric training

EXERCISES

Review

1. What are the components of health-related fitness?

2. What are the components of performance/skill-related fitness?

3. What are some of the physical benefits of participating in a fitness program?

4. What are some of the psychological benefits of participating in a fitness program?

5. What are five principles of physical training?

6. What should you be aware of when beginning a fitness program?

7. Describe the principle of specificity.

8. How do you apply the principle of overload?

9. How do you counter the principle of reversibility?

10. How would you use periodization training to prepare for the shuttle run?

11. Describe fartlek training and how it can apply to training for BFORs.

12. Describe interval training and how it can improve your 1.5-mile run.

13. Using the plyometric training technique, describe how you could train for the various components of the PREP or PARE BFORs.

Multiple Choice

1. The warm-up and cool-down components of your workout should each last ___________.
   a. 5 minutes
   b. 5–15 minutes
   c. 10–25 minutes
   d. 25–40 minutes
   e. don't need these

2. Which best describes the F in the FITT formula?
   a. one to three days per week
   b. three to five days per week
   c. two to three days per week
   d. five to seven days per week
   e. none of these

3. Intensity, type of exercise, ___________, and ___________ are the four factors involved in fitness development.
   a. time, speed
   b. frequency, distance
   c. frequency, time
   d. distance, time
   e. none of these

4. The purpose of a warm-up is
   a. to avoid tearing large-muscle groups
   b. to psychologically prepare for the workout
   c. to increase heart rate
   d. to increase internal temperature
   e. all of these

5. The most important health-related component of physical fitness is
   a. body composition
   b. cardiorespiratory endurance
   c. muscular strength
   d. muscular endurance
   e. flexibility

6. The best indicator for measuring the intensity of your workout is
   a. the total time you take to work out
   b. rapid breathing
   c. the amount you sweat
   d. your heart rate
   e. your fatigue level

7. Skill-related fitness components include
   a. aerobic and strength training
   b. speed and endurance training
   c. speed and agility
   d. flexibility and hand–eye coordination
   e. body composition and aerobic training

8. Which of the following terms refers to the ability of a muscle to exert force for only one maximum effort?
   a. muscular atrophy
   b. muscular hypertrophy
   c. muscular overload
   d. muscular strength
   e. muscular endurance

9. The maintenance of equilibrium while stationary or while moving is termed
   a. agility
   b. balance
   c. coordination
   d. poise
   e. reaction time

10. Which should be the primary advantage of good health-related physical fitness?
    a. improved work efficiency
    b. excellence in sports
    c. enjoyment of leisure
    d. prevention of disease
    e. a good appearance

11. "Speed play," known as ____________ training, refers to interval training of distances at intense levels followed by recovery periods at predetermined intervals.
    a. periodization
    b. concurrent
    c. fartlek
    d. interval
    e. plyometric

12. The ____________ training technique involves training for power or strength at the same time as endurance training.
    a. periodization
    b. concurrent
    c. fartlek
    d. interval
    e. plyometric

13. Using your body weight and minimal equipment, ____________ training involves a series of drills that involve explosive movements through countermovements to build muscular energy and power.
    a. periodization
    b. concurrent
    c. resistance
    d. interval
    e. plyometric

14. ____________ training is based on the concept that the body's energy systems can make both aerobic and anaerobic gains by training with relatively intense exercises followed by a period of recovery.
    a. periodization
    b. concurrent
    c. resistance
    d. interval
    e. plyometric

REFERENCES

Anspaugh, David J. (1996). Risk factors for cardiovascular disease among exercising versus non-exercising women. *American Journal of Health Promotion, 10*(3), 171-174.

Bouchard, C., Shephard, R.J., Stephens, T., Sutton, J.R., & McPherson, B.D. (Eds.). (1990). *Exercise, fitness, and health: A consensus of current knowledge.* Champaign, IL: Human Kinetics.

Canadian Adolescents at Risk Research Network. (2004, February). *Physical activity patterns in Canadian adolescents.* Kingston, ON: Queen's University.

Canadian Society for Exercise Physiology. (1996). *The Canadian physical activity, fitness and lifestyle appraisal: CSEP's guide to healthy living.* Ottawa: Author.

Coalition for Active Living. (2004, January). Physical activity community not surprised by troubling physical activity trends published today. Media release.

Elias, W.S., & Murphy, R.J. (1986). The case for health promotion programs containing health care costs: A review of the literature, *American Journal of Occupational Therapy, 40,* 759.

Katzmarzyk, P.T., Gledhill, N., & Shephard, R.J. (2000). The economic burden of physical inactivity in Canada. *Canadian Medical Association Journal, 163*(11), 1435-1440.

Katzmarzyk, P.T., & Janssen, I. (2004). The economic cost of physical inactivity and obesity in Canada: An update. *Canadian Journal of Applied Physiology, 29,* 90-115.

Klonoff, E.A. (1994). Predicting exercise adherence in women: The role of psychological and physiological factors. *Preventive Medicine, 23,* 257-262.

Léger, L. (1985). *SportMed Technology fitness appraisal kit: 20 metre shuttle run test with one minute stages.* Montreal: SportMed Technology.

Léger, L.A., & Lambert, J. (1982). A maximal multistage 20m shuttle run test to predict VO2max. *European Journal of Applied Physiology, 49,* 1-5.

McAuley, E., & Wall, A.E. (Eds.). (1994). Enhancing psychological health through physical activity. *Toward active living: Proceedings of the 1992 International Conference on Physical Activity, Fitness and Health.* Champaign, IL: Human Kinetics.

Ministry of Health. (2005). *The integrated pan-Canadian healthy living strategy.* The Secretariat for the Intersectional Healthy Living Network, the F/T/P Healthy Living Task Group, and the F/T/P Advisory Committee on Population Health and Health Security. Cat. No. HP10-1/2005.

Perez, C. (2003). Children who become active. *Supplement to Health Reports,* Health Canada, *14,* 17-28.

Pitts, E.H. (1996, August). The surgeon general's call to action. *Fitness Management, 12*(9), 36-38.

Plotnikoff, R., et al. (2004, December). Physical activity, smoking and obesity among Canadian school youth. *Canadian Journal of Public Health, 95*(6), 413-418.

Shephard, R.J. (1997, April). Exercise and relaxation in health promotion, *Sports Medicine, 23*(4), 211-216.

Wagner, E.H., & Lacroix, A.Z. (1992). Effects of physical activity on health status in older adults I: Observational studies. *Annual Review of Public Health, 13,* 451-469.

CHAPTER 5

Cardiorespiratory Fitness

CHAPTER OBJECTIVES

After completing this chapter, you should be able to:

- Explain why cardiorespiratory fitness is important in law enforcement.
- Understand and monitor your heart rate at rest and during exercise.
- Determine how high-intensity interval training can fit into your cardio-respiratory program to assist you in successfully completing BFOR testing.
- Determine your target heart rate zone for exercise.
- Set up a cardiorespiratory fitness program that is most suited to you.

Cardiorespiratory fitness (endurance), probably the most important component of fitness, is the ability to perform prolonged large-muscle activities at moderate to high intensity. This chapter will examine the importance of cardiorespiratory fitness in law enforcement and provide advice on creating a cardiorespiratory fitness program that will help you meet law enforcement requirements.

THE IMPORTANCE OF CARDIORESPIRATORY FITNESS IN LAW ENFORCEMENT

Cardiorespiratory fitness makes your body more efficient and helps you cope with the physical demands of your job and everyday life. The key to cardiorespiratory fitness is aerobic exercise—prolonged, rhythmic exercise that uses large-muscle groups. Examples of aerobic exercise include swimming, running, and cycling. Research by the Ontario government and the RCMP (Ontario, 1997) has demonstrated the importance of aerobic conditioning in law enforcement. The researchers found that aerobic conditioning not only facilitated foot chases but also helped officers cope with long shifts and the changing demands of the job. Both the Ontario government and the RCMP stress the importance of aerobic conditioning by incorporating a cardiovascular component in their physical readiness evaluations (PREP and PARE, respectively; see chapter 16).

THE BENEFITS OF CARDIORESPIRATORY FITNESS

As you have already read, exercise has many benefits. The following are some of the benefits of cardiorespiratory fitness:

- improved cardiorespiratory functioning, which allows the heart to meet the demands of everyday life more efficiently (blood pressure and the risk of heart disease are also reduced) (Marcus, 1998)
- reduced levels of cholesterol, triglycerides, and other potentially harmful substances in the blood, which reduces the risk of heart disease (Tucker, 1991; US Department of Health and Human Services, 1996)
- improved metabolism (metabolism is, among other things, the process whereby the body converts food into energy) (Bouchard et al., 1990)
- increased bone density, which reduces the risk of osteoporosis and improves posture, balance, and coordination, and can help reduce the risk of falls (Stevens, 1997)
- improved immune system (excessive training, however, can depress one's immune system) (Bouchard et al., 1990)
- reduced risk of developing diabetes mellitus and its associated risks (Health Canada, 2003)
- reduced risk of some cancers, including those of the colon, breast, and female reproductive organs (Vainio, 2002)
- increased energy, stamina, and resistance to physical fatigue (Bouchard et al., 1990)
- improved psychological and emotional well-being resulting from improved appearance, enhanced self-image and self-confidence, and decreased stress, anxiety, and depression (Bouchard et al., 1990; Shephard, 1997)

ASSESSING CARDIORESPIRATORY FITNESS

Your cardiorespiratory fitness affects your body's ability to maintain a level of exertion (exercise) for an extended period of time. The ability to supply energy for activities lasting more than 30 seconds depends on the consumption and use of oxygen (O_2). Most physical activities in daily life and athletics take more than 90 seconds, so O_2 consumption is critical for survival as well as performance.

Aerobic fitness consists of two main components. The first is central cardiovascular fitness (heart and lungs); the second, peripheral component is the specific muscles involved in the movement.

The central cardiovascular system will improve as long as you stress your cardiac function and ventilation system. Your improvement is limited by

- cardiac output: the amount of blood pumped per minute, which is a function of stroke volume (blood pumped per heart beat and heart rate [beats/minute])

- blood volume: dehydration or other factors affecting volume reduce the effectiveness of the cardiovascular system
- red blood cell count and O_2 carrying capacity

Peripheral adaptations require specific training to cause the muscles to adapt to the specific task (that's why cross-training on a bike will help your running but not replace the need to run). The two biggest limiting factors in peripheral aerobic fitness are:

- the ability of the muscles to remove and use oxygen from the blood
- the ability of the muscles to maintain a balanced pH (specifically, minimizing the build-up of lactic acid, thus delaying the onset of fatigue)

A person's **maximum aerobic capacity (VO_2 Max)** is a measure of his or her cardio fitness. VO_2 Max is the volume of oxygen consumed per minute. It is estimated as the point at which oxygen uptake plateaus and does not increase with further increases in workload. Once people reach their maximum aerobic capacity, they cannot continue to work at that intensity for more than a minute or two because their demand for oxygen exceeds their ability to supply oxygen.

maximum aerobic capacity (VO_2 Max)
a measure of cardio fitness; estimated as the point at which oxygen uptake plateaus and does not increase with further increases in workload

Proper testing of a person's VO_2 Max is costly and requires a controlled laboratory environment. The test is onerous and time-consuming, and therefore demands a highly motivated subject if an accurate assessment is to be obtained. As a result, simpler tests have been developed. For example, in the late 1970s the Ontario Police College, adopting the standards set by Dr. Kenneth Cooper (1982), implemented a 1.5-mile run as an indirect measure of cardiorespiratory fitness (see chapter 16 for further detail). When the Physical Readiness Evaluation for Policing (PREP) was implemented, the 20-m shuttle run replaced the run. Other tests of cardiorespiratory fitness include the Astrand-Rhyming bicycle ergometer test, the YMCA bicycle ergometer test, the Rockport Fitness Walking Test, and the Canadian Physical Fitness and Lifestyle Appraisal (CPFLA) step test.

For law enforcement applicants who do not run on a regular basis, or who are obese or otherwise in poor condition, cardiorespiratory training is of the utmost importance. You need to be physically fit to meet the demands of the PREP and PARE BFOR and other tests of occupational skills administered to law enforcement applicants. Conditioning your cardiorespiratory system will help you work toward your goals.

A word of caution: those who do not engage in regular physical activity and have joint or obesity problems or high blood pressure (144/94 or 140/90, depending on the test protocol) may require medical clearance before taking a cardiorespiratory test. Be sure to fill out the Physical Activity Readiness Questionnaire (PAR-Q) in **assignment 1.1** and talk to your fitness instructor before taking any cardiorespiratory test.

Go to **assignment 5.1** (in the appendix) and assess your readiness for participating in cardiorespiratory training.

GETTING STARTED ON CARDIORESPIRATORY TRAINING

Before you begin cardiorespiratory training, consider the frequency, intensity, duration, and type of your aerobic exercise sessions. These considerations are addressed by the FITT (frequency, intensity, time, and type) formula (table 5.1).

Although all four variables in the FITT formula are important, intensity is the key variable. The Canadian Society for Exercise Physiology (1996) identifies three techniques that allow you to effectively judge the intensity of your workout: heart rate monitoring, the Borg scale, and the talk test. Intensity can be checked during and at the end of the workout to determine whether you are at the target heart rate required.

Understanding Heart Rates

resting heart rate
your heart rate when you are in a resting state such as sleep

The first heart rate that you should be aware of is your **resting heart rate**, which you will experience during sleep or prior to getting out of bed in the morning. With exercise, you can decrease your HR as your heart and lungs become stronger. The heart is then able to pump more blood (increase *stroke volume*) throughout the body with less effort. The lungs are able to take in more oxygen (increase *maximum oxygen uptake*) with less effort, which means more blood and oxygen getting to the working muscles. Having enough oxygen going into the blood keeps the lactic acid out (removes the hydrogen ions) so that you can sustain a prolonged aerobic workout.

Resting heart rates vary between 40 and 100 beats per minute (bpm), with 70 bpm being the average. As your cardiovascular system improves, your resting heart rate decreases.

maximal heart rate
your heart rate when your heart beats at maximal effort during a sustained aerobic activity

exercising heart rate
your heart rate when your body is in motion during sustained exercise

The **maximal heart rate** is the rate at which your heart beats at maximum effort during a sustained aerobic activity. You will normally never work at 100% of your maximum unless you are doing a specific program or test in a supervised setting (for example, maximal treadmill test).

The **exercising heart rate** is the rate at which your body is in motion during sustained exercise. The goal is to stay within your target heart rate range, which is normally between 70 and 85 percent of maximal heart rate for someone who is fit.

TABLE 5.1 The FITT Formula

FITT	Health-related benefits	Performance-related benefits	High-performance-related benefits
Frequency (days/wk)	3	3–4	5+
Intensity (% of MHR)	50–60	60–85	70–90*
Time (min/day)	5–20	20–60	30–60
Type	Any rhythmic activity, including walking, cycling, jogging, swimming, and using a stair machine		

* At this intensity, there may be a risk of overtraining, which can lead to injuries and anorexia.

Heart Rate Monitoring

Heart rate monitoring—the most common technique—is easily learned. You put your index and middle fingers over either the radial artery (located on the wrist just above the base of the thumb) or the carotid artery (located on the inside and the left and right sides of the neck). Do not press too hard on the carotid artery, as this may trigger a reflex that slows the heart rate down. During exercise, the heart rate is determined by counting the beats for 10 seconds and then multiplying by 6 to get beats per minute. When you are at rest, you should count the beats for 15 seconds and then multiply by 4.

DETERMINING YOUR TARGET HEART RATE ZONE

To judge whether you are exercising at a benefit-producing intensity, you must determine your **target heart rate (THR) zone**. First, determine your maximal heart rate (MHR) by subtracting your age from 220. This gives you your MHR in beats per minute. Next, multiply your MHR by 70 percent and 85 percent. The resulting numbers are the lower and upper limits, respectively, of your THR zone. To benefit from exercise, you must exercise at an intensity that raises your heart rate into the THR zone for 30–60 minutes 3–5 times a week. Unfit people who exercise at an intensity just short of the lower limit of their THR zone will obtain some health benefits but will not improve or maintain aerobic fitness. Physical activity should include moderate activity (such as brisk walking, skating, and bike riding) with vigorous activities (such as running and playing soccer). In fact, Health Canada is encouraging all Canadians to be physically active by increasing their awareness and understanding about the benefits of physical activity and the range of opportunities to be physically active in daily life (Healthy Living Unit, 2003).

target heart rate (THR) zone
the zone that a person's heart rate must reach during exercise to improve or maintain aerobic fitness

Here's how to determine the THR for a 25-year-old:

$$\begin{aligned} \text{MHR} &= 220 - 25 = 195 \text{ bpm} \\ \text{THR zone lower limit} &= 0.70 \times 195 = 117 \text{ bpm} \\ \text{THR zone upper limit} &= 0.85 \times 195 = 166 \text{ bpm} \end{aligned}$$

Figure 5.1 shows the THR zone for ages 20 to 70. This chart is often posted on gym walls.

Go to **assignment 5.2** (in the appendix) and determine your resting heart rate and target heart rate.

The Borg scale

Developed by Gunnar A. Borg (1998), a Swedish psychologist, the **Borg scale** method does not involve counting the number of heartbeats, which can be difficult for some people while they are exercising. The Borg rating of perceived exertion (RPE) is based on how hard you feel your body is working during exercise. It is based on the physical sensations a person experiences during physical activity, including increased heart rate, increased respiration or breathing rate, increased sweating, and muscle fatigue. Although this is a subjective measure, a person's exertion rating may provide a fairly good estimate of the actual heart rate during physical activity (Borg, 1998). There is a high correlation between a person's perceived exertion rating times 10 and the actual heart rate during physical activity. For ex-

Borg scale
a method for determining the intensity of exercise, used as an alternative to heart rate monitoring

FIGURE 5.1 Target Heart Rate (THR) Zone

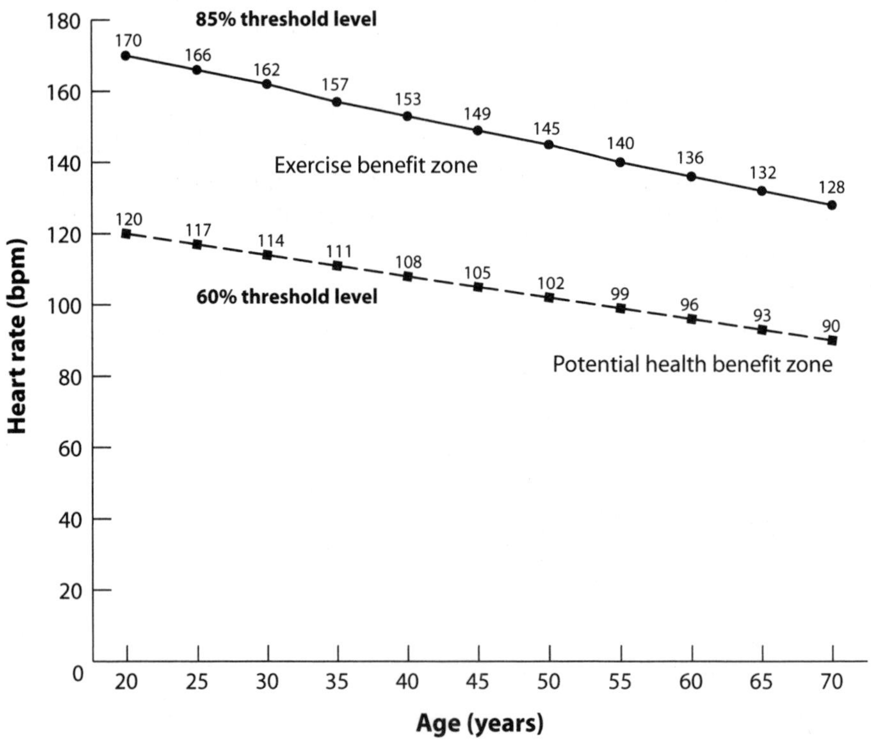

ample, if a person's rating of perceived exertion (RPE) is 12, then 12 × 10 = 120; if you were to take your heart rate, it should be approximately 120 beats per minute. Note that this calculation is only an approximation of heart rate, and the actual heart rate can vary quite a bit depending on age and physical condition.

With experience of monitoring how your body feels, it will become easier to know when to adjust your intensity. For example, a walker who wants to engage in moderate-intensity activity would aim for a Borg scale level of "somewhat hard" (12–14). If that person describes his or her muscle fatigue and breathing as "very light" (9 on the Borg scale) he or she would want to increase intensity. On the other hand, if the walker felt the exertion was "extremely hard" (19 on the Borg scale), he or she would need to slow down to achieve a moderate-intensity range. See figure 5.2.

The disadvantage of using the Borg scale is that some people underestimate or overestimate their level of exertion. It is important to regularly monitor your heart rate to ensure that your perceived exertion corresponds with the level of intensity you are trying to achieve.

To determine whether your perception is close to your actual heart rate, multiply the number that corresponds to your perception by 10. Since people just starting an exercise program may not be able to tie their intensity to a subjective perception of exertion, it is important for them to regularly check their heart rate to determine whether they are within their THR zone.

talk test
a method for determining the intensity of exercise, used as an alternative to heart rate monitoring; if a person is breathless and cannot carry on a conversation while exercising, he or she is working too hard

The Talk Test

The **talk test** is a handy guide for beginners who are concerned about their exercise intensity. A person who is active at a *light* intensity level should be able to sing while doing the activity. One who is active at a *moderate* intensity level should be able to carry on a conversation comfortably while engaging in the activity. If a person becomes winded or too out of breath to carry on a conversation, then the activity can be considered *vigorous* and the person may find it too hard to continue.

FIGURE 5.2 The Borg Scale

6	No exertion at all
7	
	Extremely light
8	
9	Very light
10	
11	Light
12	
13	Somewhat hard
14	
15	Hard (heavy)
16	
17	Very hard
18	
19	Extremely hard
20	Maximal exertion

Source: Adapted from Borg, G. (1982). Psychological bases of perceived exertion—Perceived rate of exertion. *Medicine & Science in Sports & Exercise, 14*, 344-386.

CREATING A CARDIORESPIRATORY FITNESS PROGRAM

Individuals who are enrolled in the Police Foundations Program are expected to meet certain aerobic requirements. The colleges have included only from one to three hours a week for fitness training to bring their students up to police standards. This may mean that you need to put in an additional two or three hours a week, but more likely you will be looking at putting in more hours outside of class time to achieve the goals you have set. If your fitness program offers you one hour a week of aerobic training, then, depending on your fitness level, you will have to add two to four hours of aerobic training to your weekly schedule on your own. If your fitness facility offers cycling classes, aerobics, or interval training classes, take advantage of them. Not only will they likely help to push you more, you'll have other people there to help motivate you and encourage you to test to your limits.

So what program should you follow? Your instructor may have already established a regime that he or she expects you to follow. If not, the following pages offer some simple guidelines for a training program lasting 16 weeks, which is a little longer than the length of a semester at most Ontario community colleges. The guidelines are designed for people whose fitness level is either average to good or very good to excellent. If your fitness level is poor to fair, ask your instructor to help you establish a program that is safe and effective for you and that he or she can monitor. For those of you who have already reached an excellent level of fitness, all that is required is maintenance.

Remember that an exercise program can be affected by conditions in the environment in which you exercise. For example, a run may involve

- topographical factors such as hills and sand
- obstacles such as ditches, fences, and underbrush
- meteorological and air-quality factors such as heat, humidity, cold, snow, wind, pollution, and thin air at higher altitudes
- bulky clothing or equipment that obstructs movement

You may need to adjust your running program to compensate for these factors.

HOW TO DRESS FOR WINTER RUNNING

Staying active during the winter can be an enjoyable experience. Whether you head out for a run, a walk, or a day of skiing, dressing for comfort will increase your enjoyment. Training for a career in law enforcement also means that you will have to experience the outdoors throughout the year. Here are some guidelines for dressing for Canadian winters.

Since the first layer, or base layer, is next to your skin, it is the most important layer. It should fit snugly against the skin, and never be cotton! Cotton absorbs water readily and takes forever to dry. This makes it an unsatisfactory first layer because it actually accelerates heat loss. Synthetic underwear such as polypropylene or wicking polyesters are more appropriate. These materials are more comfortable because of their ability to wick (pull moisture away from the skin) and because they are very quick to dry, often with one's own body heat.

The next layer, the insulation layer, provides warmth. The amount of insulation you need will depend on the temperature and your workout. This layer is designed to trap warm air surrounding your body. Low exertion and colder weather call for a bulkier layer than high exertion and colder weather. It is extremely important not to overheat, as this increases the moisture vapour that leaves the body. A body in motion does not need as much insulation as a body at rest. This middle layer must still wick moisture, should fit loosely over the first layer, and should be easy to remove so you can adjust to conditions.

The final layer, sometimes referred to as the element layer (the layer exposed to the elements), prevents heat loss. There are three ways a body can lose heat. The first is through *convective* heat loss, which occurs when the wind takes away the thin layer of body temperature air around us, forcing the body to expend precious energy to rewarm this lost air. The second is *conductive* heat loss, which occurs when there is contact between the body and any object cooler then itself (for example, rain or wet cotton). The third is *evaporative* heat loss, which occurs when anything we are wearing is drying out. The element layer is very important because it can prevent all three heat loss processes by keeping heat in. An outer layer should provide a combination of wind resistance, water resistance, and breathability.

Lower temperatures cause blood to be shunted away from the hands and feet to the centre of the body to keep the internal organs warm and protected. Remember that heat loss from your head alone can be as much as 50 percent at the freezing mark, so make sure that you wear a hat or at least earmuffs and mittens. Superficial warming of the hands will return blood flow to prevent tissue damage. Blood flow will not return to the feet unless the temperature of the torso is normal or slightly higher (less than 1 °C). To keep your feet warm, you must also keep the rest of your body warm at all times.

Always check the air temperature and wind chill factor before exercising in the cold. Data from the National Safety Council (www.nsc.org) suggest little danger to individuals with properly clothed skin exposed at −7 °C, even with a 50 km/h wind. A danger does exist for individuals with exposed skin when the wind chill factor (combined effect of temperature and wind) falls below −29 °C. That can be achieved by any combination of temperatures below −7 °C with a wind of 65 km/h, and temperatures below −29 °C with no wind. If you are exercising near the danger zone for skin exposure, it also is advisable to warm the air being inhaled by wearing a scarf or mask over your nose and mouth. Check with weather sites like the Weather Network (www.theweathernetwork.com) before going out.

The telltale sign of frostbite is a patch of skin that turns hard, pale, and cold. Burning, tingling, stinging, or numbing sensations may be present. The person can appear to be clumsy, which can result from impaired motor control. When the affected body part is rewarmed, a throbbing or burning pain may result. Frostbite, like burns, is classified according to the degree of tissue injury. Some minor injuries result in swelling, redness, loss of sensation, and white plaque on the skin. With more severe lesions there can be blisters that may become filled with blood. In the most extreme cases, full-thickness freezing damages bones and muscles, resulting in tissue death and loss of the affected area.

Sunny days are most enjoyable for everyone, but remember that you must protect your eyes. In winter your eyes are exposed to light from above as well as below when it is reflected from the snow. The reflection doubles the intensity of ultraviolet rays. Prolonged exposure can actually burn your eyes and eventually cause snow blindness. Symptoms can include pain in the eyes and extreme sensitivity to light. If you ever experience snow blindness, you should go inside to a dark or dimly lit room and apply cool compresses to your eyes until the pain subsides and tolerance to light returns. Remember to protect your eyes from both sun and wind with sunglasses. Sunglasses should block UVA and UVB rays between 290 and 400 nm (Weather Network, 2007).

According to the American College of Sports Science (1980), it may take up to six months to reach the maintenance phase. If you experience any discomfort or pain, inform your instructor and consult your doctor. You may have to modify your program.

Guidelines for Cardiorespiratory Fitness Training

This section offers guidelines to help you set up your fitness program. There are separate guidelines for people whose fitness level is average to good and for those whose fitness level is very good to excellent. If you feel that your fitness level is below average, consult with your instructor.

AVERAGE TO GOOD FITNESS LEVEL

1. Make sure you answered no to all the questions of the PAR-Q (in **assignment 1.1**) or have been cleared by a medical examination. Check with your instructor if you are unsure about your medical suitability to undertake a fitness program.
2. Begin and end each session with a proper warm-up and cool-down.
3. Check the intensity of your exercising by monitoring your heart rate, or use the Borg scale or talk test. If you experience aches or pains or suffer an injury, stop exercising or reduce the intensity of your exercise until you are fit to continue or have seen a doctor. Be sure to advise your instructor of the problem.

Week no.	Duration (min/day)	Intensity (% of MHR)	Frequency (days/wk)
1	15–20	65–70	3
2	15–20	65–70	3
3	20	70	3
4	20	70	3
5	25	70	3
6	25	75	3
7	25	75	3
8	30	75	3
9	30	75	3
10	35	75	3
11	35	75	3
12	40	75	3
13	40	75	3
14	40	80	3
15	40	80	3
16	40	80	3

VERY GOOD TO EXCELLENT FITNESS LEVEL

1. These guidelines apply to people who exercise at an intensity level at the upper limit of the THR zone and have been involved in high-intensity aerobic activities, including running, for a number of years. Make sure you can answer no to all the questions on the PAR-Q (in **assignment 1.1**) and have been cleared by a medical examination to participate in vigorous activities.
2. Begin and end each session with a proper warm-up and cool-down.
3. Check the intensity of your exercising by monitoring your heart rate, or use the Borg scale or talk test. If you experience aches or pains or suffer an injury, reduce the intensity of your exercise, substitute a lower-impact activity, or stop exercising until you are fit to continue or have seen a doctor. Be sure to advise your instructor of the problem.

Week no.	Duration (min/day)	Intensity (% of MHR)	Frequency (days/wk)
1	15–20	65–70	3
2	20	70-75	3
3	25	75	3
4	30	75	3
5	35	75	3
6	40	75	3
7	40	75	3
8	40	75	3
9	40	80	3
10	40	80	3
11	40	80	3
12	40	80–85	3
13	40	80–85	3
14	40	80–85	3
15	30	80–85	3
16	30	80–85	3

Note: Weeks 15 and 16 become the maintenance phase for your aerobic conditioning.

Training to Your Upper Limit

When you work at the upper limit and over these percentages, if you are not in great shape, you go into what is termed an *anaerobic threshold.* If you push too hard, your body no longer meets its demand for oxygen. You start feeling exhausted, you hyperventilate from excess amounts of lactic acid in your body, and your heart can no longer provide enough oxygen to your working muscles to sustain the demands of the task. You usually can only last a short period of time, 30 seconds to 1 minute. However, as you become more fit, you can push the range higher. As well, by training your anaerobic system, you can push the threshold through shorter and faster interval activities and thereby increase your aerobic capacity. By resting between these **high-intensity interval training (HIT)** anaerobic sessions, you enable the oxygen-rich blood to help clean out the lactic acid from your muscles and you can catch your breath before the next set.

high-intensity interval training (HIT)
a form of training to increase aerobic performance

Training for the Shuttle Run

The best way to train for the 20-m shuttle run is to practise, practise, practise. *To train to meet an acceptable level (6.5), an individual must perform aerobic activity 3–5 times per week for at least 20 minutes, working at an intensity of 75 to 85 percent of his or her maximum heart rate.*

Once a solid cardiovascular base has been established, you could train on a treadmill following the guidelines below to help build up the endurance required to meet the standards set out in the PREP.

Time frame (number of minutes)	Stage (miles per hour)
0–1	4.5
1–2	4.5
2–3	5.0
3–4	5.5
4–5	6.0
5–6	6.5
6–7	7.0
7–8	7.5
8–9	8.0
9–10	8.5
10–11	9.0
11–12	9.5
12–13	10.0
13–14	10.5
14–15	11.0
15–16	11.5

Note: In the 20-m shuttle run, it takes 6 minutes and 30 seconds to reach stage 6.5; it takes 7 minutes and 30 seconds to reach stage 7.5. Stage 6.5 is equivalent to 11 minutes and 30 seconds in the 1.5-mile run.

Remember that you are increasing intensity to prepare your body for what it will be like when doing the shuttle run. Be aware that the treadmill is not the same as running in the gym. In running, you must absorb the pounding of each step at the same time that you propel your body forward. There is also an energy cost for accelerating and decelerating the body at each end of the 20 m. Ultimately, you cannot expect to be successful by practising only on a treadmill.

To build up your endurance, you can try running to your max, recovering for about five minutes, running again to your limit, recovering for about five minutes, and then attempting the shuttle run again. Due to the short duration of the test, the shuttle run should not be considered an aerobic training session. The reality is that your cardiovascular fitness will not improve drastically with running the shuttle run for six to eight minutes.

When you are having difficulty reaching the upper stages, keep walking in your lane for about one minute, and then attempt to run the length every other beep. If you are fit enough, you may be able to stay up with the stages as long as possible. This way, you have a better understanding of the speed that you must work toward and a goal to work toward. These training effects will help your cardiorespiratory system to prepare for the demands of the tests. The physiological changes that occur as you train will prepare you to meet the demands of the different BFORs.

Many people use aerobic training to help reduce weight. Most research acknowledges that a conventional way to effectively burn body fat is to choose a particular modality (type of cardiovascular exercise) and perform it for at least 20–30 minutes at a moderate intensity level.

Often individuals feel that this is enough. However, working at a higher intensity level will burn more calories in less time. In order for this approach to be effective, the overloading process has to be progressive, which means that you need to start at an appropriate level and build from there. Once a baseline has been established, you should gradually increase speed, incline, resistance, and/or time as you become better conditioned. The body has the ability to adapt to any stressor (exercise) placed on it, which means you have to progressively overload to continue to see gains. If you run on a treadmill at 4.5 mph (the first stage of the shuttle run) for 30 minutes, most beginners will see caloric expenditure, cardiovascular conditioning, and burning of body fat at the beginning. Over time, the intensity or time (30–40 minutes) will have to increase if continued results are to be achieved.

The goal of HIT training is to keep your heart rate at a higher percentage of your maximal predicted heart rate (85–95 percent MHR). Since you can't maintain that rate for long, you have to build recovery stages into your workout (you can't run full-out the entire time). The time frames are usually done minute by minute, while adjusting speed and/or incline to affect heart rate and the rating of perceived exertion on the Borg scale. This type of training is geared to those who are in advanced cardiovascular shape and do not have any pre-existing cardiovascular conditions that limit their ability to safely exercise as outlined in chapter 1.

The suggested training regime for the shuttle run is an example of continuous increases in intensity. This example of a high-intensity workout includes changes in incline and speed to challenge your cardiovascular system, and to push those who are fitter a little further.

The idea is to increase your capacity to do work or increase the expenditure of your calories. Conditioning in this fashion can be done using treadmills, stationary bikes, elliptical machines, stair steppers, stair mills, student residence stairs, and hills.

Time (min)	Speed (mph)	Incline	RPE (1–20)
1	4	1	2
2	4.5	1	2
3	5	1	3
4	5.5	2	4
5	6	2	5
6	6.5	2.5	6
7	7	3	8
8	7.5	3	10
9	8	3.5	12
10	8.5	3	14
11	9	1	16
12	5	4	12
13	5	6	14
14	6	8	16
15	6	10	20
16	6	4	14
17	5	3	10
18	5	3	8
19	4	2	6
20	4	1	4

Effective cardio exercise is not related to calories burned during a session, but the effect the exercise has on your body during and after the session. High-intensity cardio exercise stimulates your metabolism to run at a higher level, for longer. Your metabolism will stay elevated for a longer period of time so that it burns a greater percentage of calories during the day. Change the program to suit your skills and interests.

Some students do not see aerobic training as a priority, or find it to be a frustrating experience. Their focus may be more on strength training than on aerobic training. Based on research from McMaster University (Gibala et al., 2006), sprint training can provide a time-efficient way to induce rapid physiological adaptation similar to traditional long-term endurance training, which can result in improvements in both anaerobic and aerobic performance. Examples include running full-out at your maximum aerobic capacity for one- to two-minute intervals on a treadmill, bike, or elliptical machine after completing two or three weight exercises, and then going back to do two more exercises and repeating the anaerobic interval training. It will not replace running for an extended period of time; however, it will increase your aerobic capacity as you work toward meeting the requirements for the aerobic tests (1.5-mile run, shuttle run, etc.).

Turn to **assignment 5.3** (in the appendix) and design your own cardiorespiratory training program.

KEY TERMS

maximum aerobic capacity (VO_2 Max)

resting heart rate

exercising heart rate

maximal heart rate

target heart rate (THR) zone

Borg scale

talk test

high-intensity interval training (HIT)

EXERCISES

Review

1. Why is cardiorespiratory fitness important in law enforcement?

2. Identify some of the benefits of cardiorespiratory fitness.

3. Define maximum aerobic capacity (VO_2 Max).

4. Explain why it is important to know your target heart rate (THR) zone.

5. Identify some of the conditions in the environment that can affect an exercise program.

Multiple Choice

1. The formula for determining your target heart rate zone is
   a. MHR × intensity + resting heart rate
   b. (220 – age)
   c. (220 – resting heart rate) × 60–80%
   d. (220 – age) × 60–80%
   e. none of these

2. One positive effect of cardiorespiratory fitness is
   a. your blood pressure increases
   b. it takes less time to return to pre-exercise resting heart rates
   c. your resting heart rate increases
   d. your heart's ability to pump blood decreases
   e. your resting heart rate stays elevated

3. George has a resting heart rate of 62 beats per minute (bpm) at age 25. What is his estimated maximal heart rate (MHR)?
   a. 202 bpm
   b. 205 bpm
   c. 195 bpm
   d. 190 bpm
   e. 200 bpm

4. What is George's estimated target heart rate?
   a. 100–120 bpm
   b. 120–140 bpm
   c. 117–156 bpm
   d. 127–176 bpm
   e. 150–195 bpm

5. Which of the following is *not* an aerobic exercise?
   a. jogging
   b. bicycling
   c. fitness walking
   d. tennis
   e. swimming laps

6. The best time to check your heart rate to determine the intensity of your workout is
   a. before beginning your workout
   b. immediately at the end of your warm-up
   c. immediately at the end of your cool-down
   d. immediately at the end of your cardiovascular workout
   e. five minutes after your cool-down to see if training effects have occurred

7. Which term describes the greatest amount of oxygen that can be used by your body during intense exercise?
   a. cardiorespiratory endurance
   b. maximum aerobic capacity
   c. cardiorespiratory uptake
   d. maximum endurance
   e. maximum cardiorespiratory uptake

8. Which component of the Physical Readiness Evaluation for Policing addresses cardiorespiratory fitness?
   a. pursuit and restraint
   b. victim relocation
   c. arm restraint combined with the push–pull machine
   d. shuttle run
   e. running up and down stairs

9. The best example of a situation requiring aerobic fitness in law enforcement is
   a. handcuffing a passive person
   b. chasing down someone who is resisting arrest
   c. following a vehicle in your cruiser
   d. running a 4-km run at lunch break
   e. bench pressing your body weight

10. HIT stands for
    a. high interval training
    b. heavy interval testing
    c. high-intensity interval training
    d. high intensity testing
    e. health indicator test

11. You should take your resting heart rate
    a. before you write a test
    b. after you drive to school
    c. after you finish a timed run
    d. just before you go to bed at night
    e. when you first wake up but before you get out of bed in the morning

12. Exercising heart rate can be taken
    a. while you are running
    b. before you go for a run
    c. after completing your cool-down
    d. after completing your warm-up
    e. after completing 30 curl-ups

13. Maximal heart rate refers to
    a. what your heart rate gets to every time you run
    b. the rate at which you push your heart rate during a leisure run
    c. the maximal rate your heart can pump
    d. what your heart rate is at maximal effort during a sustained aerobic activity
    e. what your heart rate is at the end of a proper warm-up

REFERENCES

American College of Sports Science. (1980). *Guidelines for graded exercise testing and exercise prescription* (2nd ed.). Philadelphia: Lea and Febiger.

Borg, G. (1998). *Perceived exertion and pain scales.* Champaign, IL: Human Kinetics.

Bouchard, C., Shephard, R.J., Stephens, T., Sutton, J.R., & McPherson, B.D. (Eds.). (1990). *Exercise, fitness, and health: A consensus of current knowledge.* Champaign, IL: Human Kinetics.

Canadian Society for Exercise Physiology. (1996). *The Canadian physical activity, fitness and lifestyle appraisal: CSEP's guide to healthy living.* Ottawa: Author.

Cooper, K. (1982). *The aerobics program for total well-being.* New York: M. Evans.

Gibala, M.J., Little, J.P., van Essen, M., Wilkin, G.P., Burgomaster, K.A., Safdar, A., Raha, S., & Tarnopolsky, M.A. (2006). Short-term sprint interval versus traditional endurance training: Similar initial adaptations in human skeletal muscle and exercise performance. *Journal of Applied Physiology, 575*(3), 901-911.

Health Canada (2003). *Responding to the challenge of diabetes in Canada. First report of the National Diabetes Surveillance System (NDSS).* Available at http://www.phac-aspc.gc.ca/ccdpc-cpcmc/diabetes-diabete/english/pubs/index.html.

Healthy Living Unit. (2003). Public Health Agency of Canada. Available at http://www.phac-aspc.gc.ca/pau-uap/fitness/about.html.

Marcus, B.H. (1998, March). Evaluation of motivationally tailored vs. standard self-help physical activity interventions at the workplace. *American Journal of Health Promotion, 12*(4), 246-253.

Ontario. Ministry of the Solicitor General and Correctional Services. (1997). *Fit to serve: Preparation for the PREP—The Physical Readiness Evaluation for Policing.* Toronto: Author.

Shephard, R.J. (1997, April). Exercise and relaxation in health promotion. *Sports Medicine, 23*(4), 211-216.

Steven, J.A., Powell, K.E., Smith, S.M., et al. (1997). Physical activity, functional limitations and the risk of fall-related fractures in community-dwelling elderly. *Annals of Epidemiology, 7*, 54-61.

Tucker, L.A. (1991, September/October). The relation between aerobic fitness and serum cholesterol levels in a large employed population. *American Journal of Health Promotion, 6*(1), 17-23.

The Weather Network (2007). TWN on TV—ski safety tips. Available at http://www.theweathernetwork.com/tv/skitips/.

US Department of Health and Human Services. (1996). *Physical activity and health: A report of the Surgeon General* (pp. 85-172). Centers for Disease Control and Prevention.

Vainio, H., & Bianchini, F. (2002). Weight control and physical activity. *IARC Handbooks of Cancer Prevention,* Volume 6. Lyon: International Agency for Research on Cancer.

CHAPTER 6

Strength and Endurance Training

CHAPTER OBJECTIVES

After completing this chapter, you should be able to:

- Explain the importance of strength and endurance training in policing.
- Explain the benefits of resistance training.
- Understand some of the basic terms and concepts associated with strength and endurance training.
- Design a strength and endurance training program to meet the job-related demands of policing.

Like cardiorespiratory fitness training, strength and endurance training (also called resistance training) is important for meeting the occupational requirements of law enforcement. In this chapter you will learn basic terms and concepts associated with strength and endurance training. Though there are different kinds of exercises for increasing strength and endurance, this chapter will focus mainly on weight training. It will also enable you to design a strength and endurance training program that is effective and safe.

THE IMPORTANCE OF STRENGTH AND ENDURANCE TRAINING

Since the late 1990s, Bona Fide Occupational Requirements (BFORs) have been the standard for assessing applicants in most of the police services in Ontario. Taking elements of the job that require endurance, strength, and stamina, these assessments have combined these components to create various BFORs that are used by policing. The upper-body strength to restrain and move people is a necessary part of law enforcement (Gledhill & Shaw, 1995; Farenholtz, 1995). For this reason, upper-body strength is one of the fitness components tested by law enforcement organizations. Candidates for law enforcement positions are subjected, for example, to upper-body strength tests involving the push–pull machine, the arm-restraint device, an 80-lb. (36-kg) bag carry, and a 150-lb. (68-kg) body drag.

Weight training has always been an integral component of training for specialized units within the emergency services. Strength, speed, quickness, and agility are keys to a successful takedown or a rescue. Many students learn the basics of weight training in high school but fail to take them further. Some have no interest in "looking big," many don't have the time to train, and others fail to research and concentrate on proper techniques for developing strength and fitness. Weight training is not just for meeting the physical demands of the job; it is an important part of remaining fit throughout your career and into retirement.

Many services have emergency response teams (ERTs), tactics and rescue units (TRUs), and provincial emergency response teams (PERTs), which require cardiovascular endurance, muscular strength and endurance, and flexibility to meet the demands of the job on a regular basis. In addition to gruelling physical training, they must learn rappelling, cover and concealment, tracking and searching, dynamic entry, high-risk vehicle assault, and urban and rural stalking (RCMP, 2001). Police services in the province of Ontario, as well as the RCMP, have specific BFOR tests for these positions. Some of the assessments last up to 30 minutes and include wearing over 50 lb. (23 kg) of equipment; involve walking, running, and crawling; and require upper-body strength to do single chin-ups and negotiate high walls.

Upper-body strength is a special concern for women entering law enforcement, many of whom fail to meet testing standards without appropriate training. Female—and male—candidates must realize that passing the tests may require a greater than usual commitment of time to training. But with the proper training, everyone has the potential to be successful.

Though strength and endurance training is important from a career perspective, it is also important for your overall well-being. It gives you more energy to perform everyday tasks, bigger muscles, more strength, better muscle coordination, and a higher proportion of lean muscle to body fat. This training also contributes to better flexibility, helps in avoiding low-back problems, and can prevent falls.

THE BENEFITS OF RESISTANCE TRAINING

In the first two to three weeks of an exercise program, muscles begin to gain strength due to the recruitment of more muscle fibres at the same time. Later, after four to six weeks, the muscle fibres increase in size (hypertrophy) through an increase in metabolic enzymes and changes in the mitochondria (Fleck & Kraemer, 1988). Additional physiological benefits from resistance training include:

- an increase in bone mineral density (Nelson et al., 1994)
- a higher resting metabolic rate (Pratley, 1994)
- positive body composition changes (Fiatarone et al., 1994)
- a reduction in the risk for metabolic syndrome (Jurca et al., 2004)
- a reduction of back pain (Risch et al., 1993)
- an improved glucose utilization, which is important for controlling diabetes (Miller et al., 1994)

A LITTLE BIT ABOUT YOUR BODY AND MUSCLES

Your body is like a car, with your muscles acting as the engine and your heart as the fuel pump. You need to look after the nutritional side as well as servicing your muscular system.

Your muscular system has more than 650 muscles. You have three types of muscle—skeletal, cardiac, and smooth. Skeletal muscle is the body's largest tissue. Skeletal muscle fibres are elongated cylinders that contain several fibres bundled into groups. These fibres are attached to bone and used to facilitate movement. These muscles are voluntary and controlled by the nervous system and brain. Cardiac muscle, found only in the heart, is responsible for the contraction of the heart. Cardiac fibres are short, branching, and completely encased by a membrane. This involuntary contraction does not tire, allowing the heart to continually contract. Smooth muscle consists of cylindrical fibres that are aligned parallel to form sheets of muscle that elicit an involuntary movement. Most smooth muscle is found around the body's organs such as the digestive tract and the circulatory and urogenital systems.

It is important to remain active because, by the age of 80, sedentary individuals will have lost up to 50 percent of their muscular strength and may require a maximal effort to carry a vacuum cleaner up a flight of stairs.

It is a myth that when you stop training regularly that your muscle will turn into fat. However, adding extra protein to your diet to enhance building larger muscles will not work either as your body is unable to store extra protein. It will either get excreted or be converted and stored as fat.

TYPES OF MUSCLE FIBRE

There are two types of muscle fibre: fast-twitch and slow-twitch (Faulkner & White, 1990). The proportion of each type in the body varies from person to person.

- *Fast-twitch fibres* build force rapidly and also use up muscular energy rapidly (often within three to four minutes). They are easily fatigued, using oxygen up very quickly. There are two types of fast-twitch fibres. *High-oxidative fast-twitch fibres* contain a large amount of myoglobin (a protein found in cardiac and skeletal muscle), which gives the muscle a dark red colour and enables the fibre to use a large amount of oxygen. *Low-oxidative fast-twitch fibres* have less myoglobin and are pale in colour (almost white). These fibres provide powerful acceleration but fatigue quickly. People with more fast-twitch fibres are better at brief, explosive activities such as 100-m sprints.
- *Slow-twitch fibres* build force slowly, use muscular energy more gradually, and are more resistant to fatigue. These fibres maintain posture at rest. They are able to work effectively using aerobic respiration (using oxygen) because they have a greater capacity for oxygen than fast-twitch fibres. People with more slow-twitch fibres are better able to endure prolonged activities such as marathons.

No matter how much of one kind or the other of muscle fibre a person has, it is possible to condition one's muscles to perform both explosive and prolonged activities.

THE BASICS OF STRENGTH AND ENDURANCE TRAINING

Strength and endurance training includes any type of exercise that requires the muscles to move, or attempt to move, against an opposing force. Strength and endurance training encompasses weight training but also a much wider range of training activities, such as push-ups and curl-ups. Most strength and endurance training programs are designed for one or both of the following purposes: to increase muscular strength or muscular endurance, and to alter body composition by increasing muscle size and decreasing the percentage of fat in the body.

Strength and endurance training trains two components of the body: the muscles and the central nervous system (CNS), which causes the muscles to fire and thus to contract. It has been well documented that gains experienced during the first six weeks of training stem primarily from CNS adaptation—the muscles learning to synchronize better with one another. Gains arising from muscular adaptation (improved muscle coordination and movement) occur later (Faulkner & White, 1990).

Basic Principles of Weight Training

THE OVERLOAD PRINCIPLE

To build muscle mass, a greater than normal load must stress the muscle. This is called the **overload principle**. The process of rebuilding and repairing stressed soft muscle tissue causes the tissue to adapt to the new level of stress. Once the tissue has adapted to the new level, additional stress must be placed on it to spur further improvement. Individuals must be cautious in increasing their training load because an abrupt increase in load may go beyond the muscle's ability to adapt, causing injury.

overload principle
the principle that muscle mass can be built up only if the muscle is subjected to a greater than normal load

GENERAL ADAPTATION

The **general adaptation** phase prepares your muscles, joints, tendons, and ligaments for intense training. It is characterized by higher repetitions, lower intensities, and short rest periods, which help the neuromuscular components synchronize so that gains can be seen.

general adaptation
the process of preparing your muscles, joints, tendons, and ligaments for intense training by educating the neuromuscular component so that gains can be seen; characterized by higher repetitions, lower intensities, and short rest periods

MUSCULAR STRENGTH AND MUSCULAR ENDURANCE

Muscular strength training is characterized by lower training volume—that is, fewer repetitions—and higher training intensity. The goal of strength training is to stress the muscular and neuromuscular systems through heavy resistance training to adapt to heavy loads. Dynamic strength training is characterized by different movement patterns at different speeds involving concentric, eccentric, and plyometric actions.

Muscular endurance training develops athletes' capacity to maintain the quality of their muscles' contractile force (strength) over a long period of time. Athletes that have good endurance levels will have the capacity to maintain productivity and speed over a longer period of time. This is important for police officers, especially those on a canine unit, who may be involved in long foot pursuits. It is also important for those officers on tactical units who must respond quickly and maintain speed while wearing approximately 50 lb. (23 kg) of gear and equipment.

REPETITIONS

A **repetition (rep)** is one complete movement of an exercise.

repetition (rep)
one complete movement of an exercise

SETS

A **set** is a group of repetitions. For example, "2 sets of 10 reps" means 2 groups of 10 repetitions each, with a rest period between each group.

set
a group of repetitions

HYPERTROPHY

Hypertrophy is the process characterized by high training volume with moderate training intensity. The goal is to build muscle mass.

hypertrophy
the process characterized by high training volume with moderate training intensity in order to build muscle mass

POWER TRAINING

Power training is the process where an athlete works to build overall body explosiveness and reactive ability. The objective is to take the strength gained in the strength phase and convert it to activity-specific power. This phase is characterized by low volume and high intensities, using Olympic and explosive lifts, as well as sport-specific plyometric exercises. High muscular power output is an indication of the ability to perform a high level of (muscle) work in a short period of time. Exercises such as heavy squats and dead lifts that target the very large, powerful muscles of the legs (quadriceps and hamstrings), the buttocks (gluteal muscles), and back (erector spinea) are examples of power exercises.

power training
the process where an athlete works to build overall body explosiveness and reactive ability by taking the strength gained in the strength phase and converting it to activity-specific power

PLYOMETRICS

Plyometrics is based on the principle that the combination of speed and strength is power. It is a method of training that enhances an individual's explosive reaction through rapid and powerful muscular contractions through stretch-shortening cycles. The maximum force that a muscle can develop is attained during a rapid eccentric contraction (lengthening; see the definition of *eccentric contraction* below).

Our muscles seldom perform only one type of contraction: A bicep curl on the way up is a concentric contraction (shortening; see the definition of *concentric contraction* below), while extending the arm is an eccentric contraction. When a concentric contraction occurs following an eccentric contraction, the force generated can be dramatically increased. At a more cellular level, if a muscle is stretched, most of the energy used to stretch it is lost in the form of heat. There is some leftover energy stored in the elastic components of the muscle. If the stored energy is then used by an opposing contraction (that is, a concentric contraction following an eccentric contraction), then a greater force is generated in those muscles (Bompa, 1999). For the most effective gains, weight training prior to plyometric training is essential to gain the greatest generation of force.

plyometrics
a method of training that enhances an individual's "explosive" reaction through rapid and powerful muscular contractions through stretch-shortening cycles; a concentric action immediately preceded by an eccentric action

Types of Muscular Action

The three common types of muscular action are isotonic, isokinetic, and isometric.

ISOTONIC ACTION

isotonic action
one of the three common types of muscular action; isotonic action occurs when a muscle contracts in response to a constant force or load applied to it; there are two types of isotonic action—concentric and eccentric

Isotonic action occurs when a muscle contracts in response to a constant force or load that is applied to it. Generally speaking, there are two types of isotonic contraction:

- *Concentric contraction* The ends of the muscle are drawn closer together (contractile force is greater than resistive force). A biceps curl on the way up is an example of an exercise that produces a concentric contraction.

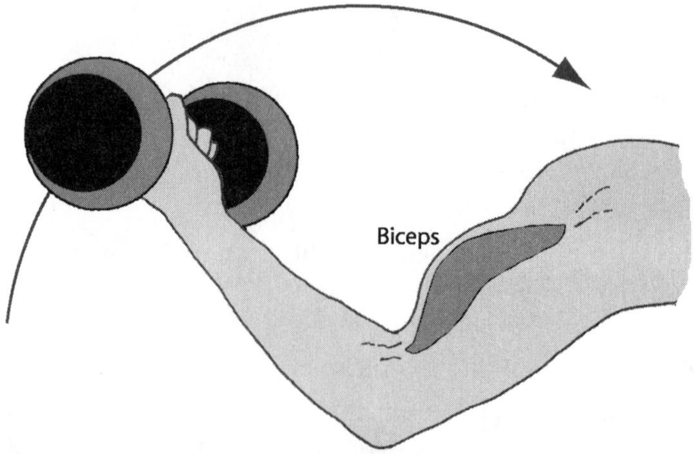

- *Eccentric contraction* The ends of the muscle are pulled farther apart (contractile force is less than resistive force). A biceps curl on the way down is an example of an exercise that produces an eccentric contraction.

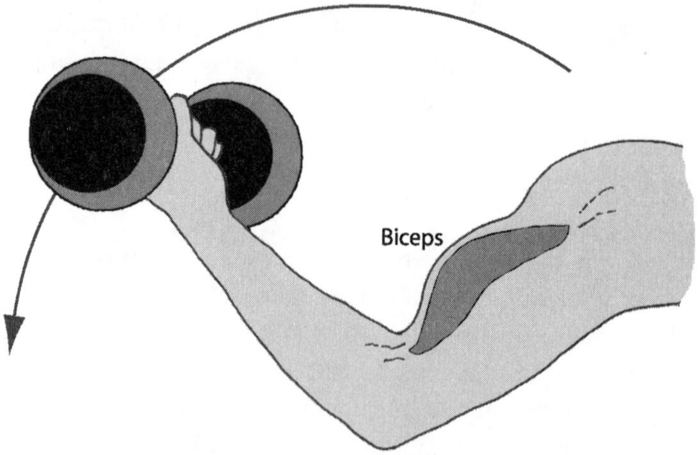

Eccentric contractions are much stronger than concentric contractions and therefore can produce greater exercise benefits. However, eccentric contractions cause more muscle soreness and present an increased risk of soft tissue damage.

isokinetic action
one of the three common types of muscular action; isokinetic action occurs during exercises involving equipment that compensates for the varying amounts of force exerted by a muscle by maintaining a constant level of resistance

ISOKINETIC ACTION

Isokinetic action is a type of isotonic action. Isokinetic exercises are performed on equipment that compensates for the varying amounts of force exerted by the muscles of an arm, leg, or other part of the body as it passes through the range of motion of an exercise. As a result, a constant level of resistance is maintained. Cybex machines are an example of equipment designed for isokinetic exercises.

ISOMETRIC ACTION

Isometric action occurs when muscle length remains constant throughout the exercise (contractile force equals resistive force). An example of an isometric exercise is the one where a person stands facing a wall, holds his or her arms out at a 90° angle, and pushes against the wall. Because isometric exercises can train only one kind of joint at a time, they are not used too much in strength and endurance training.

isometric action
one of the three common types of muscular action; isometric action occurs when muscle length remains constant, as is the case in certain exercises

Figure 6.1 illustrates the difference between isotonic and isometric actions.

FIGURE 6.1 Difference Between Isotonic and Isometric Actions

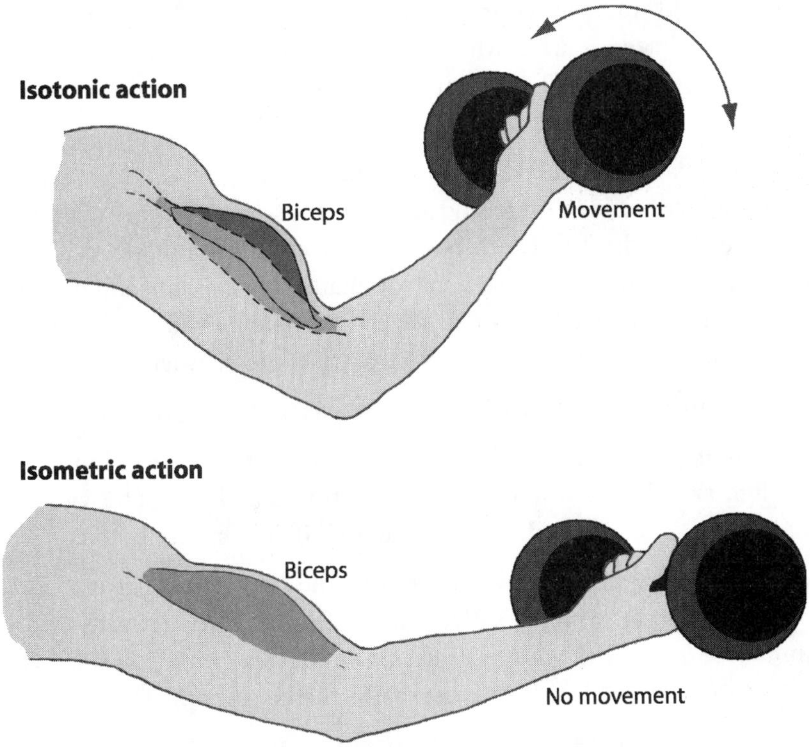

GUIDELINES FOR STRENGTH AND ENDURANCE TRAINING

As in cardiorespiratory training, you need to adhere to certain guidelines to make strength and endurance training effective, safe, and enjoyable.

Starting Out: The First Two to Three Weeks

During your first two to three weeks of training, keep these points in mind:

- For each exercise, you should do only 1–2 sets of 8–12 repetitions. After three weeks, you can gradually increase to 2–3 sets and decrease the number of repetitions. If you are a beginner, you need to pick a weight that is comfortable, with the last two or three reps becoming hard but not impossible to lift.
- Your workouts should include a total of no more than 20–25 sets. More is counterproductive, and you risk overtraining! Once you can lift your set number of reps comfortably, increase the weight slightly while reducing the number of reps.

- Small muscles such as forearm flexors recover faster than larger muscles such as the pectoralis major, and therefore can tolerate more sets without risking soreness or overtraining.
- You can exercise each muscle group two to three times a week, but remember to leave at least 48 hours between workouts involving the same muscle group.
- During your workouts, exercise the large-muscle group first so that the small muscles (which are not fatigued) can support the large muscles.
- When you weight train, always try to use the full range of motion but don't lock your knees or arms, which can put stress on the joints. Using the full range of motion will help you develop strength and maintain flexibility.
- Try to ensure that all of the major muscle groups are exercised. Also, try to achieve a balance between exercising agonists (muscles that move a joint in the desired direction) and antagonists (muscles that simultaneously resist that movement), which will help you maintain flexibility and prevent joint or soft tissue damage. For example, do alternate pushing and pulling exercises, especially in split routines (for example, presses then flies).
- Breathe out during the last two-thirds of the exertion phase of an exercise.
- Don't try to lift more than you are able to. There is less chance of injury lifting a lighter weight in a slow, controlled action than lifting a heavier weight in a fast, uncontrolled, "ballistic" action. If you are tired, stop.
- Some people feel slightly dizzy when working the large-muscle groups in the lower body, because blood is diverted to this area. If you feel this way, you should lie down with your feet raised. Do not carry on if you still feel dizzy after a few minutes or if you have had a further dizzy spell.
- Modify your workout every three weeks or so; otherwise, the muscles will adapt and your gains will level off. You can modify your workout by altering intensity (recall the FITT formula in chapter 5), the number of sets, the type and speed of muscular action, the type of exercise, and the length of rest periods between sets and workouts.
- Setting goals is a good way to stay motivated. Make sure that your goals are realistic. Remember that results take time and are sometimes very gradual. Keeping a log may help you monitor your progress.
- Remember the importance of fuelling your body with adequate nutrients and fluids, especially water.

The Frequency of Training

For your training to be effective, you must train regularly. Also, it is important to rest the muscles at least 48 hours after a workout to avoid overtraining and to allow your body to repair torn tissue. There are a number of ways to accomplish these objectives. You will likely use either the three-days-a-week routine or the four-day split routine. People at an advanced stage of training may wish to use the three-day split-phase routine described by Shipley (1998).

EXAMPLES OF DIFFERENT TRAINING PROGRAMS

Periodization Training

Periodization is an organized approach to training that involves progressive cycling of various aspects of a training program during a specific period of time to achieve specific goals (such as losing body fat or enhancing certain aspects of the body). Periodization training is the systematic variation of training specificity, intensity, and/or volume to obtain longer training and performance improvements. The aim is to develop basic hypertrophy; strengthen ligaments, tendons, and connective tissue; and build a base from which you can develop. Depending on goals (such as training for a specific test or sport), individuals will choose different programs to meet their needs or health status. The strategy is to move from higher-volume and lower-intensity programs to lower-volume and higher-intensity programs through a series of phases. Some individuals will start out in the general conditioning phase and work their way to a maintenance phase. This type of training takes into account a recovery phase, which reduces overtraining. Many websites will provide a variation on this theme. You have to decide what you want out of a program and what will work for you. For example, to train for the PREP BFOR, you need to train for the pursuit and restraint phases as well as the cardiovascular component, the shuttle run. For those starting out, table 6.1 provides general guidelines regarding sets, reps, intensity, and load and rest intervals. Many follow these until they are comfortable trying more and then move on to a specific training regime.

periodization
an organized approach to training that involves progressive cycling of various aspects of a training program during a specific period of time

TABLE 6.1 Example of Periodization Training

	General conditioning	Strength	Power	Maintenance	Active recovery
Sets	2–3	2–3	3–4	1–2	1
Reps	8–12	6–8	3–5	6–10	10–12
Intensity	Moderate	High	High	Moderate	Low
Volume (load)	High	Moderate	Low	Moderate	Moderate
Rest (between sets)	1–2 minutes	3–4 minutes	4–5 minutes	1–2 minutes	1–2 minutes

Sources: Stone, O'Bryant, & Garhmmer, 1981; Stone & O'Bryant, 1987; Bompa, 1999.

Strength Training to Develop Strength and Produce Hypertrophy in Muscles

As your body adapts to a general weight training program, you will begin to see fewer gains. In order to shock your body and begin to see more gains to your large-muscle groups, there are various forms of training that you can undertake to develop those muscles. Here are some suggestions for applying these principles:

- Begin your weight training sessions with 3–4 sets of dead lifts or squats at 85–95 percent of your **1RM**; if you don't know your 1RM, aim for 2–6 repetitions (refer to the section "Determining Load" below).
- Rest no longer than 60 seconds between sets.

1RM
one maximal repetition of weight

- Continue to do your traditional combined upper-body/lower-body routine or split routine as normal.
- Drink a carbohydrate beverage during and a carbohydrate/protein beverage after your routine to boost repair and growth of the muscle tissue.

It should be noted that increased muscle bulk from hypertrophy training does not necessarily make you stronger. Contrary to popular belief, increased muscle size does not equate with increased strength. It is the neuromuscular recruitment of the involved muscle fibres that increases strength.

A Quick Note on Performance-Enhancing Substances

There are three basic types of performance-enhancing substances associated with weight training. *Nutritional aids* include vitamins and minerals, protein and amino acid supplements, carnitine, creatine, and caffeine. *Pharmacological aids* include pain-masking drugs, anabolic steroids, prohormones, human growth hormones, and erythropoietin. *Physiological aids* include blood doping and drug masking.

Amino acids have been used by athletes to assist in the repair and building of muscle tissue and the release of growth hormone. Excessive amounts can lead to a toxic effect due to dehydration. See chapter 8 for further discussion of amino acids.

Anabolic steroids are synthetic derivatives of the male hormone testosterone. They produce retention of phosphate, potassium, and nitrogen; decrease amino acid breakdown; and increase protein synthesis. Most athletes see an increase in their muscle mass and strength, a decrease in body fat, and quicker recovery from training. There has been little consistent evidence in enhanced performance, except in lean body mass. Anabolic steroids have many harmful side effects, including liver damage, increased aggressiveness, acne, stunted growth, gynocomastia (development of breast tissue in males), high blood pressure, and sterility. In women, anabolic steroids may lead to masculinization, excessive facial hair growth, deepening of the voice, and ammenorhea (National Institute on Drug Abuse, 2006). Because the risk factors are great for those who consider steriod use as a means of gaining lean muscle mass, discussing this matter with your physician is very important before deciding to take this pharmacological aid.

VARIATIONS ON TRAINING ROUTINES

You'll find that with shift work, court time and family time some of these examples will work better for you due to your time restraints. While at school or in a specialized unit where you must train every day you work, you may be able to get in six days a week of workouts. During other times in your life, you may be restricted to two or three days a week and may only have time for a 40 minute workout. You'll have to determine at that point which program will provide you with the most benefits. Here are some examples:

- *Three-days-a-week routine* Train three non-consecutive days a week (for example, Monday, Wednesday, and Friday) and complete all exercises in your workout each time.

- *Four-day split routine* This involves training different parts of the body on different days. Ontario Police College (1994) lays out two options:

	Option A	**Option B**
Monday and Thursday	Upper body: chest, back, shoulders, and arms	Chest, shoulders, triceps, and abdominals
Tuesday and Friday	Lower body: legs and abdominals	Legs, back, and biceps

- *Three-day split-phase routine*

Day 1:	Chest, triceps, and abdominals	Day 5:	Repeat day 1
Day 2:	Back and biceps	Day 6:	Repeat day 2
Day 3:	Legs and shoulders	Day 7:	Repeat day 3
Day 4:	Rest	Day 8:	Rest

Trisets

Trisets are combinations of three exercises done with little rest in between. They can involve working the same muscle group from three different angles, working three different muscle groups, or working different areas of the same muscle from three different angles. Trisets increase training intensity by reducing the average length of rest intervals between sets. Trisets save time and raise the metabolism; however, they are associated with a higher risk of injury. They are done at about 50 percent 1RM with exercises being performed one after the other, then repeated two or three times. Rest periods are from one to three minutes. An example of a sequence for the chest and back could be decline dumbbell presses, chin-ups, incline dumbbell flies, and one-arm dumbbell rows.

trisets
combining three exercises with little rest in between; can involve working the same muscle group from three different angles, working three different muscle groups, or working different areas of the same muscle from three different angles

Split routines can involve working the upper body one day and the lower body another day. This means you can continue to work out on successive days. There are many examples of split routines. See table 6.2 for a few examples.

TABLE 6.2 Example of Trisets

	4-day routine	**5-day routine**	**5-day routine**	**6-day routine**
Monday	Upper	Chest and back	Chest	Upper
Tuesday	Lower	Legs and abs	Shoulders	Lower
Wednesday	Rest	Off	Back	Upper
Thursday	Upper	Arms and shoulders	Rest	Lower
Friday	Lower	Off	Triceps/Biceps	Upper
Saturday			Leg	Lower
Sunday				
Special note	Work abdominals each day	Work abdominals each day	Work abs and calves each day or minimum three days, but fewer sets	Work abdominals each day

Ultimately, your time restraints, interests, and goals will lead you to choose one or a combination of these programs. An example for the chest and back could be decline dumbbell presses, chin-ups, incline dumbbell flies, and one-arm dumbbell rows. Table 6.3 provides a more specific guideline for beginners depending on their goals. For each training goal, there are guidelines that help you either to build muscle strength and power or to train your muscles to last longer.

TABLE 6.3 Training Goals

Training goal	No. of exercises	No. of sets per exercise	No. of repetitions per set	Rest period between sets
Muscular endurance or muscle tone	10–12	2–3	12–18	20–30 seconds
Muscle growth	8–10	3–6	8–12	30–90 seconds
Strength and muscle growth	8–12	3–6	6–12	1–2 minutes
Power (ability to perform quick, explosive exercises)	1–6	3–5	1–5	2–5 minutes

Selecting and Arranging Exercises

A balanced program for beginners should incorporate one to three exercises for each large-muscle group, for a maximum total of 12. The order in which you complete your exercises is also important. Keep the following in mind when you exercise:

1. Do large-muscle group exercises first.
2. Always alternate between an upper-body and a lower-body exercise during your workout.
3. Push exercises should alternate with pull exercises.

How you structure your program will affect the intensity of your training, which in turn may affect the rate at which you benefit from your program.

Warming Up

Your workout must always include a proper warm-up (and cool-down). Your warm-up should consist of 5–15 minutes minimum of an aerobic activity such as light jogging or bicycling, followed by stretching. Mimic the types of exercises you will do in your workout using light weights to prepare the muscles for the workout.

Following Correct Form

The correct form in strength and endurance training is a steady, controlled execution of the exercise through the full range of motion. It is important to isolate the muscle group you are exercising. For example, if you're doing biceps curls, you need to concentrate on the biceps and not use your back. You must not bounce any weight you use. When you engage in a controlled movement you need to take at least as long extending as you do flexing (a count of two on the way up and a count of at least two on the way down). The eccentric contraction will be more effective and your muscle—not gravity—will do the work.

Proper Breathing Techniques

Your blood pressure can increase to dangerous levels if you hold your breath while weight training. It is important to exhale during the lift and continue breathing throughout the exercise to prevent your blood pressure from rising too high.

Determining Load

You also need to determine the load or weight you will lift. Several methods are available.

REPETITION RANGE METHOD

This method is appropriate for beginners and for people not involved in lifting maximum or near-maximum loads. It involves the following steps:

1. Determine the number of repetitions necessary for achieving your exercise goal (see table 6.3).
2. Through trial and error, determine the maximum load that you can lift within this repetitions range. By the third set you should begin to feel fatigue. If you cannot make it to the third set, lessen the load or do not complete the third set.
3. Work with this load as long as you remain within the desired repetition range through three sets.
4. Increase the load by 5–10 percent once you are able to perform 15 repetitions in the last set during two consecutive workouts.

PERCENT MAXIMUM METHOD

This involves determining the maximum load you can lift at a single go. Since lifting maximum loads can cause injury, this method should be used only under the supervision of your instructor or another fitness expert.

Turn to **assignment 6.1** (in the appendix) to determine your workload for your maximum bench press.

Choosing Your Training System

There are at least five training systems to choose from. Which one you choose depends on your goals and on the amount of time you have to devote to your program.

CIRCUIT TRAINING

In this system you perform a number of exercises in succession at a submaximal level, with little rest in between. This type of workout is good for muscular endurance and tone and for cardiovascular fitness.

LIGHT TO HEAVY TRAINING

As you progress through the sets, you increase the weight you are working with. This system produces a low risk of injury. The major drawback is that the muscles may tire during the earlier sets, preventing heavier lifting later.

HEAVY TO LIGHT TRAINING

As you progress through the sets, you decrease the weight you are working with. The advantage is that you may be able to lift heavier weights before the muscles tire. The disadvantage is a high risk of injury if you have not properly warmed up your muscles.

PYRAMID TRAINING

pyramid training
a system combining the light to heavy and heavy to light approaches for weight training

The **pyramid training** system combines the light to heavy and heavy to light approaches. You begin your workout with the light to heavy approach, followed by the heavy to light approach during the second half. This system is good for developing strength. It can cause injury, however, by tempting people to push too hard to finish their sets.

SUPERSET TRAINING

superset training
a system involving performing two exercises in succession, without rest; often used to exercise opposing muscle groups and results in increased strength and muscle mass of the targeted muscle group

The **superset training** system involves performing two exercises in succession, without rest. It is often used to exercise opposing muscle groups. It increases strength and muscle mass of the targeted muscle group. Its use is confined to the arms and legs. For example, leg extensions and then squats will increase the size and strength of the quadriceps muscle. In the upper arm, doing a triceps exercise followed by bench press targets the triceps muscle. If the muscle is pre-fatigued, then you will be pushing it beyond comfortable limits. This is where gains or injuries can occur.

Plyometrics

Plyometrics was designed to condition athletes to increase and develop their jumping, sprinting, and explosive power. Due to the effort required, adequate rest time is needed between exercises to recover. Individuals must be highly motivated to do this type of conditioning. Some guidelines include the following:

- Aim for a 1:5 ratio; for example, 30 seconds flat out with a 2:30 minute rest.
- Always warm up and stretch, especially your legs.
- Use explosive movements to obtain optimal results. Stay focused in order to get the most out of the workout.
- Always use correct foot placement. Aim to land with your ankle fixed.
- Aim to stay on the balls of your feet whenever possible. Avoid landing on your heels or the sides of your feet.
- Do not do circuit training more than twice a week, and remember to allow a minimum of 48 hours' rest between sessions.
- Use only your body weight when performing plyometric exercises.
- Always allow adequate recovery between reps. The importance of recovery cannot be stressed enough.

Examples of exercises include 90° jumps, lateral skating, one-leg butt kicks, ski tuck jumps, and two-foot side hops. As you become more advanced, you can try activities like decline hops, two-foot hops off a box, bench jumping, rope jumping, and depth jumps off a box. Alternating between lunges and sprints on a track also constitutes a form of plyometrics.

Designing an Appropriate Program

Comparing absolute fitness levels between males and females has been an issue for years. A high proportion of female applicants fail many entrance tests due to their size, body composition, hemoglobin levels, and muscular strength (Shephard & Bonneau, 2002). BFOR standards have tried to address these issues; however, females, and in some cases smaller males, may still be at a disadvantage if they are not training appropriately. It is important to realize that muscular strength is something that must be continually worked on throughout your career. Statistically, women tend to shy away from strength training. However, in policing it is very important that all officers have the strength when needed to do the job, whether they are physically restraining an individual, applying handcuffs, or pulling themselves over a wall while wearing a uniform, vest, and belt weighing approximately 25–50 lb. (11–23 kg).

Table 6.4 provides you with common exercises that address some of the specific areas that will help you complete the BFOR police requirements (see chapter 16). In addition to having good cardiovascular endurance, you'll need to develop upper-body strength to meet the requirements. As you practise the PREP and PARE, you will come to appreciate that technique plays a role; however, those with good strength are able to get through the protocol without injury. It will be up to you to see that you are able to meet the minimum requirements.

TABLE 6.4 Upper Beginner/Lower Intermediate Training Program

	DAY 1 chest/triceps	DAY 2 arms/shoulders/abdominals	DAY 3 legs/biceps	DAY 4 cardio/abdominals
Warm-up	Skipping (3 minutes/no breaks)	Skipping (2 minutes/no breaks)	Skipping (2 minutes/no breaks)	Skipping (2 minutes/no breaks)
	Add light cardio (5 minutes)	Add light cardio (5 minutes)	Add light cardio (5 minutes)	Add light cardio (5 minutes)
	Stretching (min. 10 minutes)	Stretching (min. 10 minutes)	Stretching (min. 10 minutes)	Stretching (min. 10 minutes)
Exercises	Bench press 3 x 15	Bent-over row pronate 2 x 12	Squats 3 x 12	30–45 minutes of continuous CV exercise (65–80% VO_2 Max)
	Incline dumbbell flies 3 x 15	Bent-over row supinate 2 x 12	Leg press 3 x 12	
	Two-handed triceps dumbbell raises 2 x 12	Seated row (bar to belly button) 3 x 15	Calf raises 3 x 12	
	One-handed triceps raise 2 x 8	Shoulder press, military press, or Arnold press 3 x 15	Leg extensions 3 x 12	
	Push-ups 3 x max	Abdominal curls or side curl-ups 2 x 35–50 (fatigue)	Biceps curl, preacher curl, or easy curl with straight bar 3 x 10	Abdominal curls or side curl-ups 2 x 35–50 (fatigue)
Rest period	30 seconds between sets; CV-based	30 seconds between sets; CV-based	45 seconds between sets	

Table 6.5 shows examples of exercises that you can use in designing your own fitness program. **Comprehensive descriptions and pictures of exercises that cover the major muscle groups are available online at www.emp.ca/fitness.** Most exercises can be easily modified to be done at home if you do not have access to a fitness facility. You will have to determine the starting weight, sets, and repetitions based on the information that you have just read, as well as on your starting fitness level and the goals you want to achieve. Although a basic program could last six to eight weeks, you might become bored after only two weeks. You can then modify your program to fit your specific needs and interests. The available equipment plays a significant role in what changes you can make to your program.

TABLE 6.5 Examples of Exercises for Designing a Weight Training Program

Major Muscle Group	Additional Muscles Used	Exercises
Trapezius		Shoulder shrugs
		Lower pulley row to neck
		Dumbbell incline shoulder raise
		Shoulder shrugs
	Biceps, shoulders	Upright row
Deltoid		Barbell incline shoulder raise
	Biceps, latissimus dorsi	Barbell rear deltoid row
		Bent-over dumbbell rear deltoid raise
	Front deltoids, forearms	Dumbbell side lateral raises
	Trapezius	Bent-over low-pulley side lateral
Pectoralis		Around the world
	Triceps, shoulders	Barbell bench press—medium grip
	Triceps, shoulders, latissimus dorsi	Bent-arm barbell pullover
		Butterfly or pec deck fly
	Muscles of the shoulder	Cable crossover
	Muscles of the shoulder	Dumbbell fly
Latissimus dorsi	Biceps, middle back	Close-grip front lats pulldown
	Middle back	Cable rows
		Pull-ups
		Straight-arm pulldown
Triceps brachii	Muscles of the chest and core	Bench dips
		Cable lying triceps extensions
		Cable triceps extension
Biceps brachii	Forearms, latissimus dorsi	Chin-ups
		Concentration curls
		Dumbbell biceps curls
		Barbell curls

continued

TABLE 6.5 Examples of Exercises for Designing a Weight Training Program *continued*

Major Muscle Group	Additional Muscles Used	Exercises
Abdominals (rectus abdominis)		Ab crunch machine
		Air bike
		Bent-knee hip raise
		Leg raises
		Cable crunch
		Cross-body crunch
		Crunch—legs on exercise ball
		Incline reverse crunch
		Abdominal ball crunch
Rhomboids (strengthens middle back)	Biceps, latissimus dorsi	Bent-over barbell row
	Biceps, latissimus dorsi	Bent-over two-dumbbell row
		Bent-over row with dumbbell
		Incline bench pull
		Lying T-bar row
Erector spinae (lower back)	Hamstrings, gluteals, upper back	Hyperextensions
	Gluteals, obliques, rectus abdominus	Superman
	Gluteals, obliques, rectus abdominus	Knee tucks
Quadriceps		Barbell full squat
	Hamstrings, gluteals, calves	Barbell dead lift
		Cable hip adduction
	Calves, gluteals	Dumbbell rear lunge
		Knee extensions
	Hamstrings, gluteus maximus	Leg press
Gluteals (maximus and medius)		Bridge
		One-legged cable kickback
	Hamstrings	Stiff-legged barbell dead lift
		Glutes kickback
Hamstrings (biceps femoris)	Glutes	Lying leg curls
		Seated leg curls
	Glutes, core	Stability ball leg curls
Brachioradialis (strengthens forearms for baton and firearms)		Wrist curl
		Dumbbell lying supination
		Palms-down dumbbell wrist curl over a bench
		Wrist roller

Turn to **assignment 6.2** (in the appendix) to start designing your strength and endurance training program.

TRAINING PROGRAMS

You will need to develop your own weight training program. You may want to emphasize endurance, or you may want to include more strength training to meet the demands of the job and BFOR standards to apply for that job. Ultimately, you will determine what fits best for you.

Tables 6.6 and 6.7 are examples of two weight training programs that were developed to show students how a program is organized. The upper beginner/lower intermediate training program is a cardiovascular-based program, but it can be used for strength depending on the weights you incorporate. The intermediate/advanced training program is a strength training program that can incorporate power. An intermediate program should not be tried if you have not done a weight training program before. Since each person has different maximal weights, table 6.6 is a shell, which can be modified and changed to reflect your personal needs and preferences. You can also replace exercises to suit your preference or availability of equipment. Table 6.7 is list of potential exercises that you can incorporate into a program.

Many gyms will have exercise instructions posted beside equipment and have qualified personnel who can provide you with instructions and suggestions to make your program fit your needs. Some people rely on free weights only; others incorporate machines with free weights; and others work with what they have at home. You will be the judge of what best suits your needs. Your instructor should be able to provide you will some guidance if you feel that one group of muscles is being worked more than another.

Upper Beginner/Lower Intermediate

This program, designed for a four-day cycle, was designed to be cardiovascular (CV) based. It is not a power-based program, although day 3 works large muscles, which could, depending on the starting weights, reflect a strength-building component. You must first determine your starting weights so that you can work toward the number of sets and reps indicated.

Intermediate/Advanced Program

This program is an example for people who have spent at least 12 weeks in a program and have advanced to being able to lift between 70 and 75 percent of their maximal weight for each exercise, six to eight reps for three sets. This program addresses gains in strength.

Turn to **assignment 6.2** (in the appendix), "Designing Your Strength and Endurance Training Program," and add to your program.

KEY TERMS

overload principle	power training	periodization
general adaptation	plyometrics	1RM
repetition (rep)	isotonic action	trisets
set	isokinetic action	pyramid training
hypertrophy	isometric action	superset training

TABLE 6.6 Intermediate/Advanced Training Program

		Week	1	2	3	4	5	6	7	8
		Reps	6–8	6–8	4–6	10–12	4–6	4–6	10–12	4–6
		% of maximal weight lifted	70%	75%	80%	75%	85%	90%	75%	80%
Day	Exercise	Sets								
1	Bench press	4								
	Fly	3								
	Crossover	2								
	Preacher curl	4								
	Hammer curl	3								
	Concentration biceps curl	2								
	Seated calf	4								
2	Lats pulldown	4								
	Wide-grip chin-up	3								
	Seated rowing	3								
	Back extension	2								
	Triceps dumbbell extension	4								
	Seated row (split rope)[a]	3								
	Close grip bicep bench	2								
3	Squat	4								
	Leg extension	3								
	Leg press	2								
	Reverse curl	3								
	Sevens[b]	3								
	Chest press	3								
	Push-up (fatigue)	3								
4	Military press	4								
	Lateral raise[c]	3								
	Frontal[d]	2								
	Shrug	4								
	Leg curl	4								
	Dip	2								
	Abs (fatigue)	2								

a Seated row (split rope): Pull the split rope straight back to the side, and extend your elbows straight back behind your back.

b Sevens: Biceps curl with easy bar with three positions: (1) start at bottom of extension and go to 90°; (2) start at 90° and bring to full flexion; (3) start at full extension and go to full flexion.

c Lateral raise: Have the dumbbells out to the side with your knees bent, and bring the dumbbells out to the side in a shoulder fly.

d Frontal: Have the dumbbells starting behind the buttocks and raise them to shoulder height out in front.

TABLE 6.7 Strength and Endurance Training Program Exercise Options

Body part	Equipment	Example of exercise
Chest	No equipment	• Push-ups • Dips
	Exercise ball, bands, tubing, free weights, medicine ball	• Chest presses • Push-ups • Barbell bench press • Dumbbell chest press on ball • Chest press with tubing • Push-ups with medicine ball
	Machines	• Bench press • Decline/incline bench press • Cable crossover • Chest fly • Decline/incline chest fly • Chest press • Pec dec • Cable crossovers
Back	No equipment	• Modified back extensions • Side leg lifts (lower back) • Prone leg lifts (lower back) • Hip extensions (lower back)
	Exercise ball, bands, tubing, free weights	• Bent over rowing (upper body) • Side leg lifts (lower body) • Good mornings • Lat pulldown • Medicine ball twists (upper body)
	Machines	• Lat pull-downs (upper back) • Lower- back extension (lower back) • Wide pull-downs (upper back) • Seated lat rows (lower back) • Pull-downs (upper back) • Dead lifts (upper back) • Hip extensions (lower back) • Rowing machine (upper + lower)
Legs	No equipment	• Leg extensions • Leg curls • Squats • Front and side lunges • Stairs • Single and double leg jumps • Vertical jumps
	Exercise ball, bands, tubing, free weights, medicine ball	• Seated calf presses • Squats • Wall squats • Front and side lunges • Calf raises • Ball squeeze and lift • Medicine ball lunge • Hamstring rolls • Seated lateral raise with hip flexion • Oblique lift
	Machines	• Leg extension • Leg curls • Squat • Lunge • Hip extension • Hip abduction • Hip adduction • Standing leg kickback • Seated calf press • Leg press • Hip flexion
Shoulder	No equipment	• Chin-ups • L-seat dips
	Exercise ball, bands, tubing, free weights	• Upright rowing • Shoulder shrugs • Dumbbell press above the head • Upright row • Seated arm raises • Behind-the-head press • Bent-over row
	Machines	• Rear deltoid rows • Lateral shoulder raise • Seated shoulder press • Front shoulder raise • Shoulder shrug • Reverse fly • Stiff arm pulldown • Rear deltoid row • Upright rowing • Low-pulley cable cross raises • Shoulder presses
Arms	No equipment	• Bicep curls • Tricep curls • Bench dips
	Exercise ball, bands, tubing, free weights, medicine ball	• Bicep curls • Tricep curls • Tricep kickbacks • Tricep presses
	Machines	• Triceps pushdown • French press • Triceps extension • Preacher curl • Reverse tricep pushdown • Standing biceps curl with pulleys • Tricep kickback • Wrist extension • Wrist curl • Reverse curl • Resisted dip • Hammer grip curls • Overhead extensions
Abdominal	No equipment	• Curl-ups • Bent knee side crunches • Crossed-leg oblique crunches • V-sits • Leg lifts • Pelvic tilts • Curl-ups
	Exercise ball, bands, tubing, free weights, medicine ball	• Medicine ball crunches • Medicine ball throws to partner
	Machines	• Reverse crunch • Resisted reverse crunch • Seated (resisted) abdominal crunch • Seated (resisted) oblique abdominal crunch • Ab crunch with attachment • Trunk rotation • Standing oblique crunch

EXERCISES

Review

1. Define "overload principle."

2. Describe how isotonic, isometric, and isokinetic actions differ.

3. Identify and distinguish between the two types of muscle fibre.

4. How should you warm up before a workout?

5. What is the difference between pyramid and superset training?

Multiple Choice

1. Which of the following is a correct safety guideline for weight training?
   a. move joints through the full range of motion
   b. exhale on exertion and inhale on the release
   c. inhale on exertion and exhale on the release
   d. arch your back while lifting heavy weights
   e. arch your back to help you lift your weights

2. During which of the following contractions does a muscle shorten as it overcomes resistance and a weight is lifted?
   a. concentric
   b. eccentric
   c. isometric
   d. isokinetic
   e. isotonic

3. During which of the following actions does muscle length remain constant?
   a. plyometrics
   b. overload
   c. isometric
   d. isokinetic
   e. isotonic

4. What is strength and endurance training also known as?
   a. weight training
   b. aerobic training
   c. cardiovascular training
   d. resistance training
   e. overload training

5. It is important to rest the muscles for a minimum of how many hours after weight training to avoid overtraining?
   a. 12
   b. 18
   c. 24
   d. 36
   e. 48

6. What is the name of the principle that states that, to build muscle mass, the muscle must be subjected to a greater than normal load?
   a. the slow-twitch principle
   b. the isokinetic principle
   c. the recovery principle
   d. the overload principle
   e. the muscle endurance principle

7. What is a group of consecutive repetitions of a resistance exercise called?
   a. a set
   b. a measure
   c. a rep
   d. a sequence
   e. a game

8. Which of the following is poor advice for strength training?
   a. warm up slowly and completely
   b. hold your breath during the lifting phase
   c. select exercises for all major muscle groups
   d. train initially for endurance if you are a beginner
   e. vary the routine to avoid boredom

9. The maximum amount of force that a muscle can generate at one time is called:
   a. power
   b. progression
   c. sticking point
   d. muscular endurance
   e. strength

10. The ability of muscle to exert force repeatedly without fatiguing is called
    a. muscular endurance
    b. muscular strength
    c. plyometrics
    d. one repetition maximum
    e. muscle capacity

11. To evaluate dynamic strength, an individual must
    a. perform as many leg press exercises as possible by pressing a heavy weight to exhaustion
    b. do three sets of 20 push-ups within five minutes
    c. perform as many sit-ups as possible in one minute
    d. perform a bench press by lifting the heaviest weight possible
    e. jump repeatedly on and off a box for one minute

12. Overload is defined as
    a. overtraining
    b. working the body harder than it is accustomed
    c. carbohydrate loading for endurance athletes
    d. periodizing exercises in a program
    e. carrying more weight than is necessary for an exercise

13. Plyometrics training involves
    a. a slow progressive repetition of an exercise
    b. a force exerted by a muscle by maintaining a constant level of resistance
    c. an organized approach to training that involves progressive cycling
    d. an explosive reaction through rapid and powerful muscular contractions
    e. a process characterized by high training volume with moderate training intensity

14. Which of the following factors does not put women at a disadvantage in entrance tests?
    a. size
    b. muscular endurance
    c. body composition
    d. hemoglobin levels
    e. muscular strength

REFERENCES

Bompa, T. (1999). *Periodization: Theory and methodology of training.* Champaign, IL: Human Kinetics.

Farenholtz, D. (1995). *Correctional Officer's Physical Abilities Test (COPAT): Physical training, conditioning, and maintenance program.* Ottawa: National Headquarters, Correctional Service of Canada.

Faulkner, J.A., & White, T.P. (1990). Adaptations of skeletal muscle to physical activity. *Proceedings of the International Conference on Exercise, Fitness, and Health* (pp. 265-275). Champaign, IL: Human Kinetics.

Fiatarone, M.A., et al. (1994). Exercise training and nutritional supplementation for physical frailty in very elderly people. *New England Journal of Medicine, 331,* 1237-1238.

Fleck, S.J., & Kraemer, W.J. (1988). Resistance training: Physiological responses and adaptations. *The Physician and Sports Medicine, 16,* 108-124.

Gledhill, N., & Shaw, C. (1995, October). *Constable Selection Project. Final report: Medical, physical, skills and abilities project.* Race Relations and Policing Unit. Toronto: Ministry of the Solicitor General and Correctional Services.

Jurca, R., LaMonte, M.J., Church, T.S., Earnest, C.P., Fitzgerald, S.J., Barlow, C.E., Jordan, A.N., Kampert, J.B., & Blair, S.N. (2004). Associations with muscle strength and aerobic fitness with metabolic syndrome in men. *Medicine & Science in Sports & Exercise, 36,* 1301-1307.

Miller, J.P., Pratley, R.E., Goldberg, A.P., Gordon, P., Rubin, M., Treuth, M.S., Ryan A.S., & Hurley, B.F. (1994). Strength training increases insulin action in healthy 50- to 65-year-old men. *Journal of Applied Physiology, 77,* 1122-1127.

National Institute on Drug Abuse. (August 2006). *Anabolic steroid abuse. Research Report Series.* Available at http://www.drugabuse.gov/PDF/RRSteroids.pdf.

Nelson, M.E., Fiatarone, M.A., Morganti, C.M., Trice, I., Greenberg, R.A., & Evans, W.J. (1994). Effects of high-intensity strength training on multiple risk factors for osteoporotic fractures. *Journal of the American Medical Association, 272,* 1909-1914.

Pratley, R.B., Nicklas, M., Rubin, J., Miller, A., Smith, M., Smith, B., Hurley, B.F., & Goldberg, A. (1994). Strength training increases resting metabolic rate and norepinephrine levels in healthy 50- to 65-year-old men. *Journal of Applied Physiology, 76,* 133-137.

Ontario Police College. Physical Training Department. (1994). *Weight training personal program design.* Toronto: Queen's Printer.

RCMP. (2001). *Emergency response team: Selection criteria.* Available at http://www.rcmp-grc.gc.ca/ert/ert2_e.htm.

Risch, S., Nowell, N., Pollock, M., Risch, E., Langer, H., Fulton, M., Graves, J., & Leggett, S. (1993). Lumbar strengthening in chronic low-back pain patients. *Spine, 18,* 232-238.

Shephard, R., & Bonneau, J. (2002). Assuring gender equity in recruitment standards for police officers. *Applied Physiology, Nutrition and Metabolism, 27*(3), 263-295.

Shipley, P. (1998). *Ontario provincial weight training program.* Toronto: Ontario Provincial Police and Ministry of the Solicitor General and Correctional Services.

Stone, M.H., O'Bryant, H.S., & Garhmmer, J. (1981). A hypothetical model for strength training. *Journal of Sports Medicine and Physical Fitness, 21,* 336, 342-351.

Stone, M.H., & O'Bryant, H.S. (1987). *Weight training: A scientific approach.* Minneapolis, MN: Burgess.

CHAPTER 7

Flexibility and Stretching

CHAPTER OBJECTIVES

After completing this chapter, you should be able to:

- Explain the benefits of stretching.
- Understand the differences among dynamic stretching, ballistic stretching, static stretching, and proprioceptive neuromuscular facilitation.
- Incorporate safe, effective stretching into your fitness program.

Flexibility is an important component of a balanced fitness program but one that is often neglected. It is achieved by incorporating stretching exercises into your fitness program. In this chapter we will look at the benefits of stretching, at stretching techniques, and at how to incorporate safe, effective stretching into your fitness program.

FLEXIBILITY

Together, muscles and bones make up what is called the *musculoskeletal system* of the body. Bones provide postural and structural support. Muscles assist the body with the ability to move (through contraction). This musculoskeletal system protects our internal organs. The point at which bones connect is called a *joint*, which is held together by *ligaments*, along with the help of muscles. Muscles are attached to bones by *tendons*.

Flexibility is the ability to move the joints freely through their full range of motion. The full range of motion is determined by the type of joint. Thus in a hinge joint such as a finger joint, the bones are connected in a way that allows movement in one plane only. But in a ball-and-socket joint such as a shoulder joint, the round head of one bone is held in the cuplike cavity of another bone, allowing the arms to move in many directions. The range of motion of most joints can be maintained or increased with proper training, but can decline quickly with disuse.

flexibility
the ability to move the joints freely through their full range of motion

Nerves connect the spinal column to the muscles. When an electrical signal crosses the neuromuscular junction, it transmits information to the muscle fibres. This stimulates the flow of calcium, which causes the actin and myosin filaments to slide across one another. When this happens, the sarcomeres in the muscle shorten all at once and the muscle fibre contracts. As the load increases, more muscle fibres are recruited by the central nervous system and a stronger force is generated by the muscles.

FAST AND SLOW MUSCLE FIBRES

The energy that produces the calcium flow in the muscle fibres comes from the *mitochondria*, the part of the muscle cell that converts glucose (blood sugar) into energy. The more mitochondria in a muscle fibre, the more energy it is able to produce.

Slow-twitch fibres (type 1 muscle fibres) are slow to contract but also slow to fatigue. They are smaller in diameter and contain more mitochondria and have more capillary flow around them, which delivers more oxygen and removes more waste products from the muscle fibres. This is why they are more resistant to fatigue. The heart has a greater number of type 1 fibres than type 2 fibres.

Fast-twitch fibres (type 2 muscle fibres) are very quick to contract and quick to fatigue. They are bigger in diameter and contain less mitochondria, with less blood flow. Waste products are slow to be removed. Type 2 fibres are activated after type 1 fibres are activated, so they are more difficult to train.

Muscle and its fibres are surrounded by connective tissues. Connective tissues are made up of tendons, ligaments, and the fascial sheaths (fascia) that cover the fibres. The more elastic connective tissue there is around a joint, the greater the range of motion in that joint.

THE BENEFITS OF STRETCHING

There are a number of reasons for incorporating stretching into a fitness program:

- Stretching enhances the body's ability to perform the exercises in one's program.
- Stretching your hamstrings, quadriceps, hip flexors, and low-back muscles regularly will help reduce the strain on your back. Flexibility training will improve your posture and help prevent low-back pain.
- Stretching reduces the risk of injury from exercising.
- Stretching increases your range of motion and helps to keep your body feeling loose and agile.
- Stretching promotes relaxation and helps to reduce stress.

Plowman and Smith (1997) identify other possible benefits of stretching:

- It can enhance physical fitness.
- It can reduce muscle tension.
- It can reduce the risk of joint sprains and muscle strains.

- It increases blood supply and nutrients to joint structures.
- It can reduce muscle soreness caused by exercise-induced injuries or explosive movements.
- It can reduce the severity of painful menstruation (dysmenorrhea).
- It can reduce resistance and tension in muscles.
- It can optimize the learning, practice, and performance of many types of skilled movements.
- It can promote the development of body awareness.

Stretching may not only help prevent injury and reduce low-back pain, but also help you recover faster (Carragee, 2005). Stretching, however, does not reduce the risk of injury or muscle soreness (Herbert & Gabriel, 2002) and there is much ongoing debate regarding when to stretch. According to Shrier (2004), stretching can cut down risks of sport or workout injury, but it may slow performance if done prior to the activity.

Muscle tissue is actually broken down during weight training. Under stress, tiny micro tears develop in the muscle fibres, contributing to the delayed-onset muscle soreness that often accompanies a strenuous workout. By bringing nutrients to the musculoskeletal system, stretching can help repair fibres and speed up the healing process. As a result, there is less muscle soreness, so you can come back stronger for the next workout.

HOW MUSCLES COOPERATE WITH EACH OTHER

When muscles cause a limb to move through the joint's range of motion, they usually act in cooperating groups:

- *Agonists* are muscles that cause the movement to occur. Through contraction they move the limb through a normal range of motion. Agonists are known as the *prime movers* since they generate the movement.
- *Antagonists* are muscles that act in opposition to the movement generated by the agonists. They return the limb to the original position.
- *Synergists* are muscles that assist the agonists, usually by neutralizing extra motion so that the movement of the agonists happens within the desired plane of motion.
- *Fixators* are the muscles that provide the support to hold the rest of the body in place while the movement occurs. They are also known as *stabilizers.*

Some commonly used agonist/antagonist muscle pairs include:

- biceps/triceps
- quadriceps/hamstrings
- pectorals/latissimus dorsi
- abdominals/spinal erectors
- forearm flexors/extensors

TYPES OF MUSCLE CONTRACTIONS

The contraction of a muscle does not imply that a muscle shortens; it only means that tension has been generated. Muscles can contract in the following ways:

- *Isometric contraction* is the state of no movement. This occurs when the muscles attempt to push or pull an immovable object (for example, pushing on a wall). The load on the muscles exceeds the tension generated by the contracting muscle.
- *Isotonic contraction* occurs when movement takes place because the tension generated by the muscle exceeds the load and it is able to push, pull, or lift an object. Isotonic contractions are divided into two types:
  - *Concentric contractions* take place when the muscle shortens against the opposing load (for example, bicep curl-up phase). The agonists (such as biceps) do all the work as they shorten.
  - *Eccentric contractions* take place when the muscle increases in length as it resists the load (for example, returning the bicep curl to the original position-down phase). The muscles that lengthen serve as the antagonists (for example, triceps).

Concentric repetitions in weight training cause muscles to shorten in length. Over time, your muscles can shorten, restricting their range of motion. This can result in a decrease in the amount of force you can generate in the muscle. Stretching of those muscles can counter the effects of concentric repetitions so that your elongated muscle can generate more force. Stretching will result in greater elasticity in your joints and connective tissue, facilitating your ability to work through a full range of motion.

STRETCHING TECHNIQUES

There are four stretching techniques: dynamic stretching, ballistic stretching, static stretching, and proprioceptive neuromuscular facilitation.

dynamic stretching
a stretching technique that involves performing movements within the full range of motion of the joint—it gradually increases reach and range of motion while the limbs are moving

ballistic stretching
a stretching technique that promotes the stretch reflex but increases the risk of injury to muscles and tendons—it requires quick, well-coordinated action–reaction movements that stretch the muscles beyond their normal range of motion

Dynamic Stretching

Dynamic stretching involves performing movements within the full range of motion of the joint. It gradually increases reach and range of motion while the limbs are moving. Kicking an imaginary soccer ball is a dynamic stretch for the hamstrings and groin muscles. Twisting side to side is a dynamic stretch for the trunk.

Ballistic Stretching

Ballistic stretching promotes the stretch reflex but increases the risk of injury to muscles and tendons. It usually involves quick, well-coordinated action–reaction movements that stretch the muscles beyond their normal range of motion. It also may involve bouncing movements during a stretch. For this reason it is not recommended, and many textbooks avoid discussing it (Ethyre & Lee, 1987). An example in law enforcement would be when you are throwing a punch and the elbow joint goes beyond the normal range of motion.

Static Stretching

Static stretching is an effective technique for improving flexibility and has gained in popularity since the mid-1980s. It involves bringing a muscle to a controlled maximum or near-maximum stretch by contracting the opposing muscle and holding the stretch for 20–30 seconds (without pain). Each stretch is repeated two or three times. Because static stretching is performed slowly, the strong reflex action that characterizes ballistic stretching does not occur.

This means that the muscle can be stretched farther and is usually helped by gravity. Static stretching increases flexibility and presents little risk of injury. It also relieves muscle soreness and helps to prevent muscle imbalance, knots, and tightness.

static stretching
a stretching technique that involves bringing a muscle to a maximum or near-maximum stretch by contracting the opposing muscle and holding the stretch for 20–30 seconds (without pain)

Proprioceptive Neuromuscular Facilitation

Proprioceptive neuromuscular facilitation (PNF) involves contracting and relaxing the muscles before stretching. Usually, the exercises require the assistance of a partner. Originally used in physiotherapy, this type of stretching has gained acceptance in the general fitness community. The two common types of PNF are as follows:

- *Contract–relax (C–R) stretching* The muscle you want to stretch is contracted and then relaxed. The now-relaxed muscle is then slowly stretched. This technique requires equipment (a towel or skipping rope) or a partner's assistance.
- *Contract–relax–antagonist–contract (CRAC) stretching* You begin by contracting and then relaxing the muscle opposite to the one to be stretched. Next, you contract the muscle to be stretched. The final action is the stretch itself. Contracting the opposite muscle promotes a reflex relaxation of the muscle to be stretched. This technique requires the assistance of a well-trained partner.

proprioceptive neuromuscular facilitation (PNF)
a stretching technique that involves contracting and relaxing the muscles before stretching

PNF is believed to be the most effective method of enhancing active flexibility, which is the active contraction and relaxation of the muscles that are being stretched (Alter, 1990, p. 10). By relaxing the muscle, PNF allows the muscle to be stretched farther. But PNF presents a higher risk of injury than static stretching, and can increase blood pressure to dangerous levels (Alter, 1990). It also has the disadvantage of often requiring a partner's assistance to avoid injury from overstretching.

GUIDELINES FOR SAFE AND EFFECTIVE STRETCHING

It is important that your warm-up begin not with stretching but with large-muscle activities such as walking or jogging, which facilitate safe stretching by increasing muscle temperature. A pre-exercise warm-up should consist of at least 5–15 minutes of light aerobic exercise followed by stretching exercises for all the major muscle groups. Performing stretching exercises at the end of your workout will increase your flexibility. Whether it's a resistance training workout or a cardiovascular workout, your body temperature will be raised, making stretching that much easier.

The FITT formula introduced in chapter 5 provides a template for you to devise a stretching routine that meets your needs:

- *Frequency* Stretch at least three times a week.
- *Intensity* Stretch to your limit, but avoid painful stretching, holding for 20–30 seconds, and repeating the stretch 2–4 times.
- *Time* Stretch at least 8–10 minutes as part of your warm-up and cool-down (some athletes stretch for as long as an hour).
- *Type* Static stretching and possibly PNF are good choices. Choose your exercises from the list you will prepare for **assignment 7.1** (in the appendix).

Here are some points to remember:

- Complete a range of stretching exercises for all the different muscle groups. Pay attention to the muscle groups that are involved most in any sport you participate in.
- Proceed slowly and avoid ballistic stretching by not bouncing.
- Breathe out as you stretch and continue to breathe as you hold the stretch.
- Use the proper movements for each exercise.
- Stretch individual muscle groups one at a time.
- Don't strain to compete with the person next to you.
- When working with a partner, ensure that he or she knows your limits.
- Stop the stretch if you begin to feel pain.

UPPER- AND LOWER-BODY STRETCHING EXERCISES

The following pages describe a stretching program that you may want to incorporate into your workout. Hold each stretch for at least 20–30 seconds.

Head Turn and Tilt

Turn your head to the left, looking over your shoulder, and hold the stretch. Repeat on the right side. Then tilt your head to the left, attempting to bring your ear toward your shoulder (do not raise your shoulder). Repeat on the right side. These exercises stretch the neck muscles.

Shoulder Stretch

Interlock your fingers and reach above your head. Your lower back should be flat or arched slightly inward.

Biceps Stretch

From a standing position, extend your right arm forward with your palm facing up. Place your left palm underneath your right elbow. Slowly straighten your right arm as much as comfortably possible, pressing your elbow down into your left hand. Hold this position for the desired amount of time and repeat this process on the left.

FIGURE 7.1 **Head Turn and Tilt**

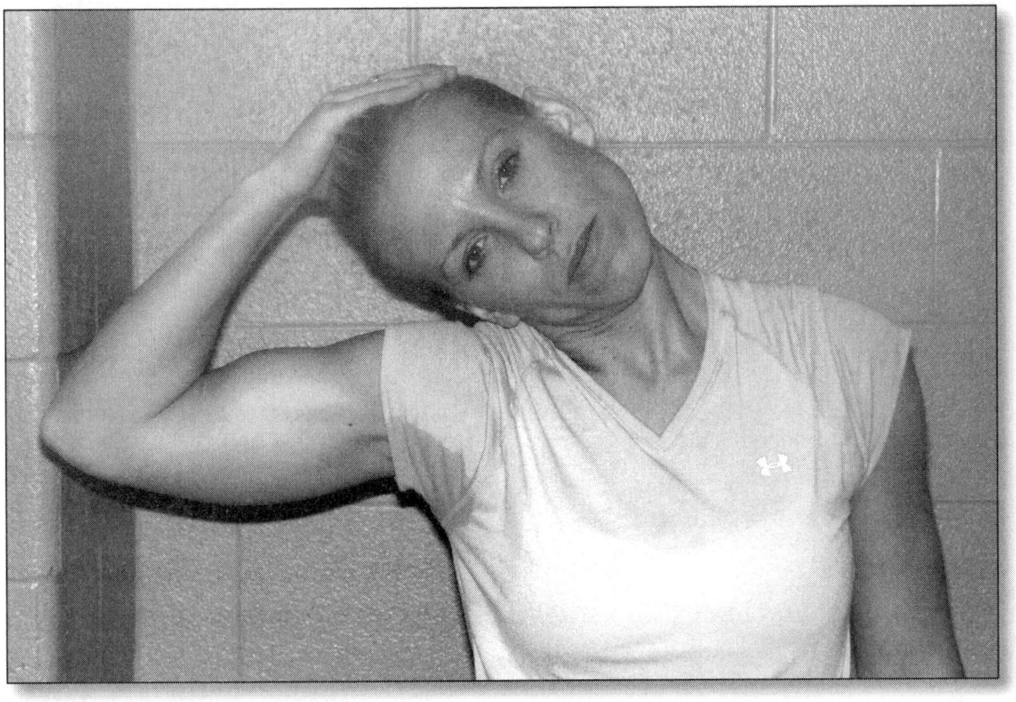

FIGURE 7.2 **Shoulder Stretch**

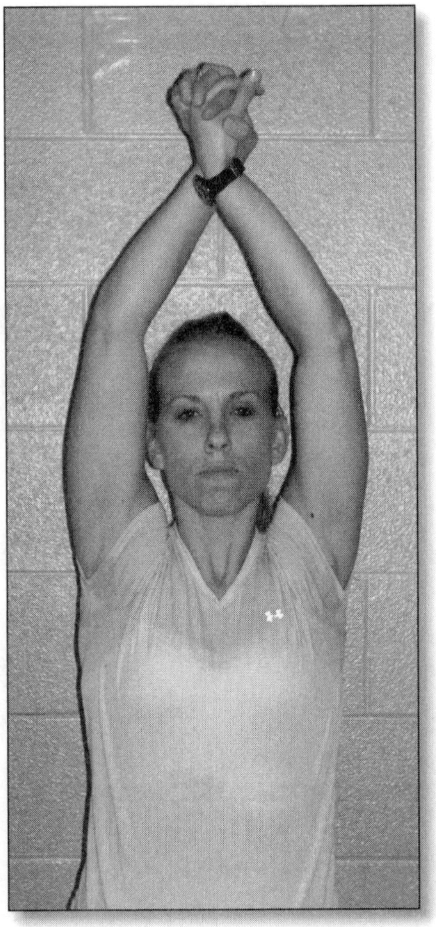

FIGURE 7.3 **Biceps Stretch**

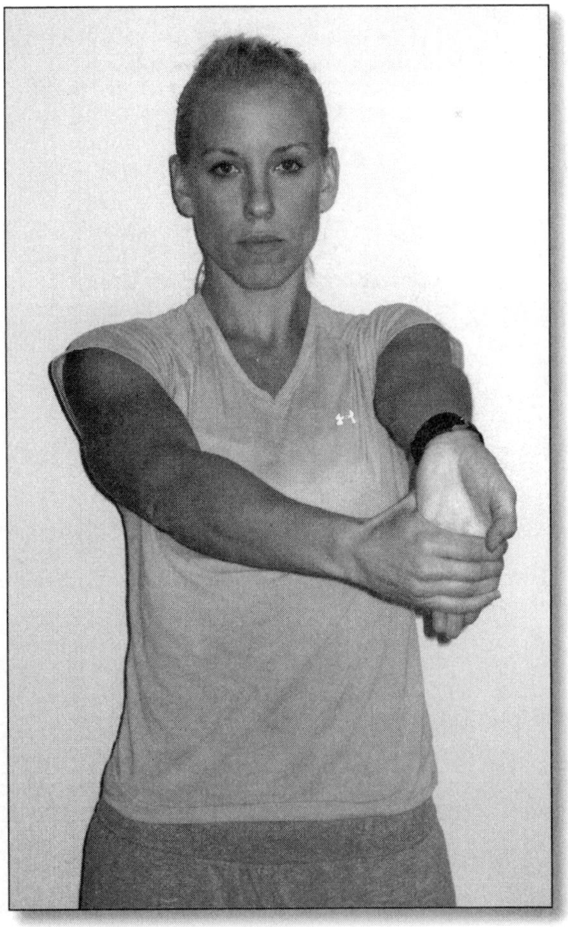

FIGURE 7.4 Triceps Stretch

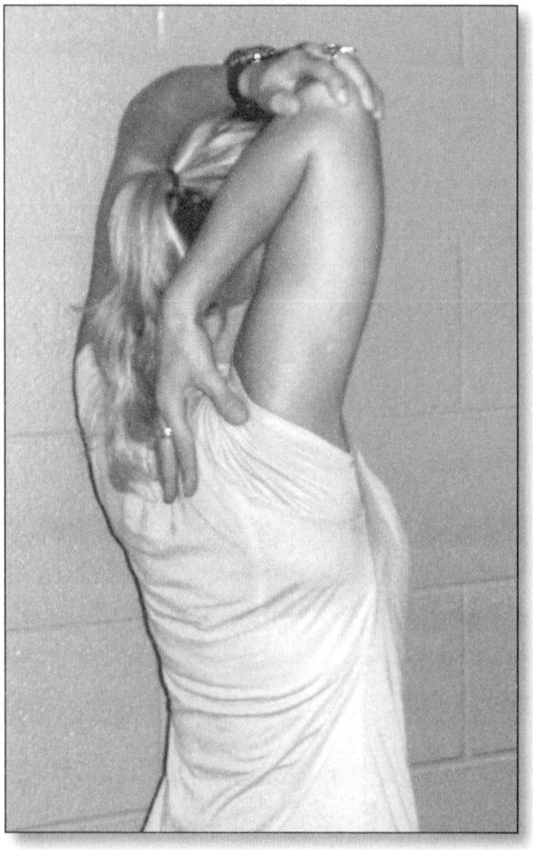

Triceps Stretch

Place your right hand behind your head and reach down your back as far as possible. With your left hand, grasp your right elbow and gently pull it behind the back of your head. Repeat with the other arm.

Front of Shoulder and Chest Stretch

In a standing position with your right foot nearest the wall and one step away from the wall, place your right hand on the wall, keeping your arm at shoulder level. Slowly turn your head toward the centre of the room until you feel mild tension in the shoulder and chest area. Hold the stretch. Relax and switch arms.

Chest Stretch

While clasping your hands behind your back, gently straighten your elbows and raise your arms as high as comfortably possible. Keep your back straight and stand in an upright position. Relax and repeat.

FIGURE 7.5 Front of Shoulder and Chest Stretch

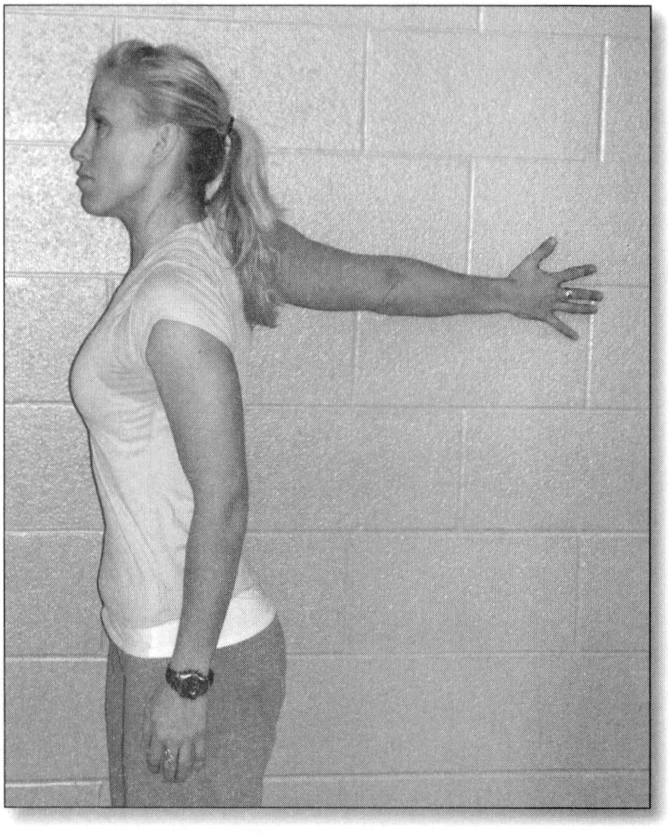

FIGURE 7.6 Chest Stretch

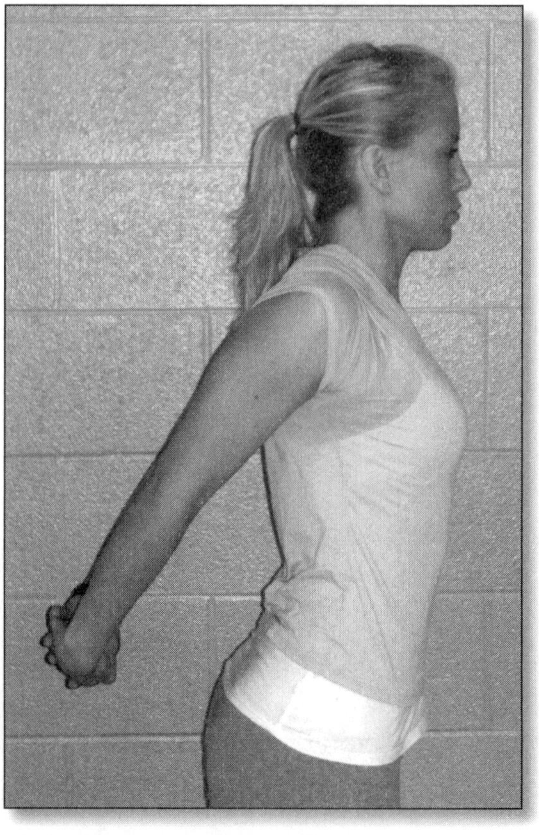

Arm Across Body Stretch

Raise your right arm in front of you to shoulder height. Reach across your body with this arm. With your left hand, come from below the right arm and grasp the right elbow. As you bring the right arm across your body with your left hand, keep the right arm parallel to the ground. Relax and switch arms.

Trunk Stretch

While standing in an upright position, bring your elbows up to shoulder height. Bend your knees slightly. Slowly twist your upper body to the right until you can look over your right shoulder. Hold this position, and then return to the original position and repeat to the left side.

Side Stretch

With feet shoulder-width apart, knees slightly bent, and your trunk in line with your legs, stretch to your left side. Extend your left arm downward to your left leg while reaching your right arm upward and outward to the left side of your body. Repeat with the other side.

FIGURE 7.9 **Side Stretch**

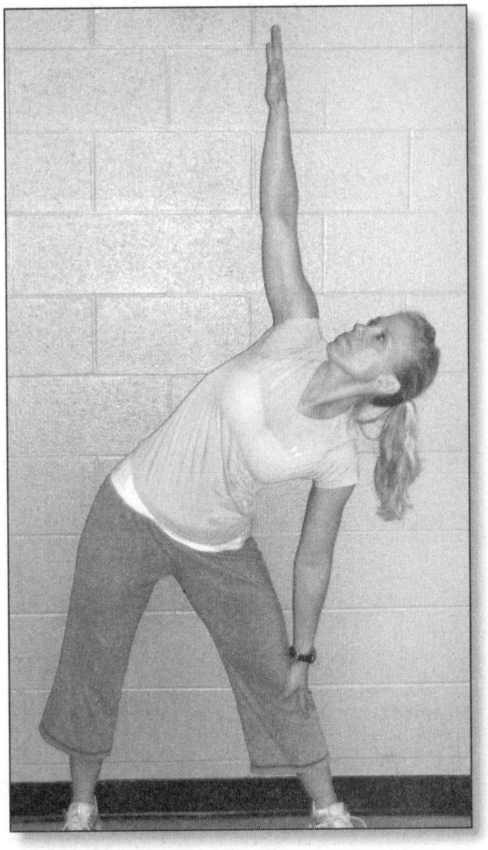

FIGURE 7.7 **Arm Across Body Stretch**

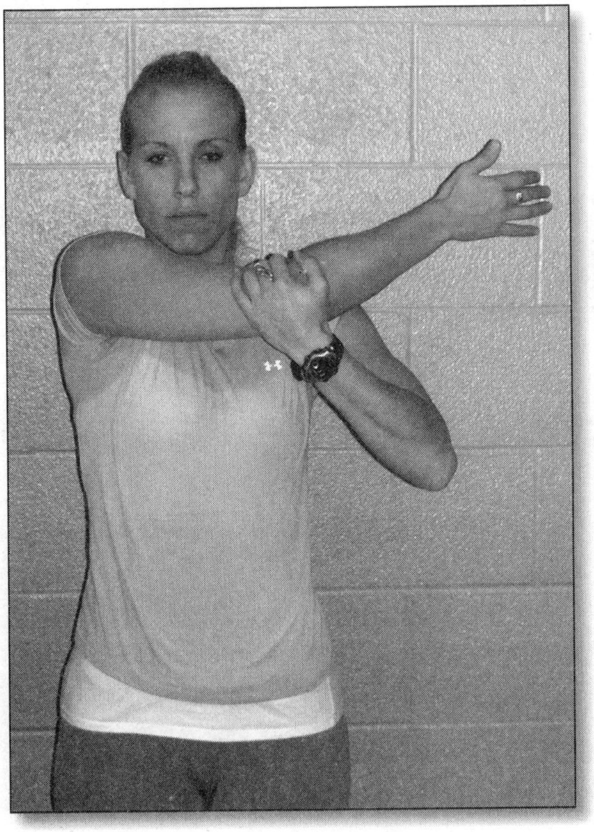

FIGURE 7.8 **Trunk Stretch**

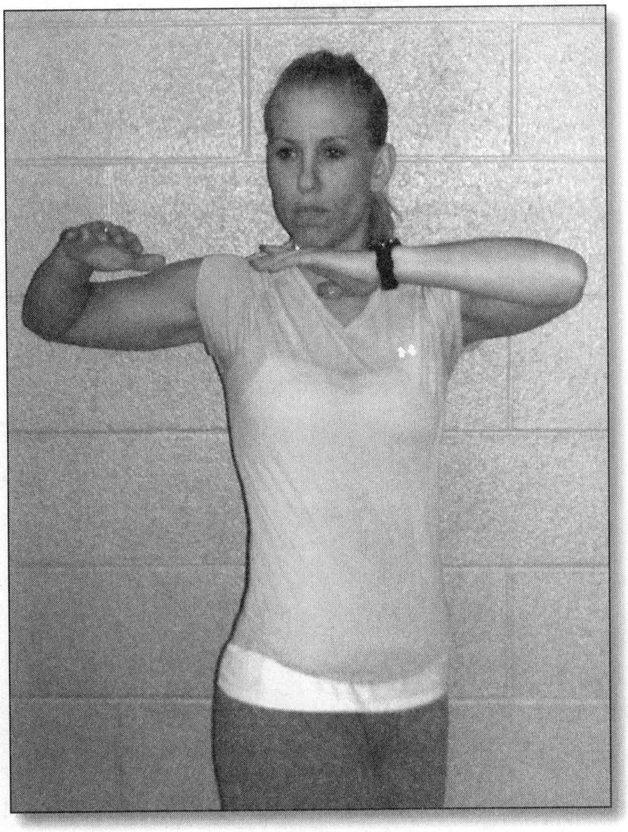

FIGURE 7.10 Hamstring Stretch

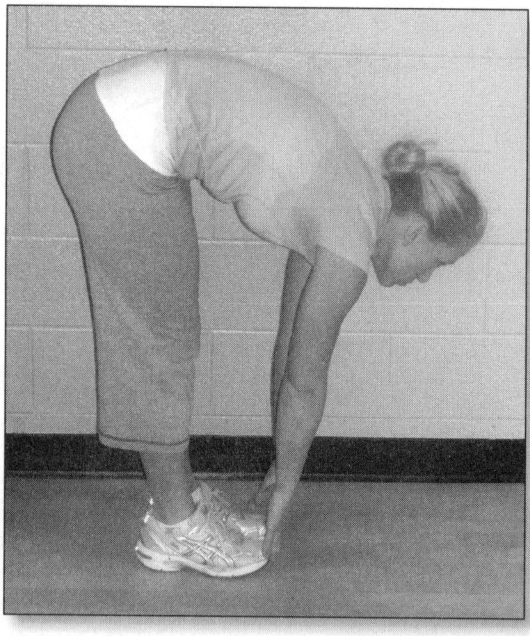

Hamstring Stretch

From a standing position, straighten your legs and slowly bend forward at the waist. Allow your hands to travel downwards along the line of your body as far as comfortably possible. At the point where you feel an intense stretch in your hamstrings, grab on to your legs and hold this position for the desired amount of time.

Back Extension Stretch—Rectus Abdominus Stretch

Lie face down with your forearms on the floor, elbows by your chest, and hands underneath your chin. Slowly raise your upper body by straightening your arms until you reach a 90° angle with the elbows. Your forearms should stay on the floor. Do not go beyond this point. Relax and repeat.

FIGURE 7.11 Back Extension Stretch—Rectus Abdominus Stretch

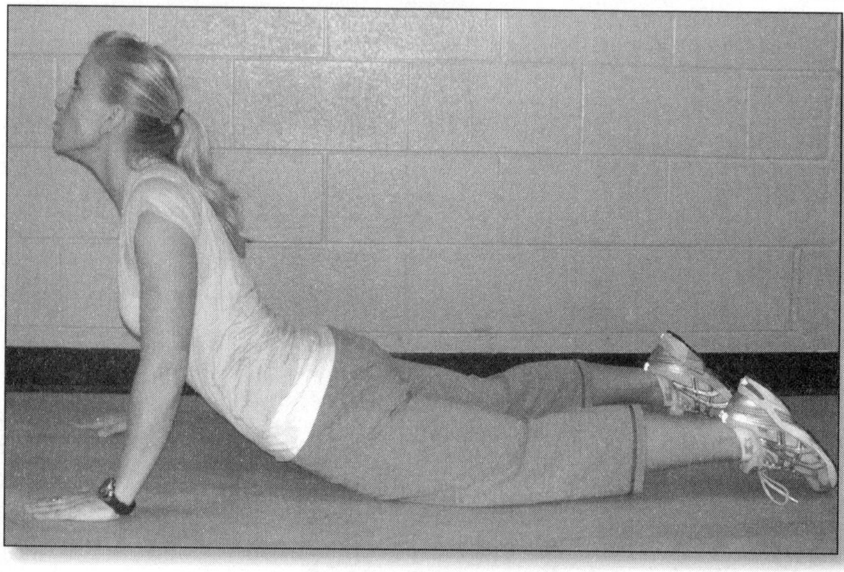

Lower-Back Stretch

Lying flat on your back, place the sole of your left foot on your right thigh. Grasp your left knee with your right hand and gently roll the knee to the right. Without your left shoulder leaving the floor, try to get the knee as close to the floor as possible. Repeat with the other side.

FIGURE 7.12 Lower-Back Stretch

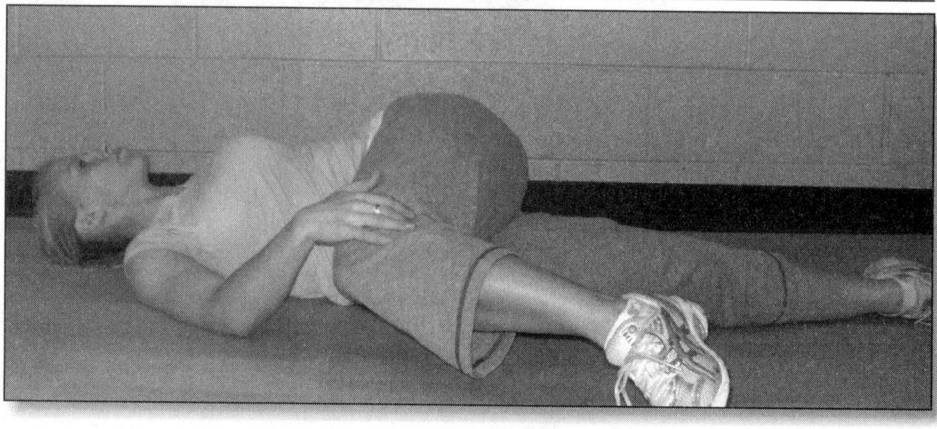

Modified Hurdle Stretch

Sit on the floor with your right leg straight out in front of you, toes pointing upward. Place your left foot against your right knee. Gradually reach forward with your upper body as far as possible. Flex from the hips. Hold, and then repeat with the left leg.

Leg Spinal Twist

Sit on the floor. Bend your left knee and place your left foot on the outside of your right knee. Keeping your right leg straight, place your right elbow on your left knee and gently rotate your trunk to the left. Look over your left shoulder. Repeat on the other side.

Groin and Inner Thigh Stretch

Stand with your feet about 2 m apart, toes pointing forward. Gradually shift all of your weight to your right leg by bending your right knee to a maximum of 90° (at a right angle to the floor). Keep your left leg straight. Place both your hands on your right knee for support. You can increase the stretch by increasing the distance between your feet. Repeat on the other side.

FIGURE 7.15 Groin and Inner Thigh Stretch

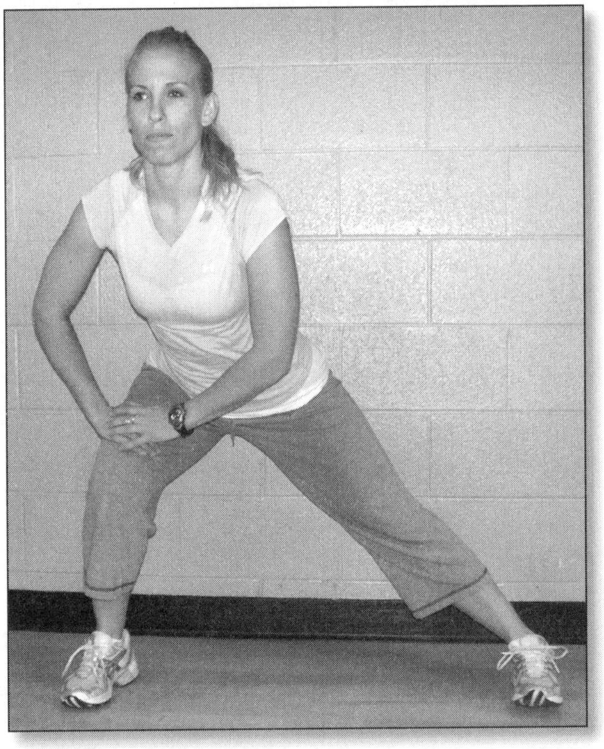

FIGURE 7.14 Leg Spinal Twist

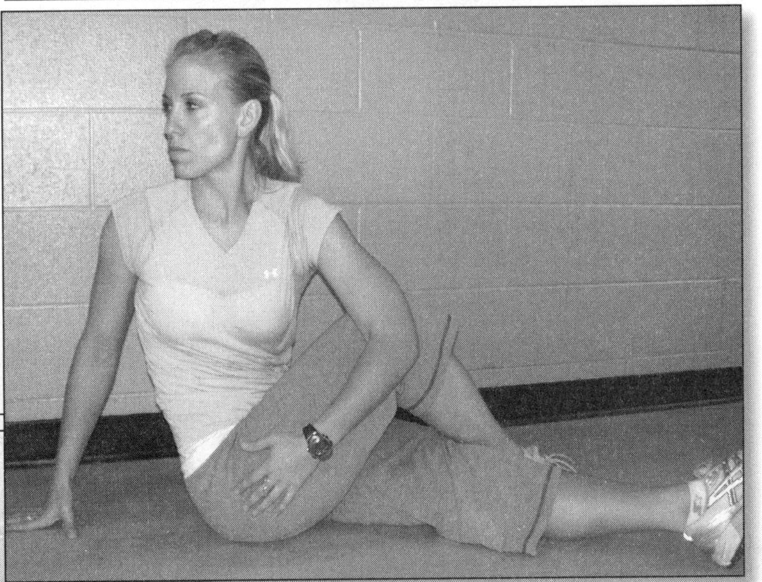

FIGURE 7.13 Modified Hurdle Stretch

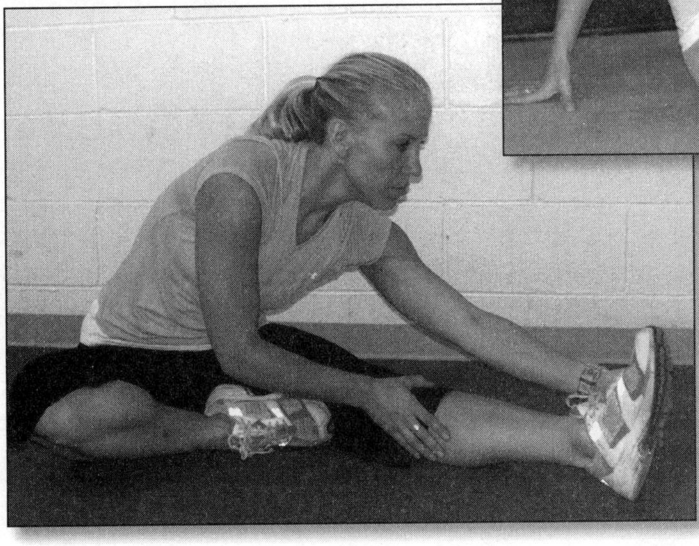

FIGURE 7.16 Groin Stretch 2 —Butterfly Adductor Stretch

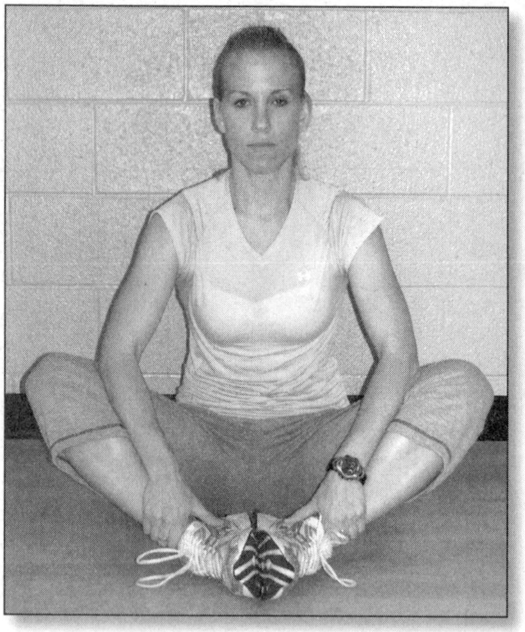

Groin Stretch 2—Butterfly Adductor Stretch

Sit down and place the soles of your feet together. Clasp your ankles with your hands so that your elbows rest on your knees. Gently push your knees down with your elbows until you feel the stretch. To stretch the lower back further, you can lower your head toward your feet. Relax and repeat.

Quadriceps Stretch

Standing in an upright position, hold on to a support with one hand (a sturdy chair, a wall, or the shoulder of a partner) for balance. With your other hand, clasp your ankle and pull your heel to your buttocks while keeping your knees together. To extend the stretch, place the bent knee behind the extended knee. Repeat with the other leg.

FIGURE 7.17 Quadriceps Stretch

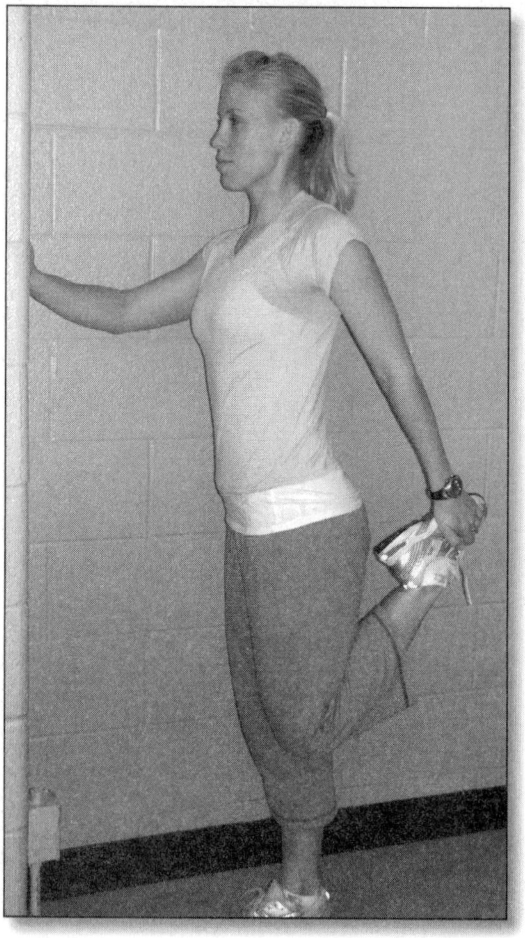

Forward Lunge

Standing, take a long step forward with your right leg and flex your right knee directly over your right foot, keeping the right foot flat on the ground. As you move forward, keep your torso in an upright position. Place your hands on your right thigh and slowly lower the hips forward and downward. Repeat with the other leg.

FIGURE 7.18 Forward Lunge

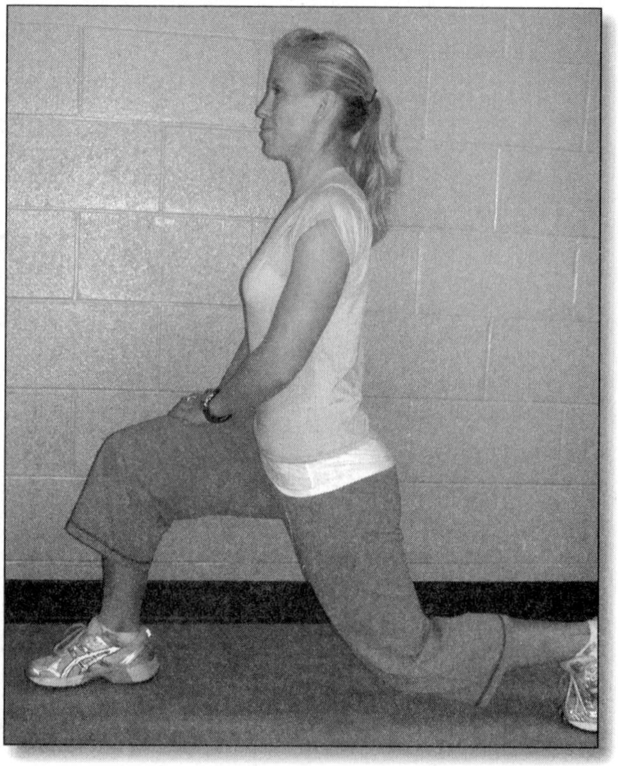

Calf and Hamstring Stretch

From a standing position, extend your right foot out to the side with your toes pointing up. Bend the left knee. Slowly reach your right arm down toward your toes and pull up on the toes to feel the stretch in the back of the thigh and calf. Repeat with the other side.

Calf Stretch

Stand an arm's length away from a wall and with your feet shoulder-width apart. Place your right foot about 0.5 m in front of your left. Keeping both heels flat on the ground, lean toward the wall by bending your right knee. Place your elbows on the wall. Your left leg should stay straight. Repeat with the left leg.

Achilles Stretch

Stand an arm's length away from a wall and with your feet shoulder-width apart. Place your elbows on the wall. Place your right foot on the back of your left knee. Keeping your left heel on the ground, bend your left knee (rather than leaning forward, you should feel like you are lowering yourself straight down). Repeat with the other leg.

FIGURE 7.19 **Calf and Hamstring Stretch**

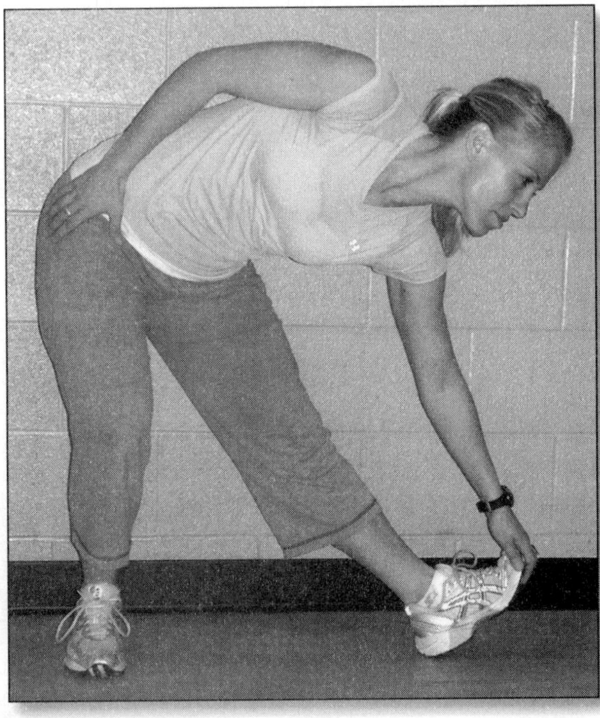

FIGURE 7.21 **Achilles Stretch**

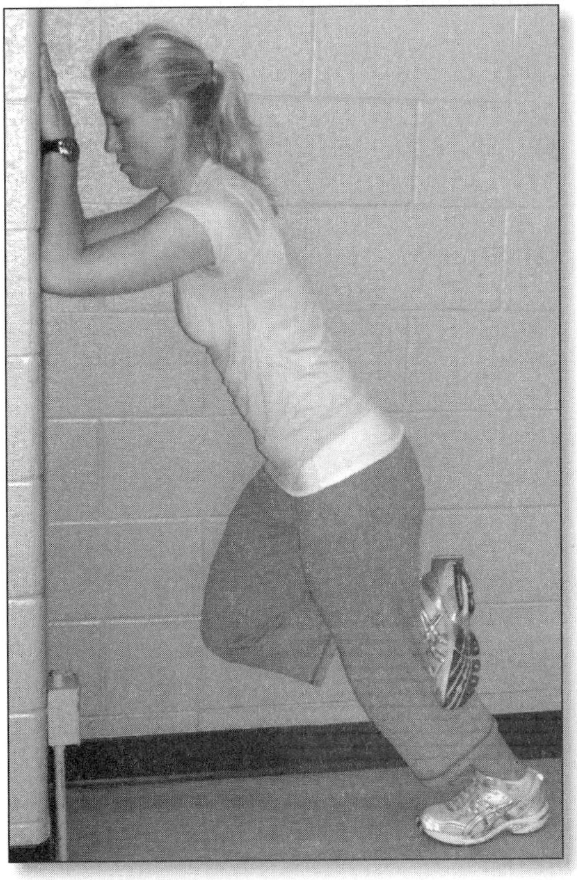

FIGURE 7.20 **Calf Stretch**

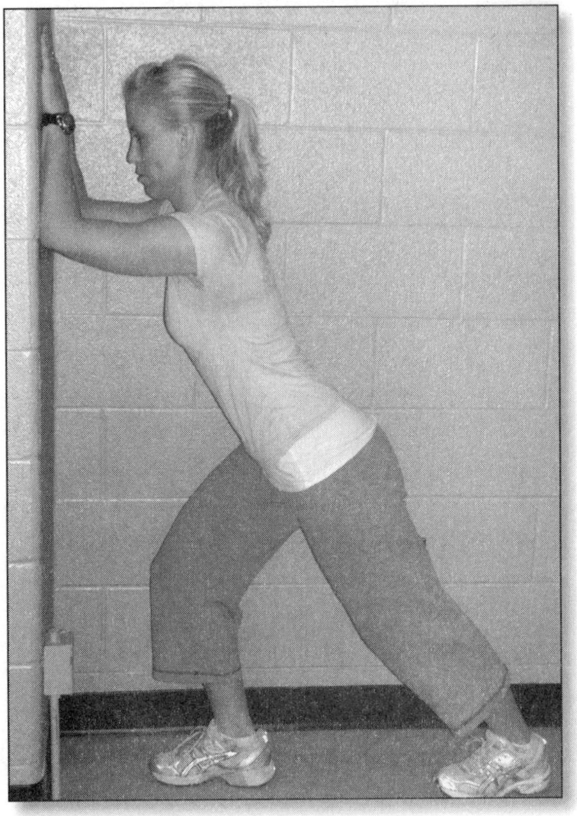

Turn to **assignment 7.1** (in the appendix) to design a stretching program.

KEY TERMS

flexibility

dynamic stretching

ballistic stretching

static stretching

proprioceptive neuromuscular facilitation (PNF)

EXERCISES

Review

1. What are some of the benefits of stretching?

2. What is static stretching? Explain its advantages.

3. What is PNF? How does it work? What are its advantages and disadvantages?

4. How often and for what length of time should stretching exercises be performed?

5. Why is flexibility so important for those in law enforcement?

Multiple Choice and True or False

1. Which of the following is a correct guideline for increasing flexibility?
   a. stretch to the point of pain and hold
   b. bounce while stretching
   c. stretch until you hear a pop
   d. warm up before beginning to stretch
   e. it's not necessary to stretch before a workout

2. Stretching for flexibility is most effective during which of the following?
   a. the warm-up
   b. the workout
   c. endurance training
   d. the cool-down
   e. doesn't really matter when

3. Dynamic stretching involves
   a. quickly moving a limb to its limits
   b. the full range of motion achieved in a slow, controlled stretch
   c. a natural response that causes a stretched muscle to contract
   d. a stretch–contract–stretch partner-assisted flexibility program
   e. alternating between a slow, controlled stretch and then a few quick stretches

4. Proprioceptive neuromuscular facilitation (PNF) involves
   a. quickly moving a limb to its limits
   b. the full range of motion achieved in a slow, controlled stretch
   c. a natural response that causes a stretched muscle to contract
   d. a stretch–contract–stretch partner-assisted flexibility program
   e. alternating between a slow, controlled stretch and then a few quick stretches

5. You should hold a stretch to the point of ____________________.
   a. pain
   b. tension
   c. locking the joint in place
   d. bouncing the joint in place
   e. full exhalation

6. Three types of stretching include static, dynamic, and ____________________.
   a. warm-up
   b. partner-assisted PNF
   c. concentric
   d. eccentric
   e. overstretching

7. The ability to move a joint or group of joints freely through their full range of motion is called
   a. ballistics
   b. flexibility
   c. stretching
   d. elasticity
   e. dynamic

8. It is best to hold a static stretch for ____________________ seconds.
   a. 10 seconds
   b. 10–20 seconds
   c. 20–30 seconds
   d. 20–60 seconds
   e. 10–30 seconds

9. Which of the following involves quick, coordinated movements that stretch the muscles while you are moving and incorporates the stretch reflex?
   a. PNF stretching
   b. ballistic stretching
   c. static stretching
   d. concentric stretching
   e. eccentric stretching

10. Which is the best advice for stretching?
   a. stretch before you warm up
   b. increase and decrease the intensity slowly during static stretching
   c. stretch until it is painful and hold it until the pain subsides
   d. start with ballistic stretches and progress to static stretches
   e. stretch only those areas that feel tight

11. The stretching technique that lengthens a muscle to an elongated position and holds that stretch for 20 to 30 seconds is known as
   a. ballistic stretching
   b. proprioceptive neuromuscular facilitation
   c. interval stretching
   d. static stretching
   e. resistance stretching

12. Ballistic stretching techniques involve the slow, gradual stretching of a muscle and its tendons.
   a. True   b. False

13. A concentric muscle action is one in which force is produced while the muscle shortens.
   a. True   b. False

14. Proprioceptive neuromuscular facilitation (PNF) involves contracting and relaxing the muscles before stretching.
   a. True   b. False

REFERENCES

Alter, M.J. (1990). *Sport stretch.* Champaign, IL: Human Kinetics.

Carragee, E.J. (2005). Persistent low back pain. *New England Journal of Medicine, 352*(18), 1891-1898.

Ethyre, B.R., & Lee, E.J. (1987). Comments on proprioceptive neuromuscular facilitation stretching techniques. *Research Quarterly for Exercise and Sport, 58,* 184-188.

Herbert, R.D., & Gabriel, M. (2002). Effects of stretching before and after exercise on muscle soreness and risk of injury: Systematic review. *British Medical Journal, 325,* 468-470.

Plowman, S.A., & Smith, D.L. (1997). *Exercise physiology for health, fitness, and performance.* Needham Heights, MA: Allyn and Bacon.

Shrier, I. (2000). Stretching before exercise: An evidence based approach. *British Journal of Sports Medicine, 34,* 324-325.

Shrier, I. (2004). Does stretching improve performance? A systematic and critical review of the literature. *Clinical Journal of Sports Medicine, 14*(5), 267-273.

PART III

Nutrition and Body Composition

CHAPTER 8

Nutrition

CHAPTER OBJECTIVES

After completing this chapter, you should be able to:

- Describe nutritional trends in Canada.
- Understand the importance of maintaining a healthy weight.
- Determine which nutrition information is valid and reliable.
- Understand portion sizes and labelling.
- Identify the six basic nutrients.
- Describe the role of water, vitamins, minerals, carbohydrates, fibre, fats, and proteins in nutrition.
- Make better food choices using *Canada's Food Guide.*
- Describe the impact of fibre, cholesterol, sodium, and caffeine on the human body.

Although Canadians are becoming increasingly aware of nutrition and the impact it has on us, approximately 5.5 million or 23 percent of Canadian adults are obese (Tjepkema, 2004). More shocking is the fact that over a quarter—26 percent—of 2- to 17-year-olds are either overweight or obese (Shields, 2004). These young people spend their time doing sedentary activities (watching TV, playing video games, using a computer) and eat vegetables and fruit infrequently.

Police officers are no exception to these statistics. After passing probation, there are few requirements for police officers to maintain a certain standard of fitness. The few exceptions are the optional Ontario Police Fitness Award (OPFA) fitness standards (given out on a yearly basis), used by some services for promotion, and the fitness requirements to enter and maintain status in specialized units (see chapter 16). There are a number of police services that will not promote cadets to constables or fourth-class constables to third-class constables if they have not met 75 percent on the OPFA standards.

It is well documented that shift work affects an officer's dietary and exercise habits. The general nutrition of police officers is poor. There is a tendency to consume high-fat fast-food meals when it is the only food available, and it's generally eaten between high-stress police calls. During shifts, officers may not eat at all, and if they do, it is through a take-out window, usually eaten quickly between calls. The diets of most officers are lacking in the nutrients found in fruits and vegetables. Compounded with the lack of meaningful exercise, some are at risk for high cholesterol, elevated triglycerides, and overall body fat, putting them at risk for heart disease and diabetes (refer to chapters 10 and 11 for more detail). This chapter will address the general concerns around nutrition, the new version of *Canada's Food Guide*, and different dietary needs.

NUTRITIONAL CONCERNS IN CANADA

It is well known that maintaining a healthy weight is good for overall health. It is a key component in preventing and controlling many diseases and conditions. However, what we know and what we practise are not always the same thing. A survey regarding Canadians' eating habits (Garriguet, 2004) found the following:

- Although a minimum of five daily servings of vegetables and fruit are recommended, 7 out of 10 children aged 4 to 8 and half of adults do not meet this minimum.
- More than a third (37 percent) of children aged 4 to 9 do not get the recommended two daily servings of milk products. By age 30, more than two-thirds of Canadians do not attain the minimum daily levels.
- According to the Institute of Medicine (2005), a US-based independent, non-governmental organization, over a quarter of Canadians aged 31 to 50 get more than 35 percent of their total calories from fat, the threshold beyond which health risks increase.
- Snacks—food and drink consumed between meals—account for more calories than breakfast, and about the same number of calories as lunch. This is a big issue for students who crawl out of bed and run to get to their first class.
- Adults in low- and lower-middle-income households are less likely than those in the highest-income households to get more than 35 percent of their daily calories from fat.
- Members of the highest income households are more likely than lower income groups to eat food prepared in a fast-food outlet.
- Each day, a quarter of Canadians, adults and children alike, eat something that was prepared in a fast-food outlet.

MAINTAINING A HEALTHY WEIGHT

A person's weight is the result of many factors, including height, genes, metabolism, behaviour, and environment. It is important that you learn how to balance your energy in (calorie intake) with your energy out (exercise). For many people, maintaining this balance means consuming fewer calories and exercising more. In addition to making healthy food choices that are lower in fats (especially saturated and trans fatty acids), cholesterol, added sugars, and salt, Canadians need to pay attention to portion sizes.

We know that those who are overweight or obese are at risk of developing the following diseases (Health Canada, 2003):

- high blood pressure (see chapter 11)
- high blood cholesterol (see chapter 11)
- type 2 diabetes (see chapter 10)
- coronary heart disease and stroke (see chapter 11)
- gallbladder disease
- arthritis
- sleep apnea and breathing problems
- some cancers, including endometrial, breast, prostrate, and colon cancer

If you are overweight or obese, simply losing as little as 10 percent of your current weight can lower your risks for the diseases listed above. It is reasonable and safe to lose one-half to one kilogram per week. Losing more per week puts you at risk for gaining the weight back. Along with making healthier eating choices, you have to make a commitment to increase your physical activity level. This involves a change in behaviour that will eventually become routine (refer to chapter 2 for a discussion on behavioural changes). Although weight-loss medication and weight-loss surgery may be options for a small percentage of the population, for most people, changing eating habits and becoming active are the keys to weight loss.

FUNCTION OF FOOD

Food provides nutrients that have a physiological and/or biochemical function in the body. There are six basic nutrients: water, vitamins, minerals, carbohydrates, fats, and proteins. Their functions are as follows:

- *To promote growth and development of muscle, soft tissues, and organs.* Protein does most of the work for growth and repair with the assistance of calcium and phosphorus in the skeletal building blocks.
- *To provide energy to the body.* Carbohydrates and fats contribute predominately, although protein will assist as a fuel source if needed.
- *To regulate metabolism.* Your body's enzymes are proteins that work with vitamins and minerals to regulate your metabolism.

BASIC NUTRIENTS

Our bodies require six kinds of nutrients to function efficiently: water (the most important), vitamins, minerals, carbohydrates, fats, and proteins. In total, these substances provide 45 essential nutrients, which our bodies assimilate through digestion. Failing to consume the appropriate nutrients in the appropriate quantities inevitably leads to ill health.

Water

Water is the transportation vehicle in the body. Our bodies are about 60 percent water. Water cools and purifies the body's tissues, participates in biochemical reactions, aids in digestion and absorption, and helps to regulate body temperature. Water helps in getting rid of waste through urine, and drinking a lot of water correlates with a lower risk of developing kidney stones and colon and bladder cancer. Water acts like a lubricant and a cushion for the joints. It protects sensitive tissue like the spine and is the fluid in the eye.

A person should drink at least eight glasses (about 2 L) of water a day. Those who are exercising, on a weight-loss program, or ill need more water. It is important to recognize the early symptoms of dehydration; a loss of just 5 percent of body fluid may result in fatigue, weakness, lethargy, dizziness, headaches, and elevated heart rate. Make sure that you drink at least 500 mL of water before any physical activity that lasts an hour or more, and make sure you consume more fluids afterward, including those that restore electrolyte balance. Electrolytes assist in heart and nerve functions, muscle control, coordination, and the body's ability to absorb fluid. The most common electrolytes are sodium, potassium, magnesium, chloride, and calcium. Sports drinks and juices are examples of these.

Vitamins

A vitamin can be defined as an essential, non-caloric, organic nutrient needed in small amounts in the diet. Vitamins act as facilitators for the other nutrients, helping in digestion, absorption, metabolism, and the building of structures in the body. Vitamins fall into two categories—fat soluble and water soluble. Fat-soluble vitamins (A, D, E, and K) are found in the fats and oils of food and are generally absorbed into the lymph system with the help of bile. They travel in the blood in association with protein carriers. Fat-soluble vitamins are stored in the liver or fatty tissue and can build up to toxic concentrations. Water-soluble vitamins are absorbed directly into the bloodstream and, instead of being stored to any great extent, are excreted in the urine. Water-soluble vitamins (B vitamins and vitamin C) can be easily leached out of food by cooking and washing with water. Although foods do not supply toxic levels of water-soluble vitamins, supplements may reach toxic levels.

Vitamins are important in many ways. For example, B vitamins, found in legumes, oats, beans, and leafy green vegetables, help convert food to energy and promote healthy skin, hair, muscles, and brain function. However, vitamin B_{12} is only found in animal sources (such as salmon, clams, and sardines) or fortified products so a strict vegetarian needs to be aware of deficiencies in B_{12}, which are linked to heart disease and stroke. Vitamin C, found in foods such as citrus fruits, tomatoes, leafy green vegetables, and sweet peppers, helps the body form collagen, a protein that is the primary component of the body's white fibrous connective tissue. Vitamin C also contributes to the formation of teeth, bones, cartilage, skin, and capillaries (narrow blood vessels), and strengthens the immune system. Table 8.1 summarizes key information about vitamins.

TABLE 8.1 Major Vitamins

	Vitamin	Major functions	Food sources	Deficiency signs and symptoms	Toxicity signs and symptoms
Fat-soluble	A	Vision, antioxidant, growth, reproduction, immune system	Fortified dairy products, liver, eggs, dark green leafy vegetables, yellow vegetables	Poor vision in dim light, blindness, anemia, diarrhea, poor growth, frequent infections	Blurred vision, growth retardation, abdominal cramping, pain in calves
	D	Bone and tooth development and growth	Fortified milk, eggs, liver, exposure to sun	Rickets (deformed bones)	Mental and physical retardation, excessive thirst, kidney stones
	E	Antioxidant, protects cell membranes	Vegetable oils, whole grains, green and leafy vegetables	Anemia, leg cramps, muscle degeneration	Discomfort, mimics the effects of anti-clotting medication
	K	Synthesis of blood-clotting proteins, assists in regulating blood calcium	Leafy green vegetables, liver, milk, cabbage-type vegetables	Hemorrhage	Jaundice, interference with anti-clotting medication
	Water-soluble vitamin B_6	Coenzyme for fat and protein metabolism, helps make red blood cells	Protein-rich foods, green and leafy vegetables, whole grains	Anemia, skin rash, irritability, muscle twitching	Depression, fatigue, nerve damage, headaches
	B_{12}	Coenzyme in new cell synthesis, maintains nerve cells	Animal products (meat, milk, cheese, eggs)	Anemia, fatigue, nerve degeneration	Unknown
Water-soluble	Thiamine	Energy metabolism, normal appetite function	Pork, liver, nuts, dried beans and peas, whole-grain cereals	Beriberi (paralysis), edema, heart failure, confusion, depression	Unknown
	Riboflavin	Energy metabolism, supports normal vision and healthy skin	Milk, yogurt, leafy green vegetables, meats, whole-grain and enriched breads and cereals	Enlarged purple tongue, hypersensitivity to light, skin rash	Unknown
	Folate	DNA production	Green leafy vegetables, oranges, nuts, liver	Anemia, depression, spina bifida in developing embryo	Unknown
	C	Antioxidant, scar tissue formation, bone growth, strengthens immune system, aids in iron absorption	Citrus fruit, dark green vegetables, cabbage-type vegetables, strawberries, cantaloupe, tomatoes	Anemia, frequent infections, bleeding gums, failure of wounds to heal	Nausea, abdominal cramps, diarrhea, gout symptoms; deficiency symptoms may appear at first with withdrawal of high doses

Source: Adapted from Sizer, F., & Whitney, E. (1997). *Nutrition: Concepts and controversies* (7th ed.), annotated instructor's edition. Belmont, CA: Wadsworth. Reprinted with permission of Brooks/Cole, a division of Thomson Learning: www.thomsonrights.com. Fax 800 730-2215.

Minerals

Minerals, which are found in all of the body's tissues and fluids, play a role in nerve function, muscle contraction, and metabolism. They are responsible for fluid and electrolyte imbalance (increased sodium concentration in response to water loss) and acid–base balance or pH (the kidneys control pH balance by excreting more or less acid). Minerals are the main components of bones and teeth. The major minerals include calcium, chloride, magnesium, phosphorus, potassium, sodium, and sulphur. Trace minerals include iodine, iron, zinc selenium, fluoride, chromium, copper, manganese, and molybdenum. We require very small amounts of minerals—an excess of any mineral can create imbalances with other minerals and be toxic.

For example, calcium (found in dairy products, kale, and soy) is the most abundant mineral in the human body. More than 99 percent of the body's calcium is stored in the teeth and bones, with the rest circulating in the blood, muscles, and interstitial fluids of the cells. In addition to promoting strong bones and teeth, calcium plays an important role in nerve transmission, muscle contraction, secretion of hormones, and the constriction and relaxation of blood vessels. Table 8.2 summarizes the key facts about minerals.

TABLE 8.2 Major Minerals

Minerals	Major functions	Food sources	Deficiency signs and symptoms	Toxicity signs and symptoms
Calcium	Builds and maintains bones and teeth, needed for muscle and nerve activity, regulates blood pressure and blood clotting	Milk products, fortified tofu and soy milk, salmon, broccoli, dried beans	Weak bone growth, rickets, stunted growth, muscle spasms, osteoporosis	Kidney stones, decreased zinc absorption
Sodium	Maintains acid–base balance inbody fluids, needed for muscle and nerve activity	Salt, cured foods, bread, milk, cheese	Muscle cramps, headaches, weakness, swelling	Hypertension, kidney disease, heart problems
Potassium	Necessary for nerve function, maintains fluid balance	Whole grains, fruits (bananas), vegetables	Muscular weakness, confusion	Heart failure, death
Magnesium	Regulates enzyme activity, necessary for nerve function	Green leafy vegetables, whole grains, nuts	Muscular weakness, convulsions, confusion	Unknown
Zinc	Component of several enzymes and the hormone insulin, maintains immune function, necessary for sexual maturation and reproduction	Meat, fish, poultry, whole grains, vegetables	Improper healing of wounds, poor growth, failure to mature sexually	Gastrointestinal problems, anemia, cardiovascular vessel diseases
Selenium	Component of an enzyme that functions as an antioxidant	Seafood, liver, vegetables and grains grown in selenium-rich soil	May protect against certain cancers and heart disease	Nerve damage
Iron	Component of hemoglobin, involved in the release of energy	Liver, red meats, and enriched breads and cereals	Anemia	Hemochromatosis—a rare iron metabolism disease

Source: Adapted from Sizer, F., & Whitney, E. (1997). *Nutrition: Concepts and controversies* (7th ed.), annotated instructor's edition. Belmont, CA: Wadsworth. Reprinted with permission of Brooks/Cole, a division of Thomson Learning: www.thomsonrights.com. Fax 800 730-2215.

Carbohydrates

Carbohydrates provide glucose (a sugar), which acts as fuel for the body. Excess glucose is stored as glycogen in the liver and muscles in small amounts and, when needed, is broken back down into glucose. Carbohydrates come primarily from plant foods—milk is the only animal source. The muscular energy needed for high-intensity exercise is obtained mostly from carbohydrates. Ingestion of carbohydrates will rapidly replenish carbohydrate stores, with the excess being converted into fat and stored in adipose tissue.

Blood glucose is the only fuel used by the cells of the central nervous system (CNS) and red and white blood cells. When glucose is depleted, ketone bodies produced by the liver can provide an alternative fuel. Ketones are acidic compounds derived from fat and certain amino acids. Normally rare in the blood, they help feed the brain when carbohydrates are not available. For the CNS to function optimally, blood glucose concentrations need to be above 4 mmol/L (millimoles per litre, the standard unit used to measure cholesterol in the blood). Normal levels are between 4 and 8 mmol/L. Below 3 mmol/L, hypoglycemia (low blood sugar) can produce symptoms of weakness, hunger, dizziness, and shivering; left too long, it may lead to unconsciousness and irreversible brain damage. Above 11 mmol/L is considered hyperglycemia. Symptoms include thirst, frequent urination, and fatigue (Canadian Diabetes Association, 2005). For more information on blood glucose, refer to chapter 10.

There are three types of carbohydrates: simple carbohydrates (sugars), complex carbohydrates (starches), and dietary fibre. Simple carbohydrates provide only quick spurts of energy. These sugars are linked to obesity, cardiovascular diseases, and reduced insulin sensitivity. Many of our processed foods contain simple sugars. Complex carbohydrates are the foundations of healthy eating. Consuming whole-grain products every day, for example, reduces the risk of heart disease and cancer (Johnson, 1999). Dietary fibre is indigestible material that aids in lowering blood cholesterol and facilitates digestion and elimination. It is discussed in more detail later in this chapter.

UNDERSTANDING THE GLYCEMIC INDEX

Regardless of what you've read or heard about the dangers of carbohydrates, they are an important part of a healthy diet. Carbohydrates provide the body with the fuel it needs for physical activity and for proper organ function. The best sources of carbohydrates—fruits, vegetables, and whole grains—deliver essential vitamins and minerals, fibre, and a host of important phytonutrients. Phytonutrients (also called phytochemicals) are compounds found in plant food (vegetables and fruit) that are not used for normal functions of the body but have a beneficial effect on health or disease. An example is flavonoids, which are found in berries, herbs, and vegetables, and are associated with a decreased risk of cancer due to their antioxidant and anti-inflammatory effects.

Carbohydrates come from a wide array of foods—bread, beans, milk, popcorn, potatoes, cookies, spaghetti, corn, and cherry pie. They also come in a variety of forms. The most common and abundant are sugars, fibres, and starches. The basic building block of a carbohydrate is a sugar molecule—a simple union of carbon, hydrogen, and oxygen. Starches and fibres are essentially chains of sugar molecules. Some contain hundreds of sugars. Some chains are straight; others branch wildly.

Carbohydrates were once grouped into two main categories: simple and complex. Simple carbohydrates include sugars such as fruit sugar (fructose), corn or grape sugar (dextrose or glucose), and table sugar (sucrose). They can be as small as one molecule or as many as two; typically, simple sugars are two molecules. Complex carbohydrates include everything made of three or more linked sugars forming chains. Starches and fibre make up complex carbohydrates. Starch is an excellent source of energy. The enzymes that break down starch chains are in the saliva and small intestine. Sugars are absorbed in the small intestine and absorbed by the bloodstream. In the cells, these molecules are combined with oxygen to create energy. In the past, simple sugars were considered bad and complex carbohydrates good, but the picture is much more complicated than that.

The digestive system handles all carbohydrates in much the same way—it breaks carbohydrates down (or tries to break them down) into single-sugar molecules, as only these are small enough to cross into the bloodstream. It also converts most digestible carbohydrates into glucose (also known as blood sugar), because cells are designed to use this as a universal energy source. Your brain can only use glucose as a source of energy. Fibre is an exception. It is put together in such a way that it can't be broken down into sugar molecules, and so it passes through the body undigested.

The glycemic index (GI) relates to the way your body's sugar levels respond to certain foods based on their effect on blood glucose levels in the first two hours of digestion. The concept was invented in 1981 by Dr. David Jenkins at the University of Toronto. Although you cannot generalize, the glycemic index concept relates to how your body digests food. Your body's response is dependent on several factors, including age, activity level, insulin levels, time of day, amount of fibre and fat in the food, how processed the food is, and what you have eaten with the food. Your rate of metabolism can determine how your body's sugar levels respond after you have eaten. It also can be dependent on how much fat and protein is consumed with the food. Cooking can also affect the glycemic level (for example, whether food is boiled, fried, or baked) (Jenkins et al., 1981; Sheard, 2004).

The glycemic index ranges from 0–100, with glucose being 100. High-glycemic foods—those that are starchy or sugary (such as simple carbohydrates)—will increase the body's sugar levels rapidly. Within 30 minutes, your body senses that energy levels are declining, which leaves you hungry again and running to the fridge (or fast-food location), even if you've just eaten loads of calories. Low-glycemic foods slowly increase sugar levels in the blood. These foods are generally lower in fat and higher in fibre, and are a rich source of vitamins, minerals, and antioxidants. A lower glycemic index suggests slower rates of digestion and absorption of the sugars and starches in the foods. This translates into a lower insulin demand, better long-term blood glucose control, and a reduction in blood lipids. Since insulin's other job is to tell your body to store fat, higher insulin levels in your blood make you more likely to convert your food to body fat rather than usable energy. Understanding the glycemic index will help you if you are trying to lose weight and help control diabetes. See table 8.3 for the glycemic index of various carbohydrates.

Knowing glycemic levels can be a useful meal-planning tool once individuals determine their responses to different foods. In general, low-glycemic foods are helpful for those who want to lose weight. Low-glycemic foods gradually increase sugar levels in the bloodstream to sustain energy levels for longer periods of time.

Since the sugars are slowly released, an individual is less likely to want to eat because energy is slowly released into the bloodstream.

If you exercise and then consume high-glycemic foods soon after a workout, it will help you recover by helping to raise low blood sugars after intense exercising. Low-glycemic foods are helpful in maintaining blood sugar levels for long periods of exercise. Many endurance athletes try to balance the consumption of high- and low-glycemic foods to maintain constant energy levels and avoid energy spikes and troughs.

TABLE 8.3 Examples of Low, Medium, and High Glycemic Index Foods

Food group	Low glycemic index foods (< 60*)	Medium glycemic index foods (60–85*)	High glycemic index foods (> 85*)
Sugars	• Fructose	• Sucrose	• Glucose
Breads and cereals	• Pumpernickel bread • All-Bran cereal • Barley • Oatmeal and oat bran	• Bagel • Bran muffins • Shredded Mini Wheats • Oatmeal (porridge) • Long grain white rice (boiled 15–25 minutes)	• White bread • French baguette • Corn Flakes • Rice Krispies • Instant white rice
Dairy products	• Milk (skim and full-fat) • Yogurt	• Low-fat ice cream	
Fruits, vegetables, and legumes	• Unripe banana • Apple, berries, apple juice • Peach (fresh), pear • Yams • Black beans • Chickpeas (garbanzo beans) • Lentils (dahl), peas • Soy beans • Peanuts	• Overripe banana • Mango • Orange juice • Papaya • Peaches in heavy syrup • New potatoes (white or red)	• Carrots • Parsnips • Baked potato (russets) • Instant potatoes • Watermelon
Processed foods	• White spaghetti noodles • Vermicelli • Tomato soup	• Popcorn • Soft drinks • Most cookies	• Jelly beans • Rice cakes

* Glycemic index scores are based on 100.

Source: Adapted from Foster-Powell, K., & Miller, M.F. (1995). International tables of glycemic index. *American Journal of Clinical Nutrition, 62*, 8715-8735.

Fibre

Dietary fibre is the term for food components (such as cellulose) that cannot be digested. All fibre-containing foods contain a combination of insoluble and soluble fibre. Dietary fibre is found exclusively in plants and is a carbohydrate.

dietary fibre
food components that cannot be digested—found exclusively in plants; the two types of dietary fibre are insoluble and soluble

Insoluble fibre is found in wheat bran and wheat bran cereals, brown rice, whole-grain foods, and fruits (such as raspberries and blackberries) and vegetables (such as broccoli and green peas). Insoluble fibre acts to promote regularity and prevent constipation.

Soluble fibre forms a gel when dissolved in water. It is found in oat bran, oatmeal, legumes (dried beans, carrots, peas, and lentils), pectin-rich fruit (apples, strawberries, and citrus fruit), and psyllium (a popular ingredient in breakfast cereals). Soluble fibre helps to control blood sugar by slowing the rate at which the sugar is absorbed, and it also helps to lower cholesterol. Soluble fibre helps to keep you feel full longer.

It is recommended that for a 2,000-calorie diet, a person should consume 30 grams of fibre per day, regardless of whether the person is male or female (National Institutes of Health, 2006). This amount, however, will vary with age and health status (such as pregnancy).

Why else is fibre important? According to Sizer and Whitney (1997):

- It promotes a feeling of fullness by absorbing water.
- It helps prevent constipation, hemorrhoids, and bacterial infection of the appendix.
- It is associated with a reduced incidence of colon cancer.
- It stimulates the muscles of the digestive tract, which helps prevent diverticulosis (inflammation of one or more pouches in the wall of the colon).
- It helps glucose regulation by slowing digestion to increase the absorption of carbohydrates.

On the other hand, consuming too much fibre can lead to certain risks, including dehydration (the fibre absorbs too much water), reduced bodily absorption of important minerals, and nutritional and energy deficiencies if the fibre replaces other foods.

THE ABCS OF NUTRITIONALLY BENEFICIAL FOODS

Antioxidants combat the oxidation of our cells. Antioxidants help repair, prevent, or limit oxidative damage (oxidation causes the loss of electrons from atoms and molecules leading to cellular damage) to our cells caused by free radicals (unstable molecules that may cause cell damage that lead to heart disease and cancer). Some of the best-known antioxidants include vitamins C and E, selenium (a trace mineral that helps reduce LDL cholesterol levels), and carotenoids (natural pigments in red, orange, and yellow hues that help protect vitamin A and cells). The better sources of antioxidants include blueberries, cranberries, blackberries, raspberries, artichokes, raisins, and prunes.

Beta-carotene is an antioxidant phytonutrient that can be converted into vitamin A when digested. Health benefits include enhancing sun protection, promoting heart health, and decreasing cancer mortality (Buijsse et al., 2005). Top dietary sources include sweet potatoes, carrots, spinach, kale, and red bell peppers.

Cruciferous vegetables contain both soluble and insoluble dietary fibre, vitamin C and other vitamins, as well as phytonutrients, which help fight cancers and cardiovascular disease. Cruciferous vegetables include broccoli, kale, Brussels sprouts, cauliflower, and cabbage.

Fats

Fats are a source of fatty acids and other substances that, in small amounts, are used to synthesize hormones and cell membranes. Fatty acids are also a fuel source. Any excess is stored as body fat that may be used for future energy needs. Without physical activity, high-fat diets lead to weight gain and sometimes obesity, which can result in an increased risk of heart disease and diabetes.

Knowing how much of which fat to include in your diet has become increasingly difficult. It's not just the amount that matters but the type that makes the difference—some fats are good at lowering the risk of certain diseases. In Canada, food labels were required to change. Manufacturers are now required to put unhealthy trans fatty acids on labels—often we were consuming them without knowing it.

Broken down, fats are a myriad of **fatty acids** (chemically, long chains of carbon molecules with hydrogen atoms attached). Fatty acids are essential for various bodily functions, including hormone production, cell growth and maintenance, and transportation and storage of fat-soluble vitamins (A, D, E, and K). They also play a role in the functioning of the immune system and, when stored in triglyceride molecules as fat, they can become a vital source of energy.

fatty acids
the fundamental constituents of fats; fatty acids can be divided into two types—saturated and unsaturated

Each gram of fat contains nine calories, no matter which fat it is. Some fats make food taste good, while other fats makes us feel full (it takes longer for them to leave the stomach). However, this is where the experts say the similarities end. Figure 8.1 outlines the percentage of saturated fat in common oils and fats.

UNDERSTANDING THE DIFFERENCES BETWEEN FATS

Fat is an important part of a healthy diet because it provides essential fatty acids and energy (calories). It also helps your body absorb vitamins A, D, and E. Fats and oils are made mostly of fatty acids. There are four main types of fatty acids: saturated fatty acids, trans fatty acids, monounsaturated fatty acids, and polyunsaturated fatty acids. Most fats and oils contain a mixture of all four types, but such mixtures usually have a higher proportion of one particular type of fatty acid.

Saturated Fats

Saturated fats (so-called because the fatty acids are completely saturated with hydrogen atoms) are solid at room temperature. Saturated fats raise your LDL cholesterol (the "bad" cholesterol) level and your risk for heart disease. You should have no more than 10 percent of your diet from saturated fats. Foods that have saturated fats include animal products (for example, poultry, the marbled fat in steak, eggs, and full-fat dairy) as well as tropical oils such as coconut, palm, and palm kernel oils. If you consume 1,800 calories a day, you should be getting a maximum of 60 grams total of fat per day and only 20 grams of saturated fats.

Trans Fatty Acids

Trans fatty acids, often called **trans fats**, are created when a vegetable oil undergoes hydrogenation, a chemical process in which hydrogen is added at high temperature to make the oil solid. The process is commonly used in food processing to prolong the shelf life of packaged products and keep them more solid and resistant to chemical change. Fried foods and fast foods tend to be higher in trans fats. Trans fats are commonly used in baked goods and snack foods, including donuts.

trans fats
unsaturated fatty acids that have been hydrogenated to give them a longer shelf life; diets high in trans fats increase the risk of diseases like atherosclerosis and coronary heart disease

Trans fatty acids raise the risk of developing heart disease by raising the so-called bad cholesterol (LDL cholesterol) and lowering good cholesterol (HDL cholesterol) (Ooman et al., 2001; Willett et al., 1993). There have been some questions raised about whether trans fatty acids raise the risk of type 2 diabetes, and they have also been implicated in some types of cancers (Adams & Standridge, 2006).

In 2005, Health Canada made it mandatory for Canadian food companies to place the amount of trans fatty acids on their Nutrition Facts labels. Prior to 2005, it appeared as "hydrogenated" or "partially hydrogenated fats" on labels. Over one-quarter of Canadians aged 31 to 50 get more than 35 percent of their total calories from fat, the threshold beyond which health risks increase (Garriguet, 2004). Americans eat about five times more saturated fat than trans fats. While trans fat is considered somewhat more harmful than its cousin, too much of either greatly increases the risk of heart disease (Neergaard, 2007).

FIGURE 8.1 Percentage of Saturated Fat in Common Oils and Fats

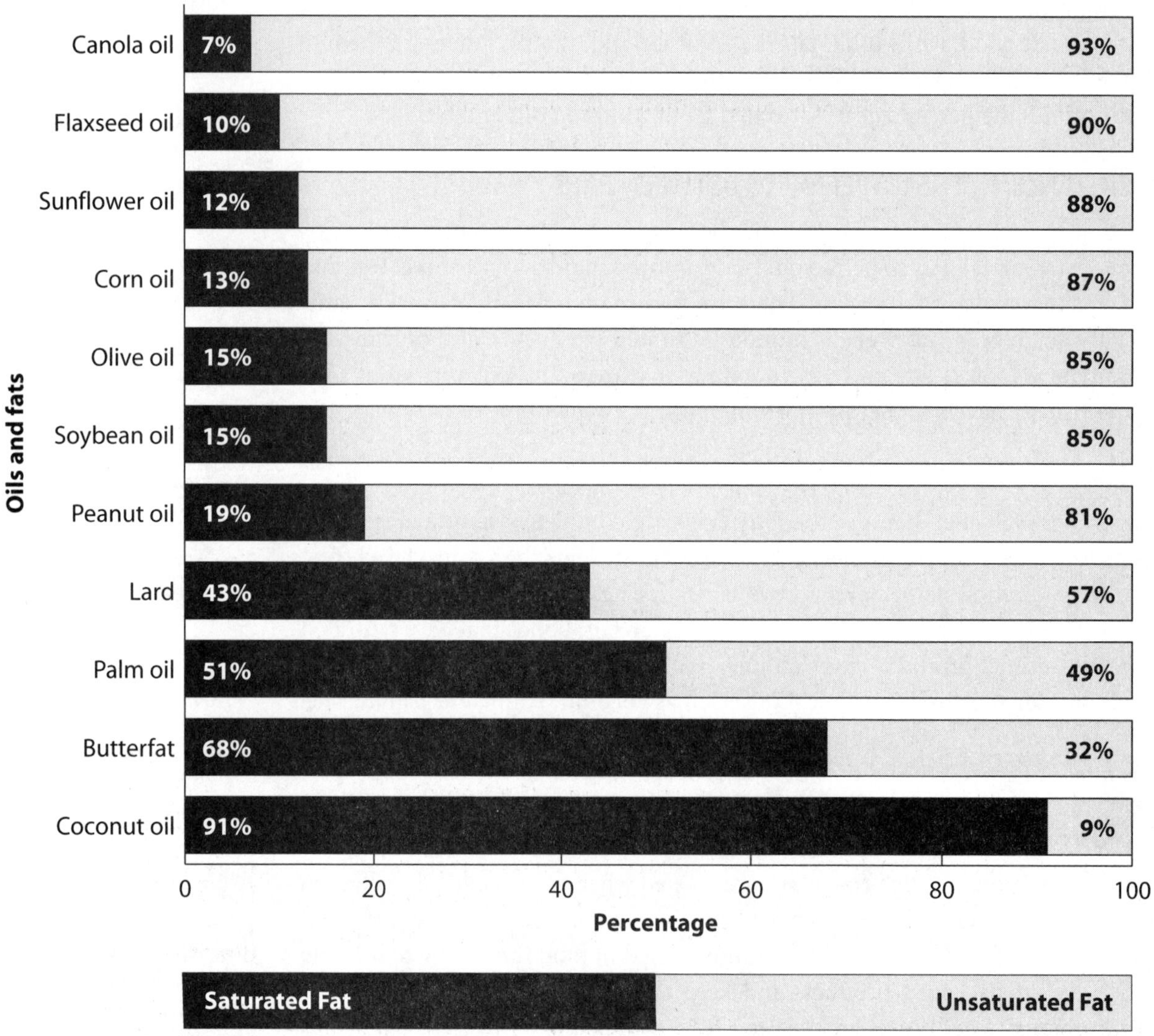

Unsaturated Fats

Unsaturated fats are not completely saturated with hydrogen atoms. They are liquid at room temperature and are subcategorized as either monounsaturated or polyunsaturated depending on which fatty acids are present in greater concentration. In general terms, monounsaturated and polyunsaturated fatty acids tend to lower the risk of heart disease.

Monounsaturated fats protect against heart disease by lowering LDL levels, and also reduce the risk of certain cancers. These fats are a part of the Mediterranean diet, which is rich in fruits, vegetables, beans, legumes, olive oil, and nuts. These contribute to lowering both heart disease and cancer. Olive, canola, and peanut oils, avocados, some margarines, and nuts (such as almonds and hazelnuts) are excellent sources of these fats.

Polyunsaturated fats are subdivided into two categories: omega-3 fatty acids and omega-6 fatty acids.

Omega-3 fatty acids are three fatty acids—eicosapentaenoic acid (EPA), docosahexaenoic acid (DHA), and alpha-linolenic acid (ALA). These fatty acids help prevent heart disease by lowering harmful triglycerides and reducing heart rhythm abnormalities, and prevent blood clotting (thus reducing the risk of a stroke or embolism). They also have anti-inflammatory properties, thus reducing inflammation in rheumatoid arthritis and colitis. They are believed to help fight wrinkles and depression. Food sources include oily cold-water fish such as salmon, mackerel, herring, and sardines for EPA and DHA. You can find ALA in flaxseeds and flaxseed oils, canola oil, soybeans and soybean oil, and walnuts, and in smaller amounts in dark green leafy vegetables.

Omega-6 fatty acids are found in linoleic acid, a second essential fatty acid. They help lower LDL cholesterol but need to be eaten in moderation, as in large quantities they can lower HDL cholesterol. Sources include safflower, sunflower, corn, soybean, and sesame oils, as well as almonds, pecans, Brazil nuts, sunflower seeds, and sesame seeds. The recommended ratio of omega-6 to omega-3 fatty acids in a healthy diet is 4:1. The conservative estimate is that Canadians are getting 10:1. The ideal number of servings of nuts per week for a good source of essential fatty acids is five (Health Canada, 2004).

UNDERSTANDING CHOLESTEROL

Cholesterol is a waxy fat-like substance that is important for normal body function. It is used for cellular function and production of hormones. Cholesterol travels through your blood packaged with other fats and proteins. When blood cholesterol is too high, it settles on the inside of the walls of blood vessels, clogging them up (see chapter 11). Twenty-five percent of our cholesterol is **dietary cholesterol** (from *exogenous* sources), while 75 percent is **blood cholesterol**, manufactured by our body (*endogenous* source). Familial hypercholesterolemia (genetic high blood cholesterol) is believed to be attributed to a mutant gene, which releases high blood cholesterol in the body and increases the risk of heart attacks. These cholesterols travel as lipoproteins (Durstine, 2006). There are two key kinds of lipoproteins:

- **Low-density lipoprotein cholesterol (LDL cholesterol)**, often referred to as "bad" cholesterol, is linked to heart disease and stroke. Although

dietary cholesterol
the cholesterol in food

blood cholesterol
the cholesterol produced by the liver

low-density lipoprotein (LDL) cholesterol
the "bad" cholesterol; it can build up in the arteries and cause health problems

approximately one-half of LDL is removed by the liver within two to six hours after its formation, the rest can travel for approximately two days with the chance of binding the arteries and veins. This form of cholesterol is decreased through diet by decreasing fat intake, increasing dietary fibre, and maintaining good body composition through aerobic activity.

high-density lipoprotein (HDL) cholesterol
the "good" cholesterol; it helps clean out undesirable LDL ("bad" cholesterol) deposits

- **High-density lipoprotein cholesterol (HDL cholesterol)** is known as the "good" form of cholesterol. It is increased through exercise, cessation of smoking, and weight reduction.

Total blood cholesterol levels should not exceed 6.2 mmol/L. LDL cholesterol should not be above 4.14 mmol/L and HDL cholesterol should be greater than 0.9 mmol/L. Many people have their cholesterol levels checked by their doctor, but many are also not aware of what levels are acceptable. RCMP officers are required to have their levels checked for their annual physicals. Although most men do not normally have this test done until they are 40 years old (and women not until 50 years old), you can ask your doctor what your levels are, and if they are high, what you can do about them. It is your right to know and make educated decisions about this part of your health and reduce your risk of cancer and cardiovascular diseases. The Dietary Guidelines for Canadians (Food and Nutrition Board, 2002) recommends keeping cholesterol consumption to less than 300 mg per day.

WAYS TO MINIMIZE YOUR RISKS AND REDUCE FAT

It is important that your diet have no more than 10 percent saturated fats and a maximum of 35 percent total dietary fat. Here are some tips to assist you:

- Avoid fried foods and high-fat bakery products.
- Follow *Canada's Food Guide* suggestions to choose lower-fat dairy products, leaner meats, and foods prepared with little or no fat.
- Read the label on packages before you buy.
- Choose soft margarines labelled as being free of trans fatty acids or made with non-hydrogenated fat.
- Fry foods less often. Try baking, broiling, and poaching instead.
- When you eat out, ask about the fat content of foods on the menu.
- Exercise at 70–85 percent of your MVO_2 for 40–90 minutes at least five times a week to reduce your risk factors associated with heart disease.

Table 8.4 categorizes food according to fat content to help you select lower-fat foods.

Proteins

amino acids
the fundamental constituents of proteins; amino acids can be divided into two types—complete (essential) and incomplete

Proteins are made up of **amino acids**, from which structural and chemical components of the body are manufactured. Adults need amino acids for health, and children and infants also need them for growth. Under certain extreme circumstances, such as starvation, amino acids may be used as fuel.

Protein is by far the most important nutrient for the body. Protein or amino acids are the main ingredient that goes into the production of antibodies, muscles, hormones, enzymes, and skin and hair cells. The human body requires 22 amino

TABLE 8.4 Learning to Choose Lower-Fat Foods

Food group	Higher-fat foods	Lower-fat foods
Dairy products	• Evaporated whole milk • Whole milk • Ice cream • Whipping cream • Sour cream • Cream cheese • Cheese (cheddar, Swiss, American) • Regular cottage cheese • Coffee creamers or non-dairy creamers • Mozzarella-filled pizza crusts	• Evaporated fat-free (skim) or reduced-fat (2 percent) milk • Low-fat (1 percent), reduced-fat (2 percent), or fat-free (skim) milk • Sorbet, sherbet, low-fat or fat-free frozen yogurt or ice cream • Imitation whipped cream made with fat-free milk • Plain low-fat yogurt • Fat-free or reduced-calorie cheeses • Low-fat (1 percent) or reduced-fat (2 percent) cottage cheese • Part-skim-milk ricotta cheese • Low-fat(1 percent) or reduced-fat (2 percent) milk powder
Cereals, grains, and pastas	• Pasta with cream sauces (alfredo, rosé) • Pasta with cheese sauce • Granola	• Rice or noodles (spaghetti, macaroni, etc.) • Pasta with red sauce (marinara) • Pasta with vegetables (primavera) • Pasta with vegetables (primavera) • Bran flakes, Rice crispies • Oatmeal • Reduced-fat granola
Meat, fish, and poultry	• Cold cuts or luncheon meats (bologna, salami, liverwurst, etc.) • Hot dogs • Bacon or sausage • Regular ground beef • Poultry with skin • Duck or goose • Oil-packed tuna • Beef (chuck, rib, brisket) • Pork (spareribs, untrimmed loin) • Frozen breaded fish or fried fish • Whole eggs • Frozen dinners (containing more than 13 grams of fat per serving)	• Low-fat cold cuts (95–97 percent fat-free luncheon meats) • Lower-fat hot dogs • Canadian bacon or lean ham • Extra-lean ground beef or turkey • Chicken or turkey without skin (white meat) • Water-packed tuna (rinse to reduce sodium content) • Beef (round, loin) with trimmed external fat • Pork tenderloin or trimmed, lean smoked ham • Fish or shellfish, unbreaded (fresh, frozen, or canned in water) • Egg whites or egg substitutes • Frozen TV dinners (with less than 13 grams of fat per serving and lower in sodium) • Turkey sausage, drained well • Vegetarian sausage (made with tofu)
Baked goods	• Croissants • Donuts, muffins • Party crackers • Cake (pound, chocolate, yellow) • Cookies	• Hard French rolls • Soft, brown whole-wheat rolls • English muffin • Reduced-fat or fat-free muffins or scones • Bagels (read nutrition labels) • Low-fat crackers (choose lower in sodium) • Saltine or soda crackers (choose lower in sodium) • Cake (angel food, white, gingerbread) • Reduced-fat or fat-free cookies (graham crackers, ginger snaps, fig bars)
Snacks and sweets	• Nuts • Ice cream (including cones or bars) • Custards or puddings made with whole milk	• Popcorn (air-popped or light microwave) • Fruit or vegetables • Frozen yogurt, frozen fruit or pudding bars • Pudding made with skim milk
Fats, oils, and salad dressings	• Regular margarine or butter • Regular mayonnaise • Regular salad dressings • Oils, shortening, or lard	• Light spread margarines • Calorie-reduced margarine such as Becel • Light mayonnaise or salad dressing • Reduced-caloric salad dressings • Herb-flavoured or wine vinegar • Non-stick cooking spray • Applesauce or fruit puree in baked goods to replace butter or oil
Miscellaneous	• Canned cream soups • Canned beans with bacon or franks • Gravy (homemade with fat) • Fudge sauce • Guacamole dip	• Canned broth-based soups • Canned baked beans in tomato sauce • Gravy mixes made with water or homemade with the fat skimmed off or removed (chilled and hardened) • Chocolate syrup • Cucumber slices or lettuce leaves • Salsa

Sources: Health Canada; Department of Health and Human Services. (n.d.). Low-calorie, lower-fat alternative foods. Retrieved from http://www.nhlbi.nih.gov/health/public/heart/obesity/lose_wt/lcal_fat.htm.

acids in order to synthesize proteins. About half of the amino acids are made by the body (known as the "non-essential" amino acids), while nine are not made by the body, so they must be obtained from food (these are known as the "essential" amino acids).

Protein is not stored in the body as such, unlike fat (in fat cells) and glucose (in muscles or the liver). Since muscles are built with protein, we need to consume and synthesize enough protein to maintain healthy, hard-working muscles as well as organs, red blood cells, cardiac muscle, and enzymes. Our bodies cannot make new cells or perform any function without protein. Our bodies need to consume approximately 0.8–1 gram of protein per kilogram of body weight over the course of the day. Consuming less than this amount may result in the body going into starvation mode and breaking down muscle instead of fat stores as a fuel source (this is why it is very important to eat breakfast, as your body assumes starvation mode after six to eight hours).

Too much protein in your diet may lead to high cholesterol, heart disease, and other diseases such as gout. A high-protein diet may put additional strain on the kidneys when extra waste matter (the end product of protein metabolism) is excreted in urine.

If not enough protein is consumed, growth failure, loss of muscle mass, decreased immunity, and weakening of the heart and respiratory systems can result, which can lead to death. Protein malnutrition can also lead to a condition known as kwashiorkor (a childhood malnutrition disease).

A nutritionally balanced diet provides adequate protein. Vegetarians must be sure to consume the proper combination of plant proteins (dry beans, lentils, legumes, nuts, soy foods, sprouted seeds, grains, spirulina, and chorella or blue-green algae) to achieve this balance. While most people who follow *Canada's Food Guide* will get enough protein in their diet, protein supplements may be useful for some individuals. The most efficient protein supplement is protein powder. Here are some guidelines to follow when looking for a protein supplement:

- As a rule of thumb, consume about the amount of protein source in a food serving that could be held in the palm of your hand (about the size of a chicken breast) three times each day.
- Make sure the protein supplement uses a natural sweetener like stevia rather than an artificial one like Aspartame.
- Make sure the protein supplement uses high-quality protein isolated from whey (extracted at low temperatures to prevent the breakdown of the amino acids themselves).
- Choose the type of supplement that's right for you. Protein supplements consist of either whole protein (such as egg, milk, or soy protein), individual amino acids, or combinations of individual amino acids. Whole protein supplements do not offer an advantage over food sources of protein, but they may offer convenience. Powders tend to be more concentrated protein sources than pills.
- Choose protein cereals made from soy, whey, and gluten that are high in fibre and protein, and low in carbohydrates and fats.
- Keep in mind that readily available instant breakfast powder mixes offer a cheaper alternative to specially marketed protein powders.

- Look at the nutritional labels for protein bars to ensure that they provide you with a healthy high-protein snack without being filled with preservatives, additives, and chemicals.
- Use tofu in soups, salads, and stir fries to provide protein without high fat.
- Use egg whites to help make simple meals.

PROTEIN SUPPLEMENTING TO BUILD MUSCLE TISSUE

The timing of protein intake is also important. Research shows that protein consumed with carbohydrates within an hour after exercise stimulates the release of insulin and growth hormone, and therefore, the growth of muscle mass (Chandler et al., 1994). Some research indicates that during the maintenance phase of body building, recommended protein intake is 1.2 grams per kilogram of body weight for maintenance of muscle mass. During the muscle-building phase, protein intake of 1.4–1.8 grams per kilogram of body weight is recommended. During the tapering or cutting phase, body builders significantly decrease their calorie intake. During this special phase of calorie and carbohydrate restriction, protein needs increase to 1.8–2.0 grams of protein per kilogram of body weight to compensate for the use of protein for energy during this hypocaloric phase (Kleiner, 2000). Research does not support protein intake in excess of 2.0 grams per kilogram of body weight. Excess protein intake is associated with dehydration and may be related to excessive urinary calcium losses and inadequate carbohydrate intake. An impairment of kidney function has also been associated with excessive protein intake (American Kidney Fund, 2002).

CANADA'S FOOD GUIDE

The first edition of *Canada's Food Guide* was introduced in July 1942 as a way to ration food during World War II while ensuring Canadians were not nutritionally deficient. There have been a number of different editions over the years to provide a practical pattern of food choices while incorporating variety and flexibility. In 2007, the new guide, *Eating Well with Canada's Food Guide*, was introduced. (For a historic perspective, see *Canada's Food Guides* from 1942 to 1992 at www.hc-sc.gc.ca/fn-an/food-guide-aliment/context/hist/fg_history-histoire_ga_e.html.) The 2007 guide translates the science of nutrition and health into practical advice for healthy eating patterns. It emphasizes healthy eating and physical activity to meet nutritional needs while reducing the risk of obesity, type 2 diabetes, heart disease, certain types of cancer, and osteoporosis.

> Get your own copy of *Canada's Food Guide* at www.hc-sc.gc.ca/fn-an/food-guide-aliment/index_e.html.

Over the last decade, prepackaged foods and fast foods have become staples in our country. With fast-food restaurants on every main street and what seems like a Tim Hortons at every major corner, access to foods high in fat, sodium, and trans fats dominate our meals when we are in a hurry. Canadians find it more difficult to provide sit-down meals and savour our food, as we are always in a hurry to go to the next activity.

Shift work, which has traditionally created barriers for access to healthy foods, has been aided in the last several years by grocery stores that stay open 24 hours to provide options to those who work at night. The marketplace is working to provide prewashed ready-to-eat vegetables, which makes it easier to include better nutritional choices in our diets. Cultural demographics in Canada are also increasing the availability of a variety of ethnically diverse food choices, which often provide healthier options.

Healthy eating patterns are based on scientific evidence to ensure Canadians are meeting their nutritional needs. These standards are called dietary reference intakes (DRIs). Table 8.5 presents the acceptable macronutrient distribution ranges (AMCDRs) for carbohydrate, protein, and fat in the diet. The 2007 guide has broken it down into three age groups and provided a larger range for each macronutrient compared with the previous (1992) guide. This means that there is more flexibility for those who are choosing different diets to meet their physical needs. For example, there is a larger range for protein, which may address athletes' needs for more protein in their diets.

TABLE 8.5 Acceptable Macronutrient Distribution Ranges

	Percentage of total calories from		
Age group	**carbohydrate**	**protein**	**fat**
1–3 years	45–65 percent	5–20 percent	30–40 percent
4–18 years	45–65 percent	10–30 percent	25–35 percent
19 years and over	45–65 percent	10–35 percent	20–35 percent

Source: Health Canada. (2007). Foods to limit. Public Works and Government Services Canada Publishing and Depository Services. Available at http://www.hc-sc.gc.ca/fn-an/surveill/index_e.html.

Canada's Food Guide recommends how many food servings people should eat from each of the four food groups, plus a small amount of added oils and fats. Recommended servings differ for different ages and there is a difference between males and females (see table 8.6). People who are very active should be encouraged to choose extra servings from the four food groups, but be sure to follow a healthy eating pattern that is low in fat, sugar, and salt. For those trying to lose weight it is very important to understand what a serving size entails (see the discussion below).

TABLE 8.6 Recommended Number of Food Guide Servings per Day

		Children			Teens		Adults			
		2–3 yrs.	4–8 yrs.	9–13 yrs.	14–18 yrs.		19–50 yrs.		51+ yrs.	
		Females and Males			*Females*	*Males*	*Females*	*Males*	*Females*	*Males*
Food group servings per day	Vegetables and fruit	4	5	6	7	8	7–8	8–10	7	7
	Grain products	3	4	6	6	7	6–7	8	6	7
	Milk and alternatives	2	2	3–4	3–4	3–4	2	2	3	3
	Meat and alternatives	1	1	12	2	3	2	3	2	3
The eating pattern also includes a small amount (30 to 45 mL or about 2 to 3 tablespoons) of unsaturated fat each day.										

Source: Health Canada. (2007). Foods to limit. Public Works and Government Services Canada Publishing and Depository Services. Available at http://www.hc-sc.gc.ca/fn-an/surveill/index_e.html.

MAKING WISE CHOICES WITH THE FOUR FOOD GROUPS

Canada's Food Guide provides the basics for making wise and healthy food choices. Whether you are at work, school, or home, you can make better choices to stay healthier (Health Canada, 2007).

Vegetables and fruit should include

- eating dark and orange vegetables daily
- enjoying naturally prepared vegetables and fruit
- eating fresh fruit and vegetables rather than juices

Grain products should include

- choosing whole-grain foods
- ensuring that grain products are low in fat, sugar, and salt

Milk and alternatives should include

- choosing low-fat milk at least two times daily
- choosing low-fat alternatives to milk, including cheeses and yogurt

Meat and alternatives should include

- considering alternatives to meat such as beans, lentils, and tofu
- choosing fish over red meat at least twice a week
- making sure the meat you choose is low in fat, sugar, and salt

UNDERSTANDING PORTION SIZES AND LABELLING

A "portion" is how much food you choose to eat at one sitting, whether cooked in your own kitchen, prepared from a package, or eaten at a restaurant. A "serving" is a measured amount of food or drink, such as a slice of bread or 250 mL of milk, which is listed on the product's nutrition facts label. Many people are not educated on what a serving is, so many are consuming multiple serving sizes. Nutritionists use serving sizes to help people understand how much of different types of foods they should eat to get the nutrients they need. In 2005, Health Canada required that all packaged food contain labels that listed nutritional content. Food labels help consumers make informed food choices. The label includes a nutrition facts table with the specific amount of food, percentage of daily values of macro- and micro-nutrients, a list of core nutrients, nutrition claims, and a list of ingredients.

Go to **assignment 8.1** (in the appendix) and do the assignment on "Portion Distortion." From the assignment, you can see that the portion size you are used to eating may be equal to two or three standard servings. If we learn more about what makes up a serving, we can monitor our eating habits to maintain a healthy weight. Table 8.7 shows examples of *Canada's Food Guide* serving sizes, and table 8.8 provides estimates of amounts of food.

TABLE 8.7 Canada's Food Guide Serving Examples

Food group	Examples of one serving
Vegetables and fruit	• 125 mL (1/2 cup) fresh, frozen or canned vegetable or fruit or 100% juice • 250 mL (1 cup) leafy raw vegetables or salad • 1 piece of fruit
Grain products	• 1 slice (35 g) bread or 1/2 bagel (45 g) • 1/2 pita (35 g) or 1/2 tortilla (35 g) • 125 mL (1/2 cup) cooked rice, pasta, or couscous • 30 g cold cereal or 175 mL (3/4 cup) hot cereal
Milk and alternatives	• 250 mL (1 cup) milk or fortified soy beverage • 175 g (3/4 cup) yogurt • 50 g (1-1/2 oz.) cheese
Meat and alternatives	• 75 g (2-1/2 oz.)/125 mL (1/2 cup) cooked fish, shellfish, poultry or lean meat • 175 mL (3/4 cup) cooked beans • 2 eggs • 30 mL (2 Tbsp) peanut butter

Source: Health Canada. (2007). Available at http://www.hc-sc.gc.ca/fn-an/food-guide-aliment/basics-base/serving-portion/index_e.html.

TABLE 8.8 Estimating Amounts of Food

Amount of food	Size estimate
3/4 cup of cereal	a small fist
1/2 cup of cooked rice, pasta, or potato	one-half baseball
1 baked potato	a fist or a bar of soap
1 muffin (equals two servings)	standard light bulb
1/2 bagel	small can of tuna
1 medium fruit	a baseball
1/2 cup (125 mL) of fresh fruit	one-half baseball
1/2 cup (125 mL) vegetables	small scoop of ice cream
1 oz (28 g) of low-fat or fat-free cheese	4 stacked dice or a pink eraser
2-1/2 oz (75 g) of lean red meat or poultry	computer mouse
2-1/2 oz (75 g) fish	eyeglass case
2 tablespoons (30 mL) of peanut butter	1 ping-pong ball
1/2 cup (60 mL) nuts	2 egg cups
1 tsp (5 mL) of vegetable oil or mayonnaise	a quarter
1/2 cup of ice cream	one-half baseball
3/4 cup frozen yogurt	a baseball
1 oz (85 g) chocolate	package of dental floss

UNDERSTANDING THE CALORIC VALUE OF NUTRIENTS

A calorie is a calorie is a calorie whether it comes from fat, protein, or carbohydrates. Also known as a **kilocalorie (kcal)**, a calorie is a measure of the amount of energy in food. An individual's energy needs are the number of calories he or she must consume to maintain health based on age, sex, weight, height, and activity level (Institute of Medicine, 2005). Just as gasoline powers your car, proper energy is required for your body. In terms of nutritional labelling, nutritional energy is recorded in kilocalories and kilojoules (kJ). Carbohydrates, fats, and proteins are the types of nutrients that contain calories and thus are the main energy sources for your body. In terms of energy density, food components have estimated energy values, while other substances found in food (water, non-digestible fibre, minerals, and vitamins) do not contribute to calculated energy density (Drewnowski, 2005). Caloric estimates are as follows:

kilocalorie (kcal)
a measure of the amount of energy in food; also referred to as a calorie; an individual's energy needs are the number of calories he or she must consume to maintain health based on age, sex, weight, height, and activity level

- *Fat* has 9 kcal/g (37 kJ/g).
- *Ethanol* (alcohol) has 7 kcal/g (29 kJ/g).
- *Protein* has 4 kcal/g (17 kJ/g).
- *Carbohydrate* has 4 kcal/g (17 kJ/g).
- *Polyols* (sugar-free sweeteners) have 2.4 kcal/g (10 kJ/g).

The calories you eat are either converted to physical energy or stored within your body as fat after your limited carbohydrates are restored. Unless you lose those stored calories either by reducing calorie intake or by increasing physical activity so that you burn more calories, this fat remains in your body. Reducing the amount of fat and saturated fat in your diet is an important way to limit your overall caloric intake. However, it is also important to reduce your overall food intake to reduce calories. Just because a product is fat-free, it doesn't mean that it is "calorie free."

NUTRIENT CONTENT CLAIMS

Terms such as "free," "low," or "reduced" in nutritional claims on labels can signal that a food has less of a certain component, such as calories, fat, saturated fat, or sodium. Such labels can help consumers moderate their intake of these components. Some labels also provide information on better options regarding fibre, vitamins, and minerals. Labelling can also help people with diabetes choose foods lower in calories, carbohydrates, and fats. Table 8.9 provides a summary of terms found on nutrition labels and their meanings.

HOW TO READ A FOOD LABEL

In Canada, it became mandatory in 2005 to use a nutrition facts table on foods. In addition to the nutrient content claims, manufacturers were allowed for the first time in Canada to place diet-related health claims on their foods. Each label must include a list of ingredients by weight. This is to help build awareness and understanding of the key features of nutrition in the foods that Canadians are eating, a matter of particular concern to those with allergies or dietary issues. By being informed of the content, people can make healthier choices. See figure 8.2 for a sample label.

TABLE 8.9 Common Nutrient Content Claims and What They Mean

Term	Meaning
Free	An amount so small, considered nutritionally insignificant
Sodium-free	Less than 5 mg sodium (per serving)
Cholesterol-free	Less than 2 mg cholesterol and low in saturated fat (includes a restriction on trans fat) Not necessarily low in total fat
Low	Always associated with a very small amount
Low-fat	3 g or less fat
Low in saturated fat	2 g or less of saturated and trans fat combined (per serving)
Reduced	At least 25 percent less of a nutrient compared with a similar product
Reduced in calories	At least 25 percent less energy than the food to which it is compared
Source	Always associated with a "significant" amount
Source of fibre	2 grams or more fibre (per serving)
Good source of calcium	165 mg or more of calcium (per serving)
Light	When referring to a nutritional characteristic of a product, it is allowed only on foods that are either "reduced in fat" or "reduced in energy" (calories)

Explanation on the label of what makes the food "light"; this may refer to sensory characteristics, such as "light in colour." Lightly salted can be used when a food contains at least 50 percent less added sodium compared with a similar product.

Source: Health Canada. (2006). Nutritional labelling. Available at http://www.hc-sc.gc.ca/fn-an/label-etiquet/nutrition/index_e.html.

FIGURE 8.2 Nutrition Label

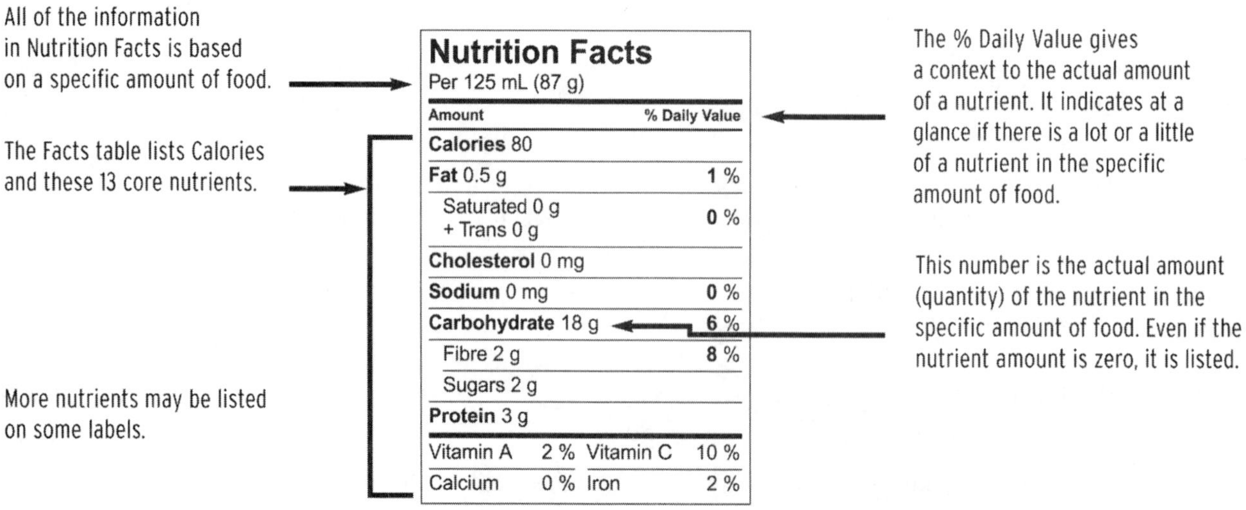
All of the information in Nutrition Facts is based on a specific amount of food.
The Facts table lists Calories and these 13 core nutrients.
More nutrients may be listed on some labels.
Nutrition Facts
Per 125 mL (87 g)
Amount
% Daily Value
Calories 80
Fat 0.5 g 1 %
Saturated 0 g + Trans 0 g 0 %
Cholesterol 0 mg
Sodium 0 mg 0 %
Carbohydrate 18 g 6 %
Fibre 2 g 8 %
Sugars 2 g
Protein 3 g
Vitamin A 2 % Vitamin C 10 %
Calcium 0 % Iron 2 %
The % Daily Value gives a context to the actual amount of a nutrient. It indicates at a glance if there is a lot or a little of a nutrient in the specific amount of food.
This number is the actual amount (quantity) of the nutrient in the specific amount of food. Even if the nutrient amount is zero, it is listed.

Source: Health Canada. (2006). Nutritional labelling. Available at http://www.hc-sc.gc.ca/fn-an/label-etiquet/nutrition/index_e.html.

Table 8.10 Guidelines for Providing Information About Foods and Making a Health Claim

To make a health claim about ...	The food ...
Potassium, sodium, and reduced risk of high blood pressure	▪ must be low in (or free of) sodium ▪ may also be high in potassium ▪ must be low in saturated fatty acids ▪ must be limited in alcohol ▪ must have more than 40 calories if the food is not a vegetable or a fruit ▪ must have a minimum amount of at least one vitamin or mineral
Calcium, vitamin D, and regular physical activity, and reduced risk of osteoporosis	▪ must be high (or very high) in calcium ▪ may also be very high in vitamin D ▪ cannot have more phosphorus than calcium ▪ must be limited in alcohol ▪ must have more than 40 calories if the food is not a vegetable or a fruit
Saturated and trans fats and reduced risk of heart disease	▪ must be low in (or free of) saturated fat and trans fat ▪ must be limited in cholesterol, sodium and alcohol ▪ must have more than 40 calories if the food is not a vegetable or a fruit ▪ must have a minimum amount of at least one vitamin or mineral ▪ must, if it is a fat or an oil, be a source of omega-3 or omega-6 polyunsaturated fatty acids
Vegetables and fruit and reduced risk of some types of cancers	▪ must be a fresh, frozen, dried or canned fruit or vegetable; fruit juice; vegetable juice ▪ must be limited in alcohol

Source: Adapted from Health Canada. (2002). Table of diet-related health claims. Nutrition labeling toolkit for educators. Food and nutrition. Retrieved from http://www.hc-sc.gc.ca/fn-an/label-etiquet/nutrition/education/nurtri-kit-trousse/te_background-le_point-08-table2_e.html.

Labels list calories and 13 core nutrients and give the percentage of the recommended daily value of each nutrient. There are some exemptions to labelling requirements (such as fresh fruit, vegetables, raw meat and poultry, individual bakery items, alcoholic beverages, coffee beans, teas, herbs and spices); however, if the food is altered in any way (such as sweeteners, vitamins, or minerals added), each item must be labelled appropriately. Standard formats make information easier to find and use.

Go to **assignment 8.2** (in the appendix) and do the assignment on nutritional labelling.

UNDERSTANDING THE ROLE OF SODIUM

Sodium is a mineral that is needed by the human body to regulate fluid balance, contraction of muscles, and conduction of nerve impulses. Salt is sodium chloride.

Food labels list sodium rather than salt content. On average, the naturally occurring sodium in foods accounts for only about 10 percent of total dietary intake, while salt added during cooking may account for 5 to 10 percent and salt added during the manufacturing process may account for as much as 75 percent. Sodium is put into foods to preserve them and provide taste. Nearly all Canadians consume more salt than they need. Salt intake is associated with higher blood pressure. Our bodies only need 1500 mg of sodium. Consuming less than 2300 mg (approximately 1 tsp of salt) of sodium per day is recommended. It is also recommended that you increase potassium-rich fruits and vegetables to reduce the risk of kidney stones and bone loss. Foods high in sodium include pizza (450–1200 mg), tomato soup (700–1,260 mg), tomato juice (340-1,040 mg) and pretzels (290–560 mg). It is important to read food labels in order to make healthier choices for sodium intake. Some tips to reduce sodium in your diet include

- choosing fresh or plain frozen foods over canned
- adding herbs, spices, and salt-free seasoning in cooking and on the table
- cooking rice, pasta, and potatoes without salt
- rinsing canned foods to remove some of the sodium
- choosing low- or reduced sodium products

The DASH Diet

The National Heart, Lung, and Blood Institute in 2001 released a eating plan called the **DASH diet**, which stands for "Dietary Approaches to Stop Hypertension." The DASH diet emphasizes fruits, vegetables, and low-fat dairy foods. It is low in saturated fat, total fat, cholesterol, and sodium for those who are at risk for cardiovascular disease. For more information, go to www.nhlbi.nih.gov/hbp/prevent/h_eating/h_eating.htm. Chapter 12 discusses this eating plan further.

DASH diet
a diet that follows *Canada's Food Guide* and the American Food Pyramid in order to reduce sodium, cholesterol, and fat in your diet

A QUICK OVERVIEW OF DIETS

When you eat less food energy than you need, your body must draw on its stores to supply it with energy. If done correctly with a balanced diet (meeting protein and carbohydrate requirements), dieting forces the body to use fat as an energy source. In order to burn fat, however, this must be a slow process so that lean body mass can be spared.

Fasting

Fasting is the act of willingly refraining from some or all food, drink, or both for a period of time. In less than a day (8–10 hours) without nutrients, the liver's glycogen stores are exhausted, as are the glucose stores in the muscle tissue. The body does not have the enzymes to convert fat to glucose. Although most of the major organs can use fat as a fuel, the nervous system can only use glucose as an energy source. To satisfy the brain's need for glucose, the body must turn protein into glucose. This affects the protein in muscles, blood proteins, liver, digestive tract lining, heart muscle, and lung tissue. This means that those trying to reduce body fat are actually reducing lean muscle tissue and depriving the body of nutrients that it needs to build enzymes, red and white blood cells, and other vital components. Fasting also slows down your metabolism, making it harder to lose weight. Ketone bodies are the product of the fat breakdown, which can provide energy to the nervous system, but can result in an imbalance in acid–base balance in the blood and a loss of minerals (Ferraris & Carey, 2000). Highly restrictive caloric diets are deficient in calcium and some fatty acids. Most people who fast experience fatigue, constipation, and nausea.

Low-Carbohydrate Diets

When deprived of sufficient carbohydrates, your body responds in a similar fashion to fasting. Low-carbohydrate diets usually result in a sizable initial weight loss, and proponents claim that you can "lose weight quickly" and "never feel hungry." Although these claims are somewhat true, they are also misleading. Severe calorie restrictions lead to loss of water and lean tissue (muscle mass). Eventually, water is regained. Ketoacidosis is the result of protein being broken down to provide energy to the nervous system. The longer a person is on a low-carb diet, the more protein the body has to use for energy. There are exclusions of food high on the glycemic index, such as white potatoes, flour, and cooked carrots. Over time, there is a nutritional deficiency due to an insufficient consumption of some food. Some research suggests that this diet may be appropriate for diabetics, as the low-fat content found in some low-carb diets may reduce risks of cardiovascular disease and obesity (Roberts & Barnard, 2003; Parillo et al., 1992).

High-Protein Diets

High-protein diets include foods rich in fat and protein. Consumption of starchy food, legumes, fruits, and sugar is prohibited. There may be substantial weight loss, but the weight is likely to be regained quickly. Loss of 2–4 kg in the first week is common (mainly due to water loss), but weight loss is slow after that. Fatigue, constipation, and high blood cholesterol levels are some of the side effects. Concerns around protein diets include the fact that they are high in saturated fats, very low in calcium (increasing the risk of osteoporosis), and low in fibre; intake is usually less than 10 grams while 25 grams per day is recommended. For the kidneys to break down protein, they produce by-products called ketone bodies, which can lead to kidney damage. Finally, high-protein diets lack many essential vitamins and minerals due to a lack of vegetables, fruits, and grains.

Vegetarianism

People choose to be vegetarians for a number of reasons. Some do it for health reasons, such as to reduce the risks of obesity, heart disease, hypertension, type 2 diabetes, and certain types of cancer (particularly colorectal cancer). Some individuals do not want to eat animals that have been slaughtered, while others find chewing red meat difficult. If planned well, vegetarian diets may be appropriate for all stages of the life cycle. Some of the nutritional benefits include a lower level of saturated fats, cholesterol, and animal protein, as well as higher levels of carbohydrates, fibre, magnesium, potassium, folate (a water-soluble B vitamin), antioxidants such as vitamins C and E, and phytochemicals (American Dietetic Association and Dietitians of Canada, 2003). There are number of variations of vegetarianism.

Although a vegetarian is a person who does not eat meat, fish, or fowl or products containing these foods, there are a number of different macrobiotic diets that follow a vegetarian diet. They include the following:

- pesco-vegetarianism, where people eat plant-based foods, dairy, eggs, and fish, but no other types of meat.
- lacto-ovo-vegetarianism, where people eat plant-based foods, dairy, and eggs, but no meat.
- veganism, where people eat only plant-based food—no dairy, eggs, or meat products.

Vegetarian diets are generally low in saturated fat and cholesterol. However, these diets run the risk of deficiencies in the following areas:

- protein—sources include soy (tofu, tempeh), whole grains, legumes, and nuts
- iron—sources include spinach, broccoli, dried beans, whole grains, dried fruit, and fortified cereals
- calcium—sources include arugula, broccoli, kale, soy, and legumes
- B vitamins—sources include legumes, oats, green leafy vegetables, and beans (B_{12} has to be obtained through animal or fortified products)
- zinc—sources include beans, oats, green peas, fortified cereals, and sunflower seeds

DRINKS THAT PEOPLE USE TO ENHANCE PERFORMANCE

There is a great deal of research around drinks that people consume in an attempt to increase their performance. The following information provides an overview of the benefits and risks of consuming them.

Caffeine: The Drug of Today

Coffee, a key source of caffeine, is the most popular and widely consumed drug in North America. It is marketed in all sorts of forms and is often served in large quantities. Caffeine is also found in a great number of carbonated and fruit drinks, including some that are specifically designed to deliver megadoses of caffeine. Habitual caffeine consumption results in addiction. Many people wake up in the morning craving the lift they get from their first cup of coffee, and police officers are no different. In order to stay alert during long shifts, many resort to consuming large quantities of caffeinated drinks.

Caffeine works by blocking the effects of adenosine, a brain chemical involved in sleep. Thinking that the body is in an emergency, the pituitary gland initiates the body's "fight or flight" response by releasing adrenalin. Adrenalin makes the heart beat faster and the eyes dilate. It causes the liver to release extra sugar into the bloodstream for energy. Caffeine also affects dopamine by making you feel that you have more energy. For this reason its use was restricted by the International Olympic Committee in the 1980s. Just 3.0 mg to 6.0 mg of caffeine per kilogram of body weight is required for the energy-enhancing effect. That's the amount in a 150 mL cup of coffee or about 375 mL of tea. If you drink more than that, your body builds up a tolerance to the energy-enhancing effect and you must consume more caffeine to get the same effect.

Some of the effects of caffeine can be viewed as beneficial in some circumstances:

- It acts as a stimulant that increases one's respiration rate, heart rate, blood pressure, and secretion of stress and other hormones (Falk et al., 1990).
- It stimulates the digestive tract, promoting efficient elimination of waste (Gordon et al., 1982).
- It gives people a "buzz" that aids mental and physical effort.

People should also be wary of excessive consumption of caffeine. Here are some key reasons:

- Caffeine has a diuretic effect that can lead to dehydration during exercise (Gordon et al., 1982).
- Some people's caffeine intake patterns fulfill all the accepted criteria for a diagnosis of drug dependence (Strain et al., 1994).
- Research has linked caffeine consumption to health risks, including fibrocystic breast disease, breast cancer, birth defects, osteoporosis, and heart palpitations (Clark, 1997; Harris & Dawson-Hughes, 1989; Joesoef et al., 1990; Willett et al., 1996).
- Excessive quantities of caffeine produce anxiety-related symptoms such as sweating, tenseness, and an inability to concentrate.
- Caffeine withdrawal can produce symptoms such as thirst, severe headaches (which may last for days), stomach aches, and a feeling of lethargy and drowsiness.

Try to limit your caffeine consumption, and be aware that caffeine is found not only in tea, coffee, and many cola drinks, but also in cocoa, chocolate, and some over-the-counter medicines. Also be aware that product labels often do not provide adequate information on caffeine content.

Sports Drinks

Athletes can choose from a number of sports drinks that offer a wide variety of nutrients including carbohydrates, electrolytes (minerals), vitamins, protein, and amino acids. Those drinks that combine carbohydrates and electrolytes are absorbed into the body quickly, help maintain fluid balance, and provide energy to working muscles. Simple sugars are used to provide quick uptake in the small intestine while helping to provide glycogen to keep muscles moving. Sodium and other electrolytes are put into drinks to help maintain fluid balance in the cells. Sodium helps to maintain blood volume. This is important because a higher blood volume translates into a lower heart rate and greater blood flow to muscle and skin (Casa et al., 2000). Examples of these drinks include Powerade and Gatorade.

Protein drinks work on the premise that providing protein during exercise will assist with muscle building. There is evidence that eating a little protein after exercise is important to help repair damaged muscles and promote training adaptations; however, there is controversy as to whether it helps during the workout (Ivy et al., 2003).

Creatine, one of the best-selling protein supplements, is a naturally occurring substance that plays an important role in energy production. Normally, our diet supplies about 1 gram of creatine per day but some people supplement creatine in hopes of enhancing athletic performance. The body converts creatine into phosphocreatine, a form of energy used by the muscles in the adenosine triphosphate or ATP cycle (the energy cycle that gains energy from the breakdown of glucose in the cells). In theory, supplemental creatine may help the body make phosphocreatine faster when it has been used up by intense activity and prevent protein catabolism (the breakdown of protein of muscles into amino acids). Most studies to date have not been able to demonstrate this during the workout (Leenders et al., 1999; Mujika et al., 2000; Astorino et al., 2005), although some have shown increased results in isometric exercise capacity and lean muscle and bone mass (Gilliam et al., 2000; Eijnde et al., 2003).

Whey protein is extracted from the liquid whey that is produced during the manufacturing of cheese or casein (the predominant phoshoprotein found in fresh milk and cheese). Both are rich in protein, vitamins, and minerals, but they also may contain growth factors (Brinkworth et al., 2002, Kuipers et al., 2002). Some research appears to support ergogenic (increasing muscular work capacity by reducing or eliminating fatigue symptoms) effects in net muscle protein synthesis (Tipton & Wolfe, 2004); however, most researchers believe that more research is needed.

Although not a steroid, protein has some negative side effects. There is an increase in water weight, which you can feel around your muscles at rest. Some people experience muscle cramps, stomach upset, diarrhea, dizziness, high blood pressure, and liver and kidney damage (Terjung et al., 2000). It is important that you consult with your physician, especially discussing all medications and supplements that you use. There are a number of medications that creatine interferes with, including non-steroidal anti-inflammatory medications like ibuprofen.

Energy Drinks

Energy drinks are the latest craze used to supply mental and physical stimulation for a short period of time. They usually contain caffeine, taurine (an amino acid), and clucuronolactone (a carbohydrate). Unlike sports drinks, which provide sugars to create energy and replenish electrolytes, these energy drinks are geared to provide you with an energy-enhancing effect. An example of an energy drink is Red Bull. Some of these drinks contain 80 mg of caffeine (that's more than three times the caffeine found in a cola drink). Some of these drinks are mixed with the stimulant ephedrine, an ingredient in many decongestants. This supplement is linked to heart problems.

Caffeine may cause heart palpitations, anxiety, and insomnia, leaving you feeling jittery and irritable. It causes kidneys to remove extra fluid leaving you dehydrated. It has been linked to heart problems and is potentially deadly. The effect of diuresis (losing more water than you gain through the drink) leads to a decrease in performance.

Hyponatremia

Hyponatremia is the result of consuming too much water during prolonged exercise, which can dilute the sodium content in your blood. In the past, water consumption for endurance athletes was based on the premise that athletes were supposed to drink as much as possible to "stay ahead" of their thirst. New guidelines recommend that they should replace as much fluid as they lose due to sweat during their event. Signs and symptoms of hyponatremia include nausea, headaches, muscle cramps, confusion, and seizures. If left untreated, hyponatremia can lead to rapid swelling of the brain, resulting in coma and death (ACSM, 2005).

HOW TO FIND THE MOST TRUSTWORTHY HEALTH INFORMATION ON THE INTERNET

As you begin to research nutritional information, being able to find trustworthy health promotion information can be overwhelming with the information that you can access from the Internet. As you research sites, here are some guidelines that you can use to help you determine the reliability and quality of the information you are reading. The checklist should include the following questions (Canadian Health Network, n.d.):

Is the resource credible?

- Is the author's name clearly stated with professional or accredited authority on the subject? Is there contact information for the author or organization?
- Is the organization that is responsible for the information reputable?
- Is medical information provided by a medical professional?
- Is evidence (scientific studies, research) provided to endorse the treatment or service?

Is the content relevant to you?

- Does the content discuss the issue you are looking for with enough detail?
- Does the site contain original content or does it only link to other sites?
- Is the information presented in a Canadian context?

Does the site reflect a broad view of health?

- Does the content of the research recognize that health has many different facets, is dynamic and changing, is unique to different demographics, and is determined by many different factors?

Is the resource timely?

- Is the information continually reviewed and updated?
- Is the date of the last update clearly marked on each item?
- If the information is only valid for a short time, is this fact clearly labelled?

Is there clear and adequate disclosure?

- Is the mandate of the research clearly shared? For example, is it a non-profit organization trying to promote nutrition, exercise, and active living, or is it a product company trying to sell you its goods?
- Is the article biased or based on a conflict of interest? Are both sides of the issue presented? (For example, promotion of a vegetarian diet should indicate that there are other dietary options or clearly state that the viewpoint is just one side of a multifaceted issue.)
- Are there commercial links or sponsorships tied to the site, or links you must access before entering the intended site?
- If a site is collecting or requesting information about you, does it tell you exactly why it wants the information? Are the site's privacy guidelines stated? If you have to register to use the site, is the reason clear and is your privacy ensured?

Are there clear caution statements?

- Does the site state that health information should not be a substitute for visiting a health professional?
- If there are fees associated with use of the resources on the site, are they clearly explained?

Is the site user-friendly?

- Is information presented in a clear manner?
- Can you contact the author/organization for additional information?

Does the site support a variety of activities?

- Does the site provide links to more information or resources available on the topic? Does the site provide an opportunity for feedback? Does the site provide screening tools, surveys, games, and activities that would help you understand the topic in greater detail?

HOW FOOD COMPANIES ARE ASSISTING CANADIANS WITH EDUCATION AND HEALTHY EATING

Food and Consumer Products of Canada (FCPC, www.fcpmc.com) speaks for companies while working with the Canadian government agencies and industry to provide support to the government's commitment for nutrition, healthy lifestyles, and workplace wellness. These companies produce products and choices and provide consumer information, advertising, and marketing that meet Canadian standards set out by Agriculture and Agri-Food Canada. Here are some of the results:

- reducing hydrogenated oils in the food supply to help consumers limit consumption of trans fatty acids

- increasing the range of products with reduced levels of calories, sugar, fat, and salt, in line with current guidelines on healthy eating
- providing portion-sized options, such as single-serve packages and child-sized portions, in line with the varied needs of consumers
- attempting to add foods that supply vitamins and minerals to create nutritionally beneficial product choices
- providing nutritional information and education so that consumers can make informed choices, including labelling on packaged foods

To help consumers interpret the nutrition information on labels, the food industry, through the FCPC, supports Healthy Eating is in Store for You (HESY), an education program developed by Dietitians of Canada and the Canadian Diabetes Association. The program educates Canadians on how to use the new nutrition facts label to make healthy food choices. You can access this website at www.healthyeatingisinstore.ca.

Many companies provide websites that offer educational nutritional information about their products and healthy recipes. Some provide fun planners for physical activities, answer health questions, and offer promotional challenges or sponsored events, games, and contests to promote healthy living. Many have specialized areas for children, and some provide links to external health or activity-based organizations.

EA Tracker

To help Canadians track their daily food and activity choices, and help them track their progress, Nestlé Canada provided funding for Dietitians of Canada to develop the Eating + Activity Tracker (EA Tracker). The tool provides personalized feedback on calories, essential nutrients, activity levels, and body mass index (BMI). You can access this website at www.dietitians.ca/eatracker.

The Long Live Kids Program

In October 2004, a national child-focused initiative was developed by Health Canada in partnership with FCPC to support a public awareness and educational program that encourages children to eat smart, move more, and become media wise. The intent was to provide an educational curriculum to schools and communities to promote healthy eating and physical activity (Long Live Kids, 2004). For more information go to http://longlivekids.ca.

The first annual Active Healthy Kids Canada report, *Dropping the Ball: Canada's Report Card on Physical Activity for Children and Youth*, was released in 2005. It raised alarm bells regarding children's health and physical activity levels. The report card found that Canadian children continued to receive failing grades on participating in physical activity. The problem was most severe among adolescents aged 12–17 years (Active Healthy Kids Canada, 2005). To read this full report, go to Active Healthy Kids Canada at www.activehealthykids.ca/Ophea/ActiveHealthyKids_v2/programs_2007reportcard.cfm.

Employee Wellness Initiatives

Many private sector companies are beginning to encourage their employees to opt for healthy food choices and engage in physical activity. Some provide flexible time schedules so that employees can participate in physical fitness programs throughout the day; nutritional counselling as a benefit option; and on-site fitness centres, weight-loss programs, and cafeteria facilities with healthy food selections. Some police services in the province have followed suit. There are a few services (Peel Regional Police Service, Waterloo Police Service, and the RCMP) that have fitness and lifestyle consultants that directly work to promote these activities.

MORE NUTRITION INFORMATION

Here are some Canadian websites that can provide you with more health and nutritional information.

- *Canadian Health Network* The Canadian Health Network (www.canadian-health-network.ca) is a national, Internet-based health information service. With content from over 500 non-profit health organizations, this site provides health information you can trust. Take a look at their collection of healthy eating resources.
- *Health Canada* Health Canada (www.hc-sc.gc.ca) is the department of the federal government responsible for helping Canadians maintain and improve their health. At this site, you will find nutrition information, including *Canada's Food Guide to Healthy Eating*, *Nutrition for a Healthy Pregnancy*, and *Nutrition for Healthy Term Infants*, as well as information on the body mass index and many more resources.
- *Dietitians of Canada* This award-winning website (www.dietitians.ca) is filled with interactive tools, tips, and fact sheets for healthy eating. Check out the Eating & Activity Tracker (EATracker) to get personalized advice about your current food choices. Cruise through the Virtual Kitchen for tips and facts about the food you eat. Take the Nutrition Challenge Quiz to test your knowledge of nutrition. The website can also help you find a nutrition professional in your area.

The bottom line comes down to making educated and healthy choices for yourself. Shift work does impact availability of foods; however, if you plan appropriately and take time to prepare meals ahead of time, you can avoid the pitfalls of poor nutrition. It is important, if you want to stay healthy, that you follow the guidelines set out by *Canada's Food Guide* and ensure that you exercise. Make sure you read and ask questions. If you need assistance to get on track with eating, do not hesitate to contact your doctor or local dietitian for advice.

KEY TERMS

dietary fibre

fatty acids

trans fats

dietary cholesterol

blood cholesterol

low-density lipoprotein (LDL) cholesterol

high-density lipoprotein (HDL) cholesterol

amino acids

kilocalorie (kcal)

DASH diet

EXERCISES

Review

1. What are the six kinds of nutrients?

2. What constitutes a balanced and healthy diet?

3. What percentages of total energy intake should come from proteins, fats, and carbohydrates?

4. Why is fibre important to your diet?

5. What is the distinction between blood cholesterol and dietary cholesterol?

6. What are some ways to reduce fat in your diet?

7. What are the benefits and risks of consuming caffeine?

8. Describe some of the changes made to the new *Canada's Food Guide*.

Multiple Choice

1. According to *Canada's Food Guide*, over half of your daily calories may come from
   a. vitamins
   b. minerals
   c. fats
   d. carbohydrates
   e. proteins

2. What is the best advice for someone participating in a regular fitness program?
   a. eat as much as you can
   b. eat more protein
   c. eat a balanced diet
   d. eat fewer carbohydrates
   e. reduce all fats

3. The guidelines in *Canada's Food Guide* do *not* include
   a. enjoying a variety of foods from each of the four food groups daily
   b. choosing higher-fat foods more often
   c. emphasizing grain products, vegetables, and fruit
   d. consuming a small amount of oils and fats
   e. limiting salt, alcohol, and caffeine

4. Carbohydrates are stored in the liver and muscles in the form of
   a. fatty acids
   b. amino acids
   c. glycogen
   d. LDL
   e. HDL

5. A good source of protein is ______________ .
   a. oranges
   b. peanuts
   c. meat
   d. strawberries
   e. squash

6. The body cannot survive without which nutrient for a prolonged period of time?
   a. carbohydrates
   b. proteins
   c. fats
   d. water
   e. minerals

7. According to *Canada's Food Guide*, one serving of Grain Products would consist of
   a. one large hamburger bun
   b. one cup of hot cereal
   c. three saltine crackers
   d. one half cup of cooked rice
   e. one toasted bagel

8. Which is *least* likely to be true of complex carbohydrates?
   a. they are high in fibre
   b. they are low in calories
   c. they are low in nutrients
   d. they are low in saturated fats
   e. they are low in amino acids

9. Which of the following is good advice for weight/fat control?
   a. eat as fast as you can so you don't think about food
   b. space meals out equally throughout the day
   c. skip lunch or breakfast if you don't feel hungry
   d. eat a large dinner and a small lunch and breakfast
   e. read a book while eating to take your mind off of food

10. "Empty calories" refers to
   a. food that does not make you fat
   b. calories with a low caloric content
   c. regurgitation of food to prevent weight gain
   d. food that is low in nutrients and high in calories
   e. the apparent inability of thin people to gain weight

11. Which of the following is true of dietary fat?
   a. it should be primarily saturated
   b. it should never be consumed by an athlete
   c. it should make up 40 percent of your total caloric intake
   d. it is an essential part of the diet
   e. it has fewer calories per gram than carbohydrates

12. How many calories are found in a 4 g serving of fat?
   a. 12 kcal
   b. 15 kcal
   c. 27 kcal
   d. 36 kcal
   e. 40 kcal

13. Complete proteins, containing all the essential amino acids, are found in
   a. legumes
   b. nuts
   c. animal products
   d. wild rice
   e. leafy green vegetables

14. Water excretion is governed by the
   a. liver
   b. kidneys
   c. brain
   d. digestive system
   e. b and c

15. Most experts agree that there is a link between excessive sodium intake and
   a. cancer
   b. hypotension
   c. blood clotting
   d. diabetes
   e. hypertension

16. Which is worst for you?
   a. butter
   b. tub margarine
   c. stick margarine
   d. low-sodium whipped butter
   e. light tub margarine

17. Four of these strategies have been clearly shown to keep blood pressure from rising. Which hasn't?
   a. cutting salt
   b. losing excess weight
   c. eating potassium-rich foods
   d. getting adequate calcium
   e. exercising regularly

18. ______________ are high in saturated fats.
   a. Corn oil and soybean oil
   b. Broccoli and cauliflower
   c. Whole milk and cheeses
   d. Bread and potatoes
   e. White and whole grain rice

19. Which of the following is the best source for omega-3 fatty acids?
   a. wheat products
   b. berries
   c. corn oil
   d. pork
   e. sardines

20. DRI stands for
   a. dietary relevance index
   b. dietary requirement index
   c. daily requirement index
   d. dietary reference intakes
   e. none of the above

REFERENCES

Active Healthy Kids Canada. (2006). Active Healthy Kids Canada: Report card on physical activity for children and youth. Available at http://www.activehealthykids.ca/Ophea/ActiveHealthyKids_v2/loader.cfm?url=/commonspot/security/getfile.cfm&PageID=19082&CFID=2471957&CFTOKEN=1936640.

Adams, S.M., & Standridge, J.B. (2006). What should we eat? Evidence from observational studies. *Southern Medical Journal, 99*(7), 744-748.

American College of Sports Medicine (ACSM). (2005). Runners must hydrate properly: Experts clarify how to balance fluid loss, intake. News release. Available at http://www.acsm.org/AM/Template.cfm?Section=Home&TEMPLATE=/CM/HTMLDisplay.cfm&FUSEFLAG=1&CONTENTID=4169.

American Dietetic Association and Dietitians of Canada. (2003). Position of the American Dietetic Association and Dietitians of Canada: Vegetarian diets. Public policy statement. *Canadian Journal of Dietetic Practice and Research, 64*(2).

American Kidney Fund. (2002). AKF warns about impact of high-protein diets on kidney health. Available at http://www.atkinsexposed.org/atkins/79/American_Kidney_Fund.htm.

Astorino, T.A., Marrocco, A.C., Gross, S.M., Johnson, D.L., Brazil, C.M., Icenhower, M.E., & Kneessi, R. J. (2005). Is running performance enhanced with creatine serum ingestion? *Journal of Strength and Conditioning Research, 19*(4), 730-734.

Buijsse, B., Feskens, E.J., Schlettwein-Gsell, D., Ferry, M., Kok, F.J., Kromhout, D., & de Groot, L.C. (2005). Plasma carotene and alpha-tocopherol in relation to 10-y all-cause and cause-specific mortality in European elderly: The Survey in Europe on Nutrition and the Elderly, a Concerted Action (SENECA). *American Journal of Clinical Nutrition, 82*(4), 879-886.

Brinkworth, G., Buckley, J.D., Bourdon, P.C., Gulbin, J.P., & David, A. (2002). Oral bovine colostrums supplementation enhances buffer capacity, but not rowing performance in elite female rowers. *International Journal of Sport Nutrition and Exercise Metabolism, 12*, 349-363.

Canadian Diabetes Association. (2005). Highs and Lows: Blood glucose levels. Available at http://www.diabetes.ca/Section_About/highs-lows.asp.

Canadian Health Network. (n.d.). How to find the most trustworthy health information on the Internet. Available online at http://www.canadian-health-network.ca. Click on English, then How to Find the Most Trustworthy Health Info on the Internet.

Casa, D.J., Armstrong, L.E., & Hillman, S.K. (2000). National Athletic Trainer's Association position statement: Fluid replacement for athletes. *Journal of Athletic Training, 35*(2), 212-224.

Chandler, R., Byrne, H., Patterson, J., & Ivy, J. (1994). Dietary supplements affect the anabolic hormones after weight training exercise. *Journal of Applied Physiology, 76*, 839-845.

Clark, N. (1997). Caffeine: A user's guide. *The Physician and Sports Medicine, 25*(11).

Department of Health and Human Services. (n.d.). Low-calorie, lower-fat alternative foods. Retrieved from http://www.nhlbi.nih.gov/health/public/heart/obesity/lose_wt/lcal_fat.htm.

Drewnowski, A. (2005). Effects of fruits and vegetables on dietary patterns and energy intakes. Digestive Health Organization. Available at http://digestivehealthorg.com/?page_id=47.

Durstine, L. (2006). Understanding blood cholesterol. *Action plan for high cholesterol.* ACSM. Available at http://www.exrx.net/Testing/LDL%26HDL.html.

Eijnde, B.O., Van Leemputte, M., Goris, M., et al. (2003). Effects of creatine supplementation and exercise training on fitness in males 55 to 75 years old. *Journal of Applied Physiology, 95*, 818-828.

Falk, B., Rosenblum, J., Shapiro, Y., Zylber-Katz, E., & Bashan, N. (1990). Effects of caffeine ingestion on the body fluid balance and the thermoregulation during exercise. *Canadian Journal of Physiology and Pharmacology, 68,* 889-892.

Ferraris, R.P., & Carey, H.V. (2000). Intestinal transport during fasting and malnutrition. *Annual Review of Nutrition, 20,* 195-219.

Finn, J.P., Ebert, T.R., Withers, R.T., Carey, M.F., Mackay, M., Phillips, J.W., & Febbraio, M.A. (2001). Effect of creatine supplementation on metabolism and performance in humans during intermittent sprint cycling. *European Journal of Applied Physiology,* 84, 238-243.

Food and Nutrition Board, Institute of Medicine. (2002). Dietary reference intakes for energy, carbohydrate, fiber, fat, fatty acids, cholesterol, protein, and amino acids (macronutrients). Washington, DC: National Academies Press. Available at http://www.nap.edu/books/0309085373/html.

Foster-Powell, K., & Miller, M.F. (1995). International tables of glycemic index. *American Journal of Clinical Nutrition, 62,* 871S-873S.

Garriguet, D. (2004). Overview of Canadians' eating habits. *Nutrition: Findings from the Canadian Community Health Survey.* Statistics Canada Catalogue no. 82-620-MIE. Ottawa: Statistics Canada.

Gilliam, J.D., Hohzorn, C., Martin, D., et al. (2000). Effect of oral creatine supplementation on isokinetic torque production. *Medicine & Science in Sports & Exercise, 32,* 993–996.

Gordon, N.F., Myburgh, J.L., Kruger, P.E., Kempff, P.G., Cilliers, J.F., Moolman, J., & Grobler, H.C. (1982). Effects of caffeine ingestion on thermoregulatory and myocardial function during endurance performance. *South African Medical Journal, 62,* 644-647.

Harris, S.S., & Dawson-Hughes, B. (1989). Caffeine and bone loss in healthy postmenopausal women. *American Journal of Clinical Nutrition, 49,* 44-50.

Health Canada. (2003). Canadian guidelines for body weight classification in adults. Catalogue no. H49-179/2003E. Ottawa: Author.

Health Canada. (2006). Nutritional labelling. Available at http://www.hc-sc.gc.ca/fn-an/label-etiquet/nutrition/index_e.html.

Health Canada. (2007). Foods to limit. Public Works and Government Services Canada Publishing and Depository Services. Available at http://www.hc-sc.gc.ca/fn-an/surveill/index_e.html.

Institute of Medicine. (2005). *Dietary reference intakes for energy, carbohydrate, fibre, fat, fatty acids, cholesterol, protein and amino acids.* Washington, DC: National Academy Press.

Ivy, J.L, Res, P.R., Spague, R.C., & Widzer, M.O. (2003). Effect of a carbohydrate-protein supplement on endurance performance during exercise of varying intensity. *International Journal of Sports Nutrition and Exercise Metabolism, 21,* 1280-1286.

Jenkins, D.A., et al. (1981). Glycemic index of foods: A physiological basis for carbohydrate exchange. *American Journal of Clinical Nutrition, 34,* 362-366.

Johnson, T. (1999, July 8). U.S. Food and Drug Administration includes whole grains in fight against heart disease and cancer. USFDA press release.

Joesoef, M.R., Beral, V., Rolfs, R.T., Aral, S.O., & Cramer, D.W. (1990). Are caffeinated beverages risk factors for delayed conception? *Lancet, 335,* 136-137.

Kleiner, S. (2000). Bodybuilding. In Rosenbloom, C. (Ed.), *Sports nutrition: A guide for the professional working with active people* (3rd ed.). Chicago: American Dietetic Association.

Kuipers, H., van Breda, E., Verlaan, G., & Smeets, R. (2002). Effects of oral bovine colostrum supplementation on serum insulin-like growth factor-I levels. *Nutrition, 18,* 566-567.

Leenders, N., Sherman, W.M., Lamb, D.R., & Nelson, T.E. (1999). Creatine supplementation and swimming performance. *International Journal of Sport Nutrition, 9,* 251-262.

Long Live Kids. (2004). Health rock. Available at http://longlivekids.ca.

Mujika, I., Padilla, S., Ibanez, J., Izquierdo, M., & Gorostiaga, E. (2000). Creatine supplementation and sprint performance in soccer players. *Medicine & Science in Sports & Exercise, 32*, 518-525.

National Institutes of Health. (2006). DASH eating plan: Your guide to lowering your blood pressure with DASH. US Department of Health and Human Services. NIH Publications No. 06-4082 Revised April 2006. Available at http://www.nhlbi.nih.gov/health/public/heart/hbp/dash/new_dash.pdf.

National Institutes of Health (n.d.) Low-calorie, lower-fat alternative foods. Department of Health and Human Services. National Heart Lung and Blood Institute. Obesity Education. Available at http://www.nhlbi.nih.gov/health/public/heart/obesity/lose_wt/lcal_fat.htm.

Neergaard, L. (2007). As foods dump trans fat, are they really getting healthier? Medbroadcast Health News. Canadian Press. Available at http://www.medbroadcast.com/channel_health_news_details.asp?news_id=12136&channel_id=1018&relation_id=0&newsletterid=7128.

Oomen, C.M, Ocké, M.C., Freskens, E.J.M., van Erp-Baart, M.J., Kok, F.J., & Kromhout, D. (2001). Association between trans fatty acid intake and 10-year risk of coronary heart disease in the Zutphen Elderly Study: A prospective population based study, *Lancet, 357*, 746-751.

Parillo, M., Rivellese, A.A., Ciardullo, A.V., Capaldo, B., Giacco, A., Genovese, S., & Riccardi, G. (1992). A high-monounsaturated-fat/low-carbohydrate diet improves peripheral insulin sensitivity in non-insulin-dependent diabetic patients, *Metabolism, 41*, 1373-1378.

Roberts, C.K., & Barnard, R.J. (2003). Low-carbohydrate diets as compared with low-fat diets. *New England Journal of Medicine, 349*(10), 1000-1002.

Sheard, N.F., Clark, N.G., Brand-Miller, J.C., Franz, M.J., Pi-Sunyer, F.X., Mayer-Davis, E., Kulkarni, K., & Geil, P. (2004). Dietary carbohydrate (amount and type) in the prevention and management of diabetes: A statement by the American Diabetes Association. *Diabetes Care, 27*(9), 2266-2271.

Shields, M. (2005). *Nutrition: Findings from the Canadian Community Health Survey.* Issue no. 1. *Measured obesity: Overweight Canadian children and adolescents.* Catalogue no. 82-620-MWE2005001. Ottawa: Statistics Canada.

Sizer, F., & Whitney, E. (1997). *Nutrition: Concepts and controversies* (7th ed.). Belmont, CA: Wadsworth.

Strain, E.C., Mumford, G.K., Silverman, K., & Griffiths, R.R. (1994). Caffeine dependence syndrome: Evidence from case histories and experimental evaluations. *Journal of the American Medical Association, 272*, 1043-1048.

Terjung, R.L., Clarkson, P., Eichner, E.R., Greenhaff, P.L., Hespel, P.J., Israel, R.G., Kraemer, W.J., Mayer, R.A., Spiret, L.L., Tarnopolsky, M.A., Wagemakers, A.J., & Williams, M.H. (March 2000). American College of Sports Medicine Roundtable: The physiological and health effects of oral creatine supplements. *Medicine and Science in Sports and Exercise, 32*(3), 706-717.

Tipton, K., & Wolfe, R. (2004). Protein and amino acids for athletes. *Journal of Sports Sciences, 22*, 65-74.

Tjepkema, M. (2005). *Nutrition: Findings from the Canadian Community Health Survey.* Issue no. 1. *Measured obesity: Adult obesity in Canada.* Catalogue no. 82-620-MWE2005001. Ottawa: Statistics Canada.

Willett, W.C., Stampfer, M.J., Manson, J.E., Colditz, G.A., Speizer, F.E., & Rosner, B.A. (1993). Intake of trans fatty acids and risk of coronary heart disease. *Lancet, 341*, 581-585.

Willett, W.C., Stampfer, M.J., Manson, J.E., Colditz, G.A., Rosner, B.A., Speizer, F.E., & Hennekens, C.H. (1996). Coffee consumption and coronary heart disease in women: A ten-year follow-up. *Journal of the American Medical Association, 275*, 458-462.

CHAPTER 9

Body Composition

CHAPTER OBJECTIVES

After completing this chapter, you should be able to:

- Understand the issues surrounding overweight and obesity in Canada.
- Distinguish between the concepts of overfat and overweight.
- Describe the three somatotypes (body types).
- Explain how basal metabolism affects body composition.
- Explain the eating disorders, including anorexia nervosa, bulimia nervosa, and the female athlete triad.
- Describe several methods for measuring body composition.

In chapter 1 you learned that weight-related problems are a health risk for many Canadians. This chapter examines obesity, eating disorders, and other weight-related issues more closely by delving into the question of what constitutes a healthy body composition.

MISGUIDED VIEWS OF THE BODY

Whereas many Canadians are justly concerned about being overweight, many others who are within a healthy weight range are obsessed with weight loss. The media equate beauty with thinness in women and muscularity in men, which contributes to the obsession with weight (Canadian Society for Exercise Physiology, 1996). As a result, problems such as anorexia, bulimia, and binge dieting arise. People struggle to maintain healthy weights. If eating better and exercising more always worked, we would not have so many diets on the market. The reality is that there are many social and environmental factors that come into play. It is not always easy to make healthy choices.

There has been a significant increase in the combined overweight/obesity rate among youth aged 12 to 17 in the last 25 years and, according to Tjepkema (2005), almost one-third (32.5 percent) of Canadians aged 18 years have a body mass index (BMI) in the overweight category. In addition, 14.9 percent have a BMI in the obese category, an increase from the 14.1 percent observed in 2000–2001 (Shields, 2005). An additional 36 percent (8.6 million) were overweight.The health consequences of excess weight include an increased risk for type 2 diabetes, cardiovascular disease, high blood pressure, osteoarthritis, some cancers, and gallbladder disease (Health Canada, 2003; Canadian Institute for Health Information, 2004). According to research estimates, the total number of deaths in Canada related to overweight and obesity from 1985 to 2000 was more than 57,000 (Katzmarzyk & Ardern, 2004). It is estimated that the direct cost of weight-related major chronic diseases on Canada's health care system was nearly $1.6 billion in 2001, and $4.3 billion if you consider indirect costs (Katzmarzyk & Janssen, 2004).

In the 1960s and 1970s insurance companies based their life and health premiums on height–weight tables. The more you weighed within a certain height class, the more you paid. The insurance companies did not take bone size into account, nor did they look at fat as a *percentage* of body weight. They simply assumed that higher weight equalled higher risk. But research in the 1990s led health experts to the idea that there are many kinds of healthy body shapes and sizes, and to the notion that each person has an "acceptable weight range." We no longer need to look simply at weight, but must turn our attention to the percentages of fat, bone, and muscle in our bodies.

Body weight is affected by our genetic makeup, our eating choices, our level of physical activity, and our social, cultural, physical, and economic environments. Where we live, learn, play, and work are all factors that affect our body weight. Consider the following data:

- Statistics Canada has determined that those with less than a secondary education eat less fruit and vegetables and have higher rates of obesity (Tjepkema, 2005).
- In terms of socio-economic status, obesity rates are higher among Canadian women in middle- and upper-middle-income households compared with highest-income households, while men in lower-middle-income households are less obese than those in highest-income households (Tjepkema, 2005).
- Physical activity levels are higher among Canadians who have a positive social support network and are in more frequent contact with their friends and family (Spanier & Allison, 2001).
- People who work in physically active jobs have a lower likelihood of being obese (King et al., 2001).
- People that were obese as children are more likely to be obese as young adults. Statistics for 2004 show that 18 percent of Canadian children and youth aged 2 to 17 years (excluding those in the territories) were overweight and 8 percent were obese (Shields, 2005).
- Neighbourhoods that have better street lighting, sidewalks, recreational facilities, and playgrounds have more physically fit individuals living in them (Addy et al., 2004).
- In terms of gender, Canadian men and women were equally likely (23 percent) to be obese in 2004; however, of the three classifications of obesity, a higher percentage of women than men were in Class III (BMI > 40) (Tjepkema, 2005).

- In 2004, off-reserve Aboriginal adults had an obesity rate 1.6 times higher (38 percent) than the Canadian average of 23 percent (Tjepkema, 2005).
- In 2004, 21 percent of Canadian children aged 2 to 5, 26 percent of those aged 6 to 11, and 29 percent of youth aged 12 to 17 were overweight or obese (Shields, 2005).
- Canadian data show that, regardless of the time since immigration, the odds of being overweight were lower among East/Southeast Asian immigrant adults than among white immigrants, and, relative to immigrant white women, the odds of being overweight were higher among long-term immigrant black and Latin American women (Tremblay, 2005).
- The connection between mental health and unhealthy weights is not restricted to obesity. Mental health problems are also associated with a number of issues surrounding eating disorders such as anorexia, bulimia, and binge eating disorders (Health Canada, 2002). Girls and women are affected more than boys and men; approximately 3 percent of women will be affected by an eating disorder. Approximately 27 percent of Ontario girls aged 12 to 18 were reported to be engaged in severe problematic food and weight behaviour (Jones, 2001). Hospitalization for eating disorders rose by 34 percent among girls under 15 from 1987 to 1999, and by 29 percent among those aged 15 to 24 over the same period (Health Canada, 2002).
- Body image is not just a women's problem. More and more studies are revealing that men are dissatisfied, preoccupied, and impaired by concerns over their appearance. One study found that the percentage of men dissatisfied with their overall appearance (43 percent) had nearly tripled in the past 25 years (Pope, Phillips, & Olivardia, 2000). There is also a growing form of male body dysmorphic disorder called muscle dysmorphia, which is a preoccupation that one's body is too small and inadequately muscular (Phillips & Castle, 2001). In reality, many men are large and muscular. Of particular concern, muscle dysmorphia may lead to potentially dangerous abuse of anabolic steroids, and studies indicate that 6 to 7 percent of high school boys have used these drugs (Pope et al., 2000). While the cause of body dysmorphic disorder is unknown and probably multi-factorial, involving genetic-neurobiological, evolutionary, and psychological factors, social pressures for boys and men to be large and muscular almost certainly contribute to the development of muscle dysmorphia (Phillips & Castle, 2001). This disorder may also go along with an eating disorder.

BODY COMPOSITION

Body composition refers to the proportion of lean tissue to fat in the body. Determining this proportion can provide an indicator of overall health and fitness in relation to weight and age. Many factors, including sex, age, heredity, activity, overall nutrition, and eating patterns, affect your body composition.

body composition
the proportion of lean tissue to fat in the body

Your body needs fat for fuel and other purposes, but if you consume too much fat and neglect physical activity, you end up with non-essential fat stored in various areas of your body. Adults over 30 tend to carry more fat on their frames than younger people do. Generally, women accumulate more fat than men do, and it tends to be distributed more evenly over the entire body (among men, the fat tends to accumulate more on the trunk and less on the extremities). Abdominal obesity is one of the six components of "metabolic syndrome"—a cluster of risk factors that increase an individual's risk of developing heart disease, diabetes, and a number of other conditions (Grundy et al., 2004).

But being overweight does not necessarily equal obesity, because many physically fit people are overweight from muscle gain (muscle is heavier than fat). Of course, people can be overweight because they carry excess fat, but it is important to distinguish between the concepts of overfat and overweight.

All fat in your body is classified as either essential or non-essential fat. Essential fat is required for normal functioning of your body. Deposits of this fat can be found in your muscles, heart, brain, spinal cord, nerves, lungs, and liver. Fat serves as an energy reserve, a regulator of body functions, an insulator against heat loss, and a protector against physical shock.

Non-essential or storage fat is stored below the surface of the skin and around major organs. Although some fat is vital for insulation and organ protection, too much can put you at health risk.

Somatotypes

somatotype
body type—there are three somatotypes: ectomorphic, mesomorphic, and endomorphic

A person's body composition is affected by his or her **somatotype** (body type). Most people have a genetic predisposition toward a specific somatotype, although it is mixed with some traits of a second somatotype. There are three somatotypes: ectomorphic, mesomorphic, and endomorphic.

- An ectomorph has a low percentage of fat in the body, small bones, a small amount of muscle, and a high metabolic rate. With this light build and slight muscular development, ectomorphs usually have a harder time gaining weight, and spend more time on strength training and less on cardiovascular training.
- A mesomorph has a low to medium percentage of fat in the body, medium to large bones, a large amount of muscle, and a medium to high metabolic rate. Many mesomorphs have a large chest and long torso, and are able to build muscle easily.
- An endomorph has a high percentage of fat in the body, large bones, a small amount of muscle, and a low metabolic rate. This body type tends to have a stocky build, wide hips, and a tendency to gain weight. Since this weight gain is more around the middle, it is harder for endomorphs to lose weight. They need to pay close attention to their diet, and focus on cardiovascular training over strength training.

Although your somatotype is inherited and cannot be changed, diet and exercise can reduce the percentage of fat in your body.

METABOLISM

Metabolism describes the chemical processes that occur within a living cell or organism, which are necessary for the maintenance of life. Some substances are broken down to yield energy for vital processes (for example, carbohydrates are broken down into glucose), while other substances are synthesized (such as muscle tissue and cells).

Basal Metabolism

Body composition is also affected by **basal metabolism**, the amount of energy a body at rest needs to maintain essential functions. The **basal metabolic rate (BMR)** is the speed at which energy is used by the body. Factors affecting the BMR include age, sex, and level of physical activity.

basal metabolism
the amount of energy a body at rest needs to maintain essential functions

basal metabolic rate (BMR)
the speed at which energy is used by the body

Your metabolism affects your ability to lose or gain weight. A high metabolic rate makes it easier to burn fat and lose weight. If your metabolism is not working properly, you will find it more difficult to keep your weight stable or to lose weight.

Cutting calories lowers your metabolic rate. Your body senses the reduction in energy intake and slows down the burning of fat to protect the fat it has. After about three months your metabolic rate levels off and you no longer lose weight. If you return to your old eating habits, your body will store more fat than it used to because the metabolic rate remains depressed. Eventually you may gain back all the weight, and even put on more weight.

When you fast for at least six to eight hours, the body protects its fat reserves by starting to break down protein instead of fat for energy. Since protein is an important constituent of muscle and other tissues, by fasting you harm key parts of the body. (The same holds true to an even greater extent in the extreme cases of anorexia and bulimia.)

The key to maintaining a healthy weight is to combine proper eating (as described in chapter 8) with a good exercise program. A program of cardiovascular exercise 30 minutes a day, every day of the week, will improve your cardiovascular system, increase your metabolic rate, and burn fat. Weight and strength training 20 minutes a day, three days a week, will increase your muscular strength and endurance, make you leaner, and have a beneficial effect on bone density.

MEASURING OVERWEIGHT AND OBESITY

Under the current Canadian guidelines for body weight classification, the term *overweight* refers to anyone with a body mass index (BMI) of 25.0 to 29.9. The term *obese* refers to someone with a BMI of 30 or more (Health Canada, 2000). BMI is used to identify weight-related health risks in individuals 18 years of age and older. Health Canada suggests that for those 65 years and older, "the normal range may begin slightly above a BMI of 18.5 and extend into the overweight range" (Health Canada, 2000, p. 10). BMI is calculated by dividing a person's body weight in kilograms by the square of his or her height in metres (Health Canada, 2000). For example, someone who is 1.8 m tall and weighs 71 kg would have a BMI of 21.9 (that is, $71/1.8^2 = 21.9$).

body mass index (BMI) measurement
a method for assessing body composition, based on weight and height

Body mass index (BMI) measurement is a popular method among health care professionals for determining whether, and to what extent, a person is overweight or obese. It is based on a weight–height ratio, and excludes considerations of frame size and muscle mass. Excluding pregnant women and those under age 18, whose rate of growth is varied, the BMI puts individuals into four categories: underweight, normal weight, overweight, and obese. The obese category is divided further.

Go to **assignment 9.1** (in the appendix) and determine your BMI.

What Does the BMI Score Mean?

For adult males and females, a BMI greater than 30.0 indicates obesity. Underweight adult males and females have a BMI of less than 18.5. Being underweight can weaken the immune system, making one more susceptible, for example, to catching cold. A very low BMI also alerts health care professionals to the possibility of anorexia or similar problems. In Canada almost one-half of Canadians are overweight or obese, while a similar proportion is in the normal weight range and a very small proportion is underweight. Canadians rank in the middle of the G7 countries in terms of the proportion of their population that is obese. See table 9.1 for an overview of body weight classifications.

Obesity is a risk factor for problems such as heart disease, hypertension, high cholesterol, diabetes, and some forms of cancer. Note, however, that a high BMI is not necessarily a problem for competitive athletes and bodybuilders (whose BMI may be high because their muscle mass is greater than average), pregnant or lactating women, children, and sedentary elderly people. Other tools are needed to assess the body composition of these groups. We do know that overweight status indicates some risk to health. Research suggests that regular physical activity can decrease the risk of several health problems. Equally, a nutritious diet has been shown to decrease some of the risks associated with being overweight.

waist circumference (WC)
an indicator of health risk associated with abdominal fat

Waist Circumference

Waist circumference (WC) is an indicator of health risks associated with excess abdominal fat. WC measurement can be used for individuals with a BMI in the 18.5–34.9 range. For BMIs equal to or exceeding 35.0, WC measurements do not provide additional information regarding the level of risk. Go to **assignment 9.2** (in the appendix) to determine your waist circumference.

Health Risk Classification

Excess fat around the waist and upper body (also described as an "apple" body shape) is associated with greater health risks than excess fat in the hip and thigh area (described as a "pear" body shape). A WC at or above 102 cm (40 inches) for men and 88 cm (35 inches) for women is associated with an increased risk of developing health problems such as diabetes, heart disease, and high blood pressure. The risk of developing health problems increases as WC increases beyond the cut-off points listed above. By looking at these two indicators, those individuals who are overweight but not obese and scored higher in the BMI will see that they are in a lower risk category. In other words, their muscle weighs more and, at this point in their lives, they are at less risk as long as they keep abdominal fat off. Take note, however, that even if the BMI of an individual is in the normal weight range, a high WC indicates some health risk. A marked weight change—either weight gain or weight loss—may place a person at risk even if he or she remains within the same BMI category. Using unhealthy practices such as restrictive eating habits to manage body weight can also increase a person's risk of health problems, even for those within the normal weight category (Health Canada, 2003). See table 9.2 for an overview of health risk classifications.

Skinfold Measurements

The Canadian Society for Exercise Physiology (1996) recommends **skinfold measurement** for determining whether people whose BMI is greater than 27 are truly overweight or overfat. Unlike BMI measurement, skinfold measurement takes body type into account. The procedure involves using calipers to measure skinfolds at five points on the body. Fitness club staff or your college fitness instructor may be available to assess your body composition this way.

skinfold measurement measurement of fat just below the skin surface at five points on the body to determine the percentage of body fat

TABLE 9.1 Canadian Guidelines for Body Weight Classification in Adults

Classification	BMI category (kg/m²)	Risk of developing health problems
Underweight	< 18.5	Increased
Normal weight	18.5–24.9	Least
Overweight	25.0–29.9	Increased
Obese		
Class I	30.0–34.9	High
Class II	35.0–39.9	Very high
Class III	≥ 40.0	Extremely high

Source: Health Canada. (2000). *Canadian guidelines for weight classification in adults.* Ottawa: Author. Adapted from World Health Organization (WHO). (2000). *Obesity: Preventing and managing the global epidemic: Report of a WHO consultation on obesity.* Geneva: Author.

TABLE 9.2 Health Risk Classification Using Both BMI and WC

		BMI		
		Normal	Overweight	Obese Class 1
WC	< 102 cm (males) < 88 cm (females)	Least risk	Increased risk	High risk
WC	≥ 102 cm (males) ≥ 88 cm (females)	Increased risk	High risk	Very high risk

Source: Adapted from National Institutes of Health (NIH). (1998). *Clinical guidelines on the identification, evaluation and treatment of overweight and obesity in adults: The evidence report.* Bethesda, MD: Author.

Waist-to-Hip Ratio Measurement

waist-to-hip ratio (WHR) measurement
a method for assessing body composition, based on the relationship between the girth of the waist and the girth of the hips

Waist-to-hip ratio (WHR) measurement is based on the relationship between the girth of the waist and the girth of the hips. Most people store excess fat either around the middle (making the body apple shaped) or on the hips (making the body pear shaped). It is generally accepted that people who carry their extra weight around the middle face a greater health risk than those who carry it on the hips. Nevertheless, obese people are more at risk than non-obese people, no matter where the excess fat is stored.

Turn to **assignment 9.3** (in the appendix) and determine your WHR.

For men, a WHR of 1.0 or greater indicates that excess fat is being carried around the middle, increasing the health risks associated with hypokinetic diseases (diseases related to lack of physical activity). For women, the crucial number is 0.8 or greater.

EATING DISORDERS

Overweight is not the only kind of weight and body image problem that occurs in our society. Western society's obsession with thinness as the ideal—especially in females, as seen in magazines, movies, and advertisements—causes many girls and women constant angst about their weight (note, however, that males can and do develop anorexia and bulimia). A preoccupation with body shape and weight, along with the extensive range of diets on the market, has led many people with poor self-image and underlying emotional problems to develop a variety of eating disorders. Approximately 3 percent of women will be affected by an eating disorder during their lifetime (Health Canada, 2002). Eating disorders carry with them a high risk of other mental and physical illnesses that can lead to death. Eating of smaller or larger portions of food than usual is common, but for some people this turns into a compulsion and their eating behaviours become extreme.

Anorexia and bulimia nervosa are often seen as "female illnesses." Although it is true that statistically more females than males are diagnosed, these disorders can and do afflict males as well. Approximately 10 percent of those with eating disorders are male (Wolf, 1991). Men who are runners, wrestlers, bodybuilders, and jockeys appear to be at higher risk than the general population.

Anorexia Nervosa

anorexia nervosa
an eating disorder in which individuals do not eat enough to maintain a healthy body weight

Anorexia nervosa is a serious medical and psychiatric disorder. People who suffer from it do not eat enough calories to maintain a healthy body weight. They usually begin at a normal or slightly above-average weight, and then starve themselves and exercise excessively to burn calories. These individuals refuse to maintain a normal body weight and have a distorted perception of the shape or size of their bodies (American Psychiatric Association, 1994). Anorexia often begins during adolescence, when many individuals have poor self-confidence and self-image.

Symptoms include extreme dieting, excessive weight loss, failure to start menses, amenorrhea (an abnormal end to menstruation), hyperactivity, intense fear of weight gain, and unusual behaviour toward food. Those affected can have dangerously low blood pressure and body temperature, chronic constipation, stunted growth, hair loss, and nail destruction. These can lead to life-threatening chemical imbalances and organ damage, which can lead to death (American Psychiatric Association, 1994; NAMI, 2003). Treatment usually involves hospitalization and behavioural therapy to help the person regain control over her or his perception of body image, eating habits, and self-esteem as it relates to friends and families.

Bulimia Nervosa

People who suffer from **bulimia nervosa** may be able to maintain a normal weight but have an intense fear of being overweight and overfat. They have a distorted body image. Bulimia is characterized by uncontrollable binge eating followed by self-induced vomiting. Many bulimics rely on laxatives and diuretics to prevent the food from being absorbed by their bodies. The majority of bulimics are women in

bulimia nervosa
an eating disorder in which individuals have an intense fear of overweight and overfat that causes binge eating followed by self-induced vomiting

WARNING SIGNS OF EATING DISORDERS

The following behaviours may indicate that a person you care about has an eating disorder:

1. a marked decrease or increase in weight that is not related to a medical condition
2. a preoccupation with food
3. unusual eating habits such as cutting up food into tiny pieces, playing with food, or hiding/disguising uneaten food
4. hiding or hoarding of large amounts of food hoarded in unusual places (for example, bedroom, closet)
5. a preoccupation with weight
6. constant dissatisfaction with weight and body size/image despite weight loss, dress size, etc.
7. negative and self-critical comments about body shape, size, and physical appearance
8. behavioural changes including isolation, depression, irritability, or loss of trust in friends
9. frequent trips to the washroom, especially after meals
10. smell of vomit in the washroom or on the breath
11. abuse of laxatives, diet pills, or diuretics
12. excessive exercising or multiple, daily trips to the gym
13. wearing of baggy clothes used to mask weight loss

Help is available, for you and the person you care about. Contact:

- HealthyOntario.com
  www.healthyontario.com/features/eating_disorders.htm
- What's Eating You?
  www.whatseatingyou.com

their late teens or early 20s who have suffered a critical incident. They have difficulty handling emotions like depression, loneliness, and anger. They also have low self-esteem and tend to come from families with high expectations. The eating disorder may be an attempt to gain control over one part of their life.

Symptoms include a cycle of uncontrollable eating binges followed by self-purging, use of laxatives and diuretics, menstrual irregularities, fluctuations in weight, dental decay, salivary gland enlargement, bowel problems or digestive complaints, and feelings of guilt and depression (Stice, 2002; Jacobi et al., 2004; American Psychiatric Association, 1994). Treatment includes drug therapy and psychotherapy to treat depression and emotional problems and to change eating patterns.

While these behaviours may be contained to a single episode, many relapse continually. Those who have substance use disorders are at higher risk for long-term health problems (Keel et al., 1999). Long-term physical effects include heart conditions, electrolyte imbalance, and kidney failure, which can lead to death. Even one acute episode can result in psychological, social, and health problems, including depression, alcohol dependency, and anxiety disorders (Lewinsohn et al., 2000; American Psychiatric Association Work Group on Eating Disorders, 2000; Sullivan et al., 1998). These eating disorders are usually not public issues, resulting in the mistaken impression that others (such as, family members) are to blame.

Binge Eating Disorder

binge eating disorder (BED)
an eating disorder associated with obesity, where the person alternately eats obsessively and then diets and restricts eating; the disorder is diagnosed if the person does not follow the binge eating with compensatory behaviours such as vomiting, excessive exercise, or laxative abuse

Binge eating disorder (BED) is diagnosed if the binge eating is not followed by compensatory behaviours such as vomiting, excessive exercise, or laxative abuse. This disorder is associated with obesity. BED usually starts during adolescence or young adulthood. Men are more likely to be affected by BED than by other eating disorders. Individuals with BED who are obese must contend with negative societal attitudes toward obesity. As a result, many become isolated and lose self-esteem. They are hungry because they have been dieting or restricting their eating in response to that hunger. Many overeat to comfort themselves, to avoid uncomfortable situations, or to numb their feelings. They feel that they are out of control and unable to stop eating.

Female Athlete Triad

female athlete triad
an eating disorder among female athletes defined by three conditions: disordered eating, amenorrhea, and osteoporosis

The **female athlete triad** was first described in the early 1990s. It is defined by three conditions: disordered eating, amenorrhea, and osteoporosis. Although researchers are still determining to what extent this condition occurs, Yeager et al. (1993) believe that a large percentage of women who are suffering from it are not diagnosed. The concern is not only for the performance of these athletes but also for their future health.

DISORDERED EATING

The first part of the female athlete triad is the precipitating event for the triad (Yeager et al., 1993). "Disordered eating" refers to a broad spectrum of abnormal eating behaviours (Sanborn et al., 2000). At the severe end of the spectrum are athletes who meet the diagnostic criteria for anorexia or bulimia. At the other end of the spectrum are athletes who are consuming fewer calories than their body requires.

They may appear to be eating a healthy diet, but they are not consuming enough calories. Whichever end of the spectrum applies to a woman, this mismatch of energy needed versus what she is consuming creates an energy drain on the endocrine system, which in turn leads to the second and third parts of the triad.

AMENORRHEA

Amenorrhea is the cessation of menstrual periods for three or more consecutive cycles. It is the result of insufficient estrogen production by the ovaries. Missing periods is a warning sign that something is not right in the female body. Confirmation by medical diagnosis is important and should not be ignored. Women who do not menstruate for more than three or four months can lose bone strength.

Amenorrhea is associated with a condition known as *anorexia athletica*, in which people exercise excessively because they believe this will control their bodies and give them a sense of power, control, and self-respect. These excessive behaviours may lead to amenorrhea. Some of the symptoms include over-exercise, being fanatical about weight and diet, taking time away from school, work, and relationships to exercise, a focus on the outcome of exercising rather than the fun of participating, a belief that self-worth is dependent on physical results, being disappointed with training outcomes, and saying things like, "It's okay to exercise this much because I'm an athlete" (National Eating Disorder Information Centre, 2005).

OSTEOPOROSIS

Osteoporosis is another consequence of inadequate estrogen. Yeager et al. (1993) describe osteoporosis in the female athlete triad as "premature bone loss or inadequate bone formation." They point out that the failure to build bone at a normal rate or losing bone density at a young age leads to short- and long-term problems, including stress fractures and early bone mineral density loss. After the age of 30, women can expect to lose an average of 0.5 percent of bone density per year, a rate that accelerates to 2 percent after menopause (Yeager et al., 1993). Without estrogen, these young athletes may never be able to maximize bone mineral density.

Treatment for female athlete triad takes multiple approaches. In addition to medical diagnosis and supervision, the athlete requires nutritional education and some form of counselling to deal with the disorder.

It is important for athletes not to skip meals and snacks in order to maintain enough energy for competition. Snacking on foods such as bagels, cheese, unsalted nuts and seeds, raw vegetables, fruit, and granola bars will aid in acquiring the required amount of iron, calcium, and protein. It is also important for female athletes to keep track of their menstrual periods and to discuss any irregularities with a physician.

If you recognize the symptoms of any eating disorder in yourself or a friend, do not hesitate to do something about it. There are excellent counselling services available that can help individuals get back on track and get the proper medical attention. As a police officer, while you are not qualified to make diagnoses, you can watch for signs that should not be ignored. These may include physical or sexual abuse, emotional abuse (teasing and harassment), perfectionism, rigidity, and substance abuse and elite performance in competitive sports in which body shape and size are factors.

KEY TERMS

body composition

somatotype

basal metabolism

basal metabolic rate (BMR)

body mass index (BMI) measurement

waist circumference (WC)

skinfold measurement

waist-to-hip ratio (WHR) measurement

anorexia nervosa

bulimia nervosa

binge eating disorder (BED)

female athlete triad

EXERCISES

Review

1. What issues surround overweight and obesity in Canada?

2. Describe the three somatotypes.

3. Explain the terms *body mass index* and *waist-to-hip ratio.*

4. Determine the BMI for an adult female who is 1.70 m tall and weighs 55.0 kg. Comment on the result.

5. Why is fasting a poor way to lose weight? What is a more appropriate way to modify body weight?

6. How are eating disorders not just physical problems?

7. What methods are available to assess your body composition?

Multiple Choice

1. The following signs all indicate an eating disorder except
   a. unusual eating behaviours such as cutting up food into very small pieces, playing with food, or hiding or disguising food that is uneaten
   b. disordered eating, amenorrhea, and osteoporosis
   c. an intense fear of being overweight and overfat
   d. satisfaction with body weight and body shape or size
   e. uncontrollable binge eating followed by self-induced vomiting

2. What is one health risk associated with obesity?
   a. diabetes
   b. glaucoma
   c. nerve disorder
   d. indigestion
   e. hernia

3. Which of the following is true about overweight?
   a. it is defined as "excessive abdominal fat"
   b. it is possible to be obese and not overweight
   c. overweight and obesity mean the same thing
   d. it is possible to be overweight but not obese
   e. overweight is the same as being underweight

4. Which of the following is a characteristic of anorexia nervosa?
   a. intense fear of fat
   b. denial of appetite
   c. avoidance of food
   d. excessive exercising
   e. all of the above

5. The female athlete triad is characterized by
   a. disordered eating, amenorrhea, and osteoporosis
   b. disordered eating, dismenorrhea, and weight gain
   c. weight gain, amenorrhea, and excessive exercise
   d. weight gain, amenorrhea, and osteoporosis
   e. none of the above

6. The body mass index (BMI) is determined by
   a. skinfolds
   b. body weight
   c. body height
   d. body weight and body height
   e. body weight and skinfolds

7. The three somatotype bodies are
   a. ectomorphic, endomorphic, and mesomorphic
   b. ectomorphic, endomorphic, and mendomorphic
   c. ectomorphic, mesomorphic, and cytomorphic
   d. endomorphic, mesomorphic, and octomorphic
   e. endomorphic, mesomorphic, and mendomorphic

8. A high BMI may indicate
   a. a low immune system
   b. overweight
   c. anorexia
   d. a healthy body
   e. none of the above

9. The waist-to-hip ratio (WHR) provides an estimate of
   a. fatness
   b. location of regional fat deposition
   c. cholesterol
   d. athletic potential
   e. the percentage of fat in your body

10. Bulimia nervosa is associated with all the following except
    a. fear of becoming obese
    b. restricted eating patterns
    c. periods of binging and purging
    d. high levels of physical activity
    e. suffering from a critical incident

11. The body mass index measures
    a. the relationship between height and weight
    b. bioelectrical impedance
    c. girth (or circumference) at various body sites
    d. anorexia nervosa
    e. percentage of body fat

12. An eating disorder characterized by excessive preoccupation with food, self-starvation, and/or extreme exercising to achieve weight loss is known as
    a. bulimia nervosa
    b. anorexia nervosa
    c. binge eating disorder
    d. social physique anxiety
    e. satiety

13. Jadie is 1.65 m tall and weighs 60 kg. Her BMI is approximately
    a. 20
    b. 21
    c. 22
    d. 23
    e. 24

REFERENCES

Addy, C.L., et al. (2004). Associations of perceived social and physical environmental supports with physical activity and walking behavior. *American Journal of Public Health, 94*(3), 440-443.

American Psychiatric Association. (1994). *Diagnostic and statistical manual of mental disorders* (4th ed.). Washington, DC: Author.

American Psychiatric Association Work Group on Eating Disorders. (2000). Practice guidelines for the treatment of patients with eating disorders. *American Journal of Psychiatry, 157*, 1-39.

Canadian Institute for Health Information. (2004). *Improving the health of Canadians.* Ottawa: Author.

Canadian Society for Exercise Physiology. (1996). *Canadian standardised test of fitness interpretation and counselling manual.* Ottawa: Author.

Grundy, S. M., et al. (2004). Definition of metabolic syndrome: Report of the National Heart, Lung, and Blood Institute/American Heart Association Conference on Scientific Issues Related to Definition. *Circulation, 109*(3), 433-438.

Health Canada. (2000). *Canadian guidelines for weight classification in adults.* Ottawa: Author.

Health Canada. (2002). *A report on mental illnesses in Canada.* Catalogue no. 0-662-32817-5. Ottawa: Author.

Health Canada. (2003). *Canadian guidelines for body weight classification in adults.* Ottawa: Author.

Jacobi, C., Hayward, C., de Zwaan, M., Kraemer, H., & Agras, W.S. (2004). Coming to terms with risk factors for eating disorders: Application of risk terminology and suggestions for a general taxonomy. *Psychological Bulletin,130*(1), 19-65.

Jones, J.M., Bennett, S., Olmsted, M.P., et al. (2001). Disordered eating attitudes and behaviours in teenaged girls: A school-based study. *Canadian Medical Association Journal, 165*(5), 547-552.

Katzmarzyk, P.T., & Ardern, C.I. (2004). Overweight and obesity mortality trends in Canada, 1985–2000. *Canadian Journal of Public Health, 95*(1), 16-20.

Katzmarzyk, P.T., & Janssen, I. (2004). The economic costs associated with physical inactivity and obesity in Canada: An update. *Canadian Journal of Applied Physiology, 29*(1), 90-115.

Keel, P.K., Mitchell, J.E., Miller, K.B., Davis T.L., & Crow, S.J. (1999). Long-term outcome of bulimia nervosa. *Archives of General Psychiatry, 56*, 63-69.

King, G.A, Fitzhugh, E.C., Bassett, D.R., McLaughlin, J.E., Strath, S.J., Swartz, A.M., & Thomson, D.L. (2001). Relationship of leisure-time physical activity and occupational activity to the prevalence of obesity. *International Journal of Obesity and Related Metabolic Disorders, 25*, 606-612.

Lewinsohn, P.M., Striegel-Moore, R.H., & Seeley, J.R. (2000). Epidemiology and natural course of eating disorders in young women from adolescence to young adulthood. *Journal of the American Academy of Child Adolescent Psychiatry, 30*, 1284-1292.

National Alliance on Mental Illness (NAMI). (2003). Anorexia nervosa. Available at http://www.nami.org/Content/ContentGroups/Helpline1/Anorexia_Nervosa.htm.

National Eating Disorder Information Centre (NEDIC). (2005). *Anorexia athletica.* Available at http://www.nedic.ca/knowthefacts/definitions.shtml.

Phillips, K.A., & Castle, D.J. (2001). Body dysmorphic disorder in men. *British Medical Journal, 323*, 1015-1016.

Pope, H.G., Phillips, K.A., & Olivardia, R. (2000). *The Adonis complex: The secret crisis of male body obsession.* New York: Free Press.

Sanborn, C.F., Horea, M., Siemers, B.J., & Dieringer, K.I. (2000, April). Disordered eating and the female athlete triad. *Clinics in Sports Medicine, 19*(2), 199-213.

Shields, M. (2005). Overweight Canadian children and adolescents. *Nutrition: Findings from the Canadian Community Health Survey.* Catalogue no. 82-620-MWE2005001. Ottawa: Statistics Canada.

Spanier, P.A., & Allison, K.R. (2001). General social support and physical activity: An analysis of the Ontario Health Survey. *Canadian Journal of Public Health 92*(3), 210-213.

Stice, E. (2002). Risk and maintenance factors for eating pathology: A meta-analytic review. *Psychological Bulletin, 128*(5), 825-848.

Sullivan, P.F., Bulik, C.M., Fear, J.L., & Pickering, A. (1998). Outcome of anorexia nervosa: A case-control study. *American Journal of Psychiatry, 155*, 939-946.

Tjepkema, M. (2005). Measured obesity: Adult obesity in Canada. *Nutrition: Findings from the Canadian Community Health Survey.* Catalogue no. 82-620-MWE2005001. Ottawa: Statistics Canada.

Tjepkema, M. (2006). Adult obesity. *Health Reports, 17*(3), 9-25.

Tremblay, M.S. (2005). Obesity, overweight and ethnicity. *Health Reports, 16*(4), 23-34.

Wolf, N. (1991). *The beauty myth: How images of beauty are used against women.* New York: William Morrow.

World Health Organization. (2000). *Obesity: Preventing and managing the global epidemic: Report of a WHO consultation on obesity.* Geneva: Author.

Yeager, K.K., Agostini, R., Nattiv, A., & Drinkwater, B. (1993). The female athlete triad: Disordered eating, amenorrhoea, osteoporosis. *Medicine and Science in Sports and Exercise, 25*(7), 775-777.

PART IV

Understanding and Managing Potential Health Problems

CHAPTER 10

Diabetes

CHAPTER OBJECTIVES

After completing this chapter, you should be able to:

- Understand the facts around diabetes disease.
- Describe the three types of diabetes.
- Describe signs and symptoms associated with diabetes.
- Describe the complications associated with diabetes.
- Explain the risk factors associated with diabetes.
- Describe lifestyle modifications that officers who have diabetes must make in order to perform shift work.

Diabetes is a chronic disease in which your body cannot properly use glucose for energy. **Glucose**, a component of carbohydrates and the main source of energy for the brain, comes from foods such as breads, cereals, pasta, rice, potatoes, fruits, and some vegetables. To use glucose for energy, your body needs insulin, a hormone secreted by beta cells in the pancreas. When your body has little or no insulin, the glucose builds up in your blood instead of being used for energy. This causes high blood glucose levels.

diabetes
a chronic disease in which your body cannot properly use glucose for energy

glucose
a simple form of sugar that acts as fuel for the body

High blood sugar is associated with diabetes. Normal glucose levels are between 4.0 and 7.0 mmol/L when fasting and between 5.0 and 10.0 mmol/L two hours after eating (Canadian Diabetes Association, 2003). When blood glucose levels are consistently above 10 mmol/L a person is hyperglycemic, which can lead to serious medical conditions (discussed below). As a police officer, this can have an impact on your career and on your ability to drive a cruiser.

Low blood sugar is also associated with diabetes. When blood glucose levels are between 2.5 and 4.0 mmol/L, a person is hypoglycemic (discussed below). At this level, individuals need to be aware that they should not drive or operate machinery as their responses are impaired. Below this level (2.5 mmol/L), individuals are severely hypoglycemic and may experience loss of consciousness or seizures. If diabetics cannot control their blood glucose levels, their licence may be taken away (for more information, go to www.diabetes.ca/section_about/aboutdriveguide.asp).

Diabetes is the seventh leading cause of death in the world among adults aged 60 years and over (Public Health Agency of Canada, 2006). In 1999–2000, about 5.1 percent of the Canadian population aged 20 and over (approximately 1.2 million people) had been diagnosed with diabetes (Murphy et al., 2005). As age increases, so does prevalence of the disease, with more men being affected than women (Health Canada, 2003). Rates among Aboriginal peoples are almost triple the rate of the general population (Diabetes Division, 1999). Canadian adults with diabetes are twice as likely as those without the disease to die prematurely (Health Canada, 2003). In 2004, academic research estimated that there will be a 76.5 percent increase in the number of people living with diabetes between 2004 and 2016 (Canadian Diabetes Association, 2004). However, the prevalence of diabetes in Ontario had increased so much between 1995 and 2005 that it has already exceeded the predicted global rate set for 2030, while the mortality rate fell by 25 percent from 1995 to 2005 (Lipscombe & Hux, 2007). Of great concern is the proportion of children and adolescents who are overweight. The proportion in Ontario has tripled in the past 30 years, and the evidence clearly indicates that overweight children tend to become overweight adults, thus increasing their risk of developing type 2 diabetes in their lifetime.

The gap between the death rates of diabetics and non-diabetics is greater in younger age groups. For example, a 35-year-old Canadian with diabetes is four times more likely to die than one without diabetes, whereas an 85-year-old Canadian with diabetes is just 1.4 times more likely to die than one without diabetes (Health Canada, 2003).

TYPES OF DIABETES

There are three types of diabetes (Canadian Diabetes Association, 2007c): type 1 diabetes, type 2 diabetes, and gestational diabetes.

type 1 diabetes
type of diabetes that occurs when the pancreas no longer produces insulin or produces very little

Type 1 diabetes occurs when the pancreas either no longer produces insulin or produces very little. About 10 percent of people with diabetes have this type. Type 1 diabetes usually begins in the first two decades of life. In this form of diabetes, the immune system destroys the insulin-producing cells of the pancreas. A combination of genetic factors and environmental stressors such as viruses are believed to trigger this form of diabetes. Treatment requires a strict diet, planned physical activity, home blood glucose testing several times a day, and multiple daily insulin injections. This form of diabetes has huge implications for an individual's state of health. The pain and discomfort due to blood glucose monitoring and needle injections often lead to anxiety and fear. In fact, one report indicated that 45 percent of insulin users avoided injections due to anxiety (Zambanini et al., 1999). Fatigue is also a symptom. Type 1 diabetes can result in a drastic reduction in one's quality of life, and shortens the average lifespan by 15 years (Health Canada, 2002).

type 2 diabetes
type of diabetes that occurs when the pancreas cannot produce enough insulin or the body is unable to use the insulin effectively

Type 2 diabetes (formerly known as adult-onset diabetes mellitus) occurs when the pancreas cannot produce enough insulin or the body is unable to use the insulin effectively. About 90 percent of diabetics have this type. Type 2 diabetes usually develops in obese individuals over the age of 40. This form of diabetes is now widely considered to be one of the components of a group of disorders called "metabolic syndrome," which includes insulin resistance, high cholesterol, lipid disorders, obesity, high blood pressure, a high risk of blood clotting, and disturbed blood flow to many organs (Health Canada, 2000). Obesity, physical inactivity, poor diet, and stress significantly increase the risk of type 2 diabetes. The disease may be controlled by diet, exercise, and medication taken orally. In addition, some require insulin injections. Weight loss can also help to bring blood sugar into the normal range, as approximately 80 percent of people who develop type 2 diabetes are overweight (US Department of Health and Human Services, 2001). Life expectancy is also reduced in people with type 2 diabetes.

The mechanisms of type 2 diabetes are not fully understood. However, some experts believe it happens in three stages (American Diabetes Association, 2007):

- The first stage is called *insulin resistance.* Although insulin can attach to the liver and muscle receptors, this stage prevents insulin from moving glucose from the blood into the cells.
- The second stage is called *postprandial hyperglycemia,* which occurs when the pancreas cannot produce enough insulin and there is an abnormal rise in blood sugar after a meal.
- The third stage is termed *fasting hyperglycemia,* a state of elevated glucose levels most of the time. Elevated glucose impairs and possibly destroys beta cells, thereby stopping insulin production and causing full-blown diabetes.

Gestational diabetes is a temporary condition that occurs during pregnancy (generally after the 24th week) and resolves after delivery. Hormonal changes associated with pregnancy and the growth demands of the fetus increase insulin needs to two to three times the normal level. Gestational diabetes occurs in 2–4 percent of all pregnancies (American Diabetes Association, 2004; Stone et al., 2000). It increases the risk to both mother and child of developing type 2 diabetes. Women who gain over 14 kg (30 pounds) during pregnancy have an increased risk. Gestational diabetes may result in an increased incidence of very large babies, respiratory distress syndrome, low blood calcium, neonatal hypoglycemia (low blood sugar) and pre-eclampsia (toxemia of pregnancy).

gestational diabetes a temporary condition in which hormonal changes associated with pregnancy and the growth demands of the fetus increase insulin needs to two to three times the normal level; generally occurs after the 24th week of pregnancy and resolves after delivery

CHILDREN AND DIABETES

Although type 1 can develop in children only a few months old, it is rare for children under five years to develop diabetes. The incidence increases with age through childhood and adolescence, and then decreases during adulthood. Type 2 diabetes is on the rise. One of the biggest risk factors is being overweight. Over 26 percent of children between 2 and 17 are either overweight or obese, with 8 percent being obese (Tjepkema & Shields, 2004). One of the most significant issues is unrecognized hypoglycemia, which may be disruptive to children's performance and participation in physical activity (Pacaud, 2002). This may lead to metabolic control problems. Education, regular monitoring, and lifestyle choices can help regulate metabolism.

COMPLICATIONS ASSOCIATED WITH DIABETES

Diabetes results in premature death and a reduction of functional health. This is attributed to the complications associated with consistently high blood glucose levels over a prolonged period of time. Many aspects of quality of life may be affected by diabetes. Diabetics often suffer from the pain and discomfort from insulin injections, as well as anxiety and fatigue. Chronically high levels of blood glucose may lead to heart disease and stroke, retinopathy, kidney disease, amputation, nerve disease (including erectile dysfunction), and other complications.

Due to the chronic nature of the disease, and the degree of complications associated with it, diabetes is an expensive disease to treat, both in terms of health care costs and the toll it takes on quality of life. In end-stage organ (kidney) failure, diabetes plays a pivotal role. Complications of diabetes are caused by persistently high blood glucose levels, blood pressure, and cholesterol; months and years of elevated levels can damage the blood vessels and nerves, increasing the risk for heart disease, blindness, nerve and kidney damage, and skin complications such as bacterial and fungal infections and diabetic dermopathy. Over time, all of these complications due to diabetes may lead to diabetic retinopathy, diabetic neuropathy, renal (kidney) failure, and diabetic foot.

DIABETIC DERMOPATHY

Diabetic dermopathy, also known as shin spots or pigmented pretibial patches, is a skin condition usually found on the lower legs of people with diabetes. It is thought to result from changes in the small blood vessels that supply the skin and from minor leakage of blood products from these vessels into the skin. Many diabetics have difficulty with their feet and must keep them clean and dry and look after the quality of their toenails.

In 2003, people with diabetes comprised 6 percent of Ontario's population, yet accounted for 32 percent of heart attacks, 43 percent of heart failure cases, 30 percent of strokes, 51 percent of new kidney dialysis patients, and 70 percent of amputations (Institute for Clinical Evaluative Sciences, 2003), in addition to costing our health care system over $1 billion each year in direct costs.

Complications affect all types of diabetes (Canadian Diabetes Association, 2006a). They include:

- *Depression,* which is twice as common in people with diabetes as in the general population. About 25 percent of patients with diabetes have symptoms of depression, and major depression is present in at least 15 percent of those afflicted.
- *Heart disease and stroke.* People with diabetes are at very high risk for these conditions. In fact, up to 80 percent of people with diabetes will die as a result of a heart attack or stroke. Compared with the general population, diabetics have problems at a younger age and die from these events at rates much higher than people without diabetes (three times higher for men and five times higher for women).
- *Digestive problems,* which are relatively common among people with diabetes. Constipation affects 60 percent of people with diabetes. Diabetes is also linked to diarrhea, and is one of the most common causes of gastroparesis (delayed emptying of the stomach), which affects up to 75

percent of people with diabetes. Gastroparesis can cause bloating, loss of appetite, vomiting, dehydration, heartburn, nausea, an early feeling of fullness when eating, weight loss, erratic blood glucose levels, reflux, and spasms of the stomach wall.

- *Dental problems.* Diabetes can contribute to dry mouth and a burning sensation on the tongue, which can lead to irritation of the lining of the mouth. If blood glucose levels are poorly managed, toothaches, bleeding of the gums, infection of the gum and bone tissues, and delayed healing responses may result.
- *Compromised men's sexual health.* Diabetes causes damage to the walls of the blood vessels, which affects circulation and blood flow. Fifty percent of men will experience erectile dysfunction (ED) within 10 years of a diagnosis of diabetes. In fact, in up to 12 percent of men with diabetes, ED is the first sign that leads to the diagnosis of diabetes.
- *Thyroid disorders,* which are experienced more frequently by people with diabetes than by the general population. The thyroid is a butterfly-shaped gland in the lower neck (just beneath the skin in the front of the windpipe) that regulates the body's metabolism. Approximately one-third of people with type 1 diabetes have thyroid disease. An overactive thyroid (hyperthyroidism) may increase insulin requirements, while an underactive thyroid (hypothyroidism) may decrease insulin requirements.
- *Diabetic retinopathy and other eye conditions.* Diabetic retinopathy is a disease that affects the retina. It is the most common cause of blindness in people under age 65. About one in four people with diabetes experiences this problem. Those that develop diabetes are also more likely to develop cataracts at a younger age and are twice as likely to develop glaucoma. Almost all people who have had diabetes for more than 30 years will have retinopathy in various stages of progression (Janghorbani et al., 2001). It is the leading cause of adult blindness in Canada (Health Canada, 2003). Diabetes causes the arteries in the retina to weaken and begin to leak, forming dot-like hemorrhages. Vision may begin to blur, floaters (blood leaking into the retina) may drift in front of the eyes, and vision may decrease. With abnormal vessel growth and scar tissue, some people develop retinal detachment (separation of the sensory and pigment layers) and glaucoma (increased intra-ocular pressure causing irreversible optic nerve damage).
- *Neuropathy (damage to sensory nerves) of the extremities,* which can lead to loss of sensation, making people more prone to injury. Numbness and tingling in the feet is often the first sign, though symptoms vary depending on the nerve(s) and the part of the body affected. Because of poor circulation, wounds heal slowly or ineffectively. Some people suffer from pressure sores. Gangrene and amputation are more common in people with this complication.
- *Diabetic foot,* which is a complication that can result in infection in the skin, muscles, or bones of the foot, resulting in poor circulation and neuropathy. The immune system is compromised, which can lead to the loss of sensation in the foot, reduced blood circulation, poor wound

healing, death of the tissue, severe infection, gangrene, and potentially amputation. Approximately 15 percent of individuals with diabetes will develop foot ulceration at some point in their life (American Podiatric Medical Association, 2007) and half of all leg amputations occur in people with diabetes (Foster & Edmonds, 2001).

- *Diabetic nephropathy*, which is the most common cause of chronic kidney failure. In individuals with this condition, the kidneys lose the ability to filter out waste products, leading to a buildup of waste products in the blood and ultimately end-stage renal disease (ESRD). Early intervention can prevent or delay the advance of diabetic kidney disease.

RISK FACTORS ASSOCIATED WITH DIABETES

Some of the risk factors for developing diabetes include the following (Canadian Diabetes Association, 2007b):

- *Being 40 years of age or older.*
- *Being overweight.* A BMI greater than 27 indicates a risk for developing type 2 diabetes and other health problems, including cardiovascular disease and premature death (CCDPC, 2003).
- *Having an apple-shaped figure.* Individuals who carry most of their weight in the trunk of their bodies tend to have a higher risk of diabetes than those of similar weight with pear-shaped bodies (excess fat carried mainly in the hips and thighs). A waist measurement of more than 100 cm (39.5 inches) in men and 95 cm (37.5 inches) in women suggests an increased risk (CCDPC, 2003).
- *Having a sedentary lifestyle.* Lack of exercise and sitting for long periods of time can lead to being overweight, which increases the risk of diabetes and impedes glucose uptake.
- *Belonging to a high-risk group.* People of Aboriginal, Hispanic, Asian, or African descent are three to five times more likely than the general population to develop diabetes. Aboriginal people in particular suffer a greater risk and burden of poor health compared with other Canadians. Of special note, diabetes also develops at an earlier age among First Nations people, and in recent years, type 2 diabetes has been diagnosed in children (First Nations and Inuit Regional Health Survey National Steering Committee, 1999). Almost one-third of First Nations women with diabetes report getting the diagnosis during pregnancy (Dean, 1998). Factors that pose a risk to Aboriginal populations are lifestyle and heredity. The relatively recent shift from traditional diets high in animal protein to "modern urban diets" high in carbohydrates, combined with decreased physical activity, has resulted in high levels of obesity that compound pre-existing risks for diabetes. Type 2 diabetes, in particular, is increasingly prevalent, as is its main risk factor—excess body weight. Rates of diabetes in Aboriginals have escalated from 9.3 percent in 1995 to 15 percent in 2002 (Public Health Agency of Canada, 2005).

- *Family history.* The genetic link for type 2 diabetes is stronger than the genetic link for type 1. Having a parent or sibling with the disease particularly increases risk (CCDPC, 2003).
- *History of diabetes during pregnancy.* Nearly 40 percent of women who have diabetes during their pregnancy go on to develop type 2 diabetes later, usually within 5 to 10 years of giving birth. Giving birth to a baby that weighs more than 4 kg (9 pounds) is another symptom of gestational diabetes (CCDPC, 2003).
- *Dyslipidemia (high cholesterol) or other fats in the blood.* More than 40 percent of people with diabetes have abnormal levels of cholesterol and similar fatty substances that circulate in the blood. These abnormalities appear to be associated with an increased risk of developing cardiovascular disease among persons with diabetes.
- *Impaired glucose tolerance.* If blood sugar control and reaction to sugar loads are considered abnormal, there is a higher risk of developing type 2 diabetes within five years and developing cardiovascular disease (CCDPC, 2003).
- *High blood pressure.* Up to 60 percent of people with undiagnosed diabetes have high blood pressure (CCDPC, 2003).

WHAT HAPPENS WHEN YOU ARE HYPOGLYCEMIC OR HYPERGLYCEMIC?

Insulin shock is another term used for hypoglycemia or low blood sugar. Symptoms include shakes, sweating, trembling, dizziness, moodiness (irritability), confusion, blurred vision, and hunger. In severe cases, low blood sugar may cause you to pass out. It is common in those who take too much insulin, skip meals, drink too much alcohol, and exercise too vigorously. Treatment includes providing the individual with something to ingest that contains a high amount of glucose; this will increase blood sugar levels adequately in order to improve mental status. Such treatment can include tablets made of glucose or dextrose (these can be obtained at health food stores), fruit juices such as orange juice and apple juice, milk, 100 mL of regular soda, or table sugar (10–15 grams or 2–3 teaspoons) with water. Bystanders should not try to administer fluids by mouth to someone who is unconscious, since this may cause the person to vomit and choke.

Hyperglycemia is a condition caused by greater than normal glucose in the blood. Symptoms include increased thirst, frequent urination, dry mouth, nausea, vomiting, shortness of breath, and fatigue. Prolonged high levels can lead to ketoacidosis, which results when fat is used as the energy source rather than glucose, resulting in ketones (a chemical byproduct of the breakdown of fat) in the urine. This is more common in type 1 diabetes, and can lead to serious dehydration and coma. Symptoms of ketoacidosis include a slightly sweet breath odour (which smells like nail-polish remover), extreme dryness of the mucous membranes, weight loss, increased thirst and urination, weakness, abdominal pains, generalized aches, nausea and vomiting, and breathlessness (Canadian Diabetes Association, 2007a).

SYMPTOMS OF DIABETES

Some of the symptoms of diabetes include the following (Canadian Diabetes Association, 2007b):

- unusual thirst
- frequent urination
- unusual weight loss or weight gain
- extreme fatigue or lack of energy
- blurred vision
- frequent or recurring infections
- cuts and bruises that are slow to heal
- tingling or numbness in hands or feet

Note, however, that many people who have type 2 diabetes display no symptoms.

LIVING WITH DIABETES AND SHIFT WORK

In the province of Ontario, there are medical conditions that may constitute grounds for disqualification to be hired as a police constable. If a candidate is dialysis-dependent, this is considered a disqualification. If an individual is insulin-dependent, the applicant will be referred to a specialist to determine if he or she meets the medical standards for driving (in accordance with the driving fitness guidelines of the CMA and the Canadian Diabetes Association). Those candidates who are non-insulin-treated diabetics and do not have an understanding of how to control insulin levels through diet, medication, and exercise may be considered ineligible as well. (To learn more about medical requirements, refer to *Self Assess! Medical Requirements for Candidates* at www.mcscs.jus.gov.on.ca/english/publications/policing_services/Self_assess_2006.pdf.)

Shift work can be hard on everyone, but it can be especially challenging for those with diabetes. One of the biggest changes in recent years regarding diabetes management is taking responsibility for your own care. Shift work will increase your risk of a hypoglycemic incident. This pattern of work influences the body's circadian rhythms, which regulate daily processes such as hunger and fatigue, thus disrupting your body's internal clock and affecting blood glucose control from physical and mental stress.

Putting a plan in place will help you deal effectively with diabetes. In particular, you should do the following (Canadian Diabetes Association, 2006b; Diabetes UK, 2006):

- Prepare a written plan that you can share with your supervisor, which includes a medical plan and personal health identification.
- Wear personal health identification (such as a medical alert bracelet).
- Bring quick accessible food that you can consume following a check of your blood glucose level.

- Have regularly planned meals. Snacking and strict adherence to certain mealtimes may not be as critical for people on regular or intermediate action or premixed insulins; however, they are very important for somebody on insulin and pills (taken in place of injections).
- Have your blood glucose meter with you in your cruiser. When you are driving for work or operating machinery (such as snowmobile patrol or water patrol), it is best that you check your levels every couple of hours to know how much insulin you need rather than risk a hypoglycemic reaction.
- Take regular rest breaks.
- Engage in physical activity, which is very important even if you are working the night shift.
- Manage your stress. Stress can increase your body's production of hormones that block the effects of insulin, causing your blood sugar to rise. As well, prolonged stress may lead to depression.

Despite all the latest advancements in the treatment of diabetes, there are still complications that may preclude you from policing. Those that have foot problems may find it difficult to wear steel-toed boots on cold concrete for 12-hour shifts. Retinopathy may impair your vision, making it difficult to work as a patrol officer. Finally, shift rotation can be stressful. It is best to have shifts that rotate every two to three days and move "forward" (from morning to afternoon to night). The stress of shift work can be further compounded by adding court days to regular shifts.

CONCLUSION

Remember that *you* have to take care of you. Research suggests that lifestyle and type 2 diabetes are closely linked. This means that you can help to prevent or delay the onset of the disease. A healthy diet, weight control, exercise, and stress management are important preventive steps.

With early diagnosis, you can manage diabetes fairly well. It is important that you learn as much about the disease as you can in order to make healthier life choices, and be sure to get tested every three years after you reach age 45.

You need to know what, when, and how much to eat in order to manage your blood sugar levels. You may need to add pills and/or insulin to your lifestyle changes to achieve your blood glucose target. You must also maintain a healthy weight, especially if you have type 2 diabetes. Exercise is known to lower blood sugar and enhance overall fitness. This will also help to keep your blood pressure at or below 130/80 and your cholesterol level down.

Here are some additional suggestions to help prevent, delay, or manage the disease:

- If you smoke, make a serious effort to quit.
- See an eye specialist on a regular basis to check for signs of eye disease.
- Exercise proper foot care, have your feet checked regularly by your physician, and keep your vaccinations up to date.

- Speak to a specialist if you are feeling overwhelmed or depressed about how diabetes is negatively affecting you.
- If your extremities feel numb or you experience "pins and needles," advise your physician.
- Have your urine tested regularly for early signs of kidney disease.
- Have your teeth cleaned twice a year.
- Consult your physician if you experience sexual dysfunction.
- Manage your stress.

Stay healthy by asking your doctor the right questions. Be a proactive patient who is informed.

APPENDIX: DIABETES DICTIONARY

Since this chapter only provides an overview of diabetes, I encourage you to learn more about the disease and how it may affect your life. The Diabetes Dictionary is adapted from www.diabetes.ca with permission of the Canadian Diabetes Association.

adult-onset diabetes
The former term for non–insulin-dependent, or type 2, diabetes. Although this type of diabetes usually occurs after 40 years of age, it may develop at younger ages.

amputation
The surgical removal of a limb or part of a limb. People with diabetes may be at increased risk for gangrene due to nerve damage in the legs and feet, which may require amputation.

autoimmune disease
A disorder in which a person's own antibodies destroy body tissues, such as the beta cells in the pancreas.

blood glucose meters
Hand-held machines designed to test blood glucose levels. A drop of blood from your finger is placed on a small strip of material, which is then inserted into the meter for analysis, and the result is displayed. Blood glucose meters allow people with diabetes to play an active role in monitoring their own blood glucose levels.

blood pressure
The pressure exerted by blood flow on artery walls. People with diabetes should aim for a blood pressure of 130/80 or lower. High blood pressure (hypertension) can cause health problems such as heart attacks, strokes, and kidney problems.

body mass index (BMI)
A unit of measurement used to describe weight in relation to height (kg/m^2) for people 18 years of age and older. Classifications include *underweight* (<18.5), *normal weight* (18.5–24.9), *overweight* (25–29.9), and *obese* (>30).

cataract
A grey-white film that can cover the lens of the eye, obscuring vision. Cataracts tend to occur in people over 50 years of age, but can occur at a younger age and advance more rapidly in the presence of diabetes. If left untreated, cataracts can cause blindness.

coma
A state of unconsciousness. In diabetes, it may result from a variety of causes, including severe hypoglycemia or ketoacidosis.

diabetes
A condition in which the body either cannot produce insulin or cannot effectively use the insulin it produces. (See gestational diabetes; type 1 diabetes; type 2 diabetes)

diabetic retinopathy
A disease in which the small blood vessels (capillaries) in the back of the eye (retina) may bleed or form new vessels. This condition usually occurs in people with long-standing diabetes. Regular eye examinations are an important part of diabetes management.

dialysis
A method of removing waste products and excess water from the body when the kidneys no longer function adequately.

familial occurrence
The pattern of a disease within a family. Family and twin studies have shown that type 2 diabetes is far more likely to run in families than type 1 diabetes.

gangrene
The death of body tissues, which is usually due to loss of blood supply to the affected area, followed by bacterial invasion.

gestational diabetes
A condition that develops during pregnancy due to a deficiency of insulin during pregnancy that disappears following delivery. Women who have had gestational diabetes are at a high risk of developing type 2 diabetes later in life.

glucagon
A hormone produced by the pancreas that stimulates the liver to produce large amounts of glucose. It is given by injection for hypoglycemia and generally restores blood sugar within 5 to 10 minutes.

glucose
A simple form of sugar that acts as fuel for the body. It is produced during digestion of carbohydrates and carried to the cells in the blood.

glycogen
Main carbohydrate storage material, which is stored in the liver and muscles for use when energy is required.

glycosuria
An increased amount of sugar in the urine. It is usually an indication of an elevated blood glucose level.

hyperglycemia
A condition caused by greater than normal levels of glucose in the blood. Symptoms include thirst, frequent urination, and fatigue.

hyperlipoproteinemia
The presence in the blood of greater than normal amounts of certain lipids and other fatty substances.

hypertension
The medical term for high blood pressure.

hypoglycemia
A condition in which blood glucose levels drop too low. Symptoms may include shakes, sweating, trembling, hunger, dizziness, moodiness, confusion, and blurred vision.

impotence
A form of sexual dysfunction in which a man is unable to achieve an erection.

insulin
A hormone produced by the beta cells of the pancreas in response to increased levels of glucose in the blood.

insulin lipodystrophy
The loss of fatty tissue that can occur as a result of repeated insulin injections in the same area.

insulin pump
A portable, battery-operated device that delivers a specific amount of insulin through a small needle inserted under the skin. It can be programmed to deliver constant doses throughout the day and/or deliver extra insulin as required.

insulin receptors
Areas on the outer walls of a cell that permit insulin to bind to the cell. When cells and insulin bind together, the cell is able to take glucose from the bloodstream and use it for energy.

insulin shock
Another term for hypoglycemia or low blood sugar.

ischemia
An inadequate supply of blood to body tissues or organs. It can occur if blood vessels are narrowed or constricted.

islets of Langerhans
The endocrine clusters of cells in the pancreas that produce insulin, glucagons (a hormone that responds to a low concentration of glucose in the blood), and pancreatic polypeptide (which suppresses pancreatic secretions and stimulates gastric secretions).

juvenile-onset diabetes
The former term for insulin-dependent, or type 1, diabetes.

ketoacidosis
A severe complication of diabetes that occurs when there is too little insulin in the blood to allow blood glucose to be used for energy; in response, the body begins to burn fat for energy and produces large amounts of ketones, which poison the body and may lead to diabetic coma.

ketones
Chemicals produced by the liver when the body cannot use glucose and must break down fat for energy. Ketones can poison and even kill body cells. When ketones build up, the body gets rid of them in the urine. Ketones that accumulate in the body over long periods of time can lead to serious illness and coma.

mmol/L
The abbreviated form of millimoles per litre, a term used to describe how much glucose is present in a specific amount of blood.

nephrologist
A medical doctor who specializes in the care and treatment of people with kidney diseases.

nephropathy
Any disease of the kidneys.

neuropathy
Inflammation or degeneration of the peripheral nerves.

obesity
An abnormal increase in the proportion of fat cells. Obesity may be accompanied by other signs of poor health and is a risk factor for type 2 diabetes.

ophthalmologist
A medical doctor who specializes in treatment and care of the eyes.

oral agents
Medications, taken by mouth, for the treatment of type 2 diabetes.

oral glucose tolerance test (OGTT)
A test of the body's ability to metabolize carbohydrates. It is performed by giving a standard dose of glucose and measuring the blood and urine for glucose at regular intervals.

pancreas
An oblong flattened organ located deep in the abdomen that is part of the digestive and endocrine systems. It secretes various substances such as digestive fluid, insulin, and glucagons.

podiatrist
A health professional who diagnoses and treats disorders of the feet.

type 1 diabetes (or insulin-dependent diabetes)
Occurs when the pancreas no longer produces insulin or does not produce enough of it. The body needs insulin to use sugar as an energy source. Type 1 diabetes usually develops in childhood or adolescence, and affects 10 percent of people with diabetes.

type 2 diabetes (or non-insulin-dependent diabetes)
Occurs when the pancreas does not produce enough insulin to meet the body's needs or the insulin is not metabolized effectively. Type 2 diabetes usually occurs later in life, and affects 90 percent of people with diabetes.

ulcer
A crater-like lesion of the skin or mucous membrane, often as a result of inflammatory processes.

urine tests
Tests that measure substances, such as blood glucose or ketones, present in the urine.

vascular disease
A disease of the blood vessels.

KEY TERMS

diabetes

glucose

type 1 diabetes

type 2 diabetes

gestational diabetes

EXERCISES

Review

1. What is the prevalence of diabetes in Canada?

2. Describe the difference between type 1 and type 2 diabetes.

3. What are five risk factors associated with type 2 diabetes?

4. What are five of the signs or symptoms of diabetes?

5. How does shift work affect diabetes?

6. Describe five ways to regulate your blood sugar levels.

7. What are three severe complications of diabetes?

8. How can you moderate diabetes risks?

Multiple Choice and True or False

1. What symptom(s) may indicate that you should get checked for diabetes?
   a. your feet swell up
   b. you feel more energized than usual
   c. you may be extra thirsty and lose weight quickly
   d. you gain weight and are hungry
   e. you experience heart palpitations

2. How often should you test your blood glucose?
   a. it depends on the individual
   b. every 24 hours
   c. every couple of hours
   d. before you eat
   e. when you first get up and when you go to bed

3. What does diabetes have to do with your nerves?
   a. it makes them more aware of your surroundings
   b. it affects the transmission of nerve impulses
   c. it interferes with blood flow to the tissues
   d. it has nothing to do with your nerves
   e. it sends feedback to the brain

4. What is the greatest risk factor for diabetes?
   a. poor lifestyle choices
   b. ethnic background and genetic susceptibility
   c. eating too much sugar
   d. smoking and drinking
   e. exercising too much

5. What does diabetes have to do with erectile dysfunction?
   a. it is not involved in sexual dysfunction
   b. no one really understands the link
   c. nerve damage affects the blood flow to the penis
   d. it prevents the dysfunction
   e. blood flow to the groin is decreased

6. What does diabetes have to do with dental care?
   a. diabetes is unrelated to dental care
   b. diabetes can cause gum disease and teeth problems
   c. dentists want to be involved in your health care
   d. diabetes affects the alignment of your teeth
   e. diabetes medication promotes good dental health

7. What is diabetes ketoacidosis?
   a. the name of a diabetic research project
   b. a life-saving condition
   c. a form of indigestion caused by too much acid
   d. the breakdown of protein to use as an energy source in place of glucose
   e. the breakdown of fat to use as an energy source in place of glucose

8. What do diabetes pills do?
   a. they treat pancreas problems
   b. they help keep blood glucose in the target range
   c. they help to keep you regular
   d. they reduce pain
   e. they help digestive enzymes

9. How does diabetes affect your eyes?
   a. lack of insulin interferes with brain signals to the eyes
   b. lack of insulin reduces energy levels to the brain
   c. high blood glucose levels can damage blood vessels in the retina
   d. low blood glucose levels can cause cornea damage
   e. low blood glucose causes headaches behind the eyes

10. Who should check your blood glucose levels?
    a. only your doctor
    b. your doctor and a diabetic educator
    c. you
    d. you, your doctor, and a diabetic educator
    e. you don't have to check your levels outside of a medical checkup

11. How does diabetes affect your feet?
    a. it causes athlete's foot
    b. it causes feet to become very sweaty
    c. it causes blisters on the feet
    d. it affects the arch in your foot
    e. it causes nerve damage to the feet

12. Can children and young people develop type 2 diabetes?
    a. yes, but mostly adults develop type 2 diabetes
    b. yes, but they grow out of it
    c. no, only adults get type 2 diabetes
    d. no, because they exercise too much
    e. yes; children first develop type 1, which then becomes type 2

13. How does diabetes affect your kidneys?
    a. it affects the liver rather than the kidneys
    b. high blood glucose levels can affect the kidneys' filter system
    c. insulin gets blocked in the kidneys
    d. fat cells get blocked by the kidneys
    e. protein cells get blocked by the kidneys

14. Why is it important to check blood glucose levels with diabetes?
    a. regular checks don't change the condition of the disease
    b. regular checks ensure that blood glucose remains at a normal level
    c. regular checks ensure that you don't need to take insulin
    d. regular checks take your blood glucose levels down
    e. regular checks ensure you have enough fluids in your body

15. How is type 2 diabetes controlled?
    a. through insulin injections
    b. you don't need to do anything
    c. exercise and diet alone
    d. insulin, exercise, diet, and healthy lifestyle choices
    e. through a high carbohydrate diet

16. You can help prevent or delay type 2 diabetes.
    a. True
    b. False

17. If you have diabetes in your family, are you at risk?
    a. you definitely will get diabetes
    b. you aren't at any risk for diabetes
    c. if one person has diabetes, everyone will have diabetes
    d. you are at low risk for developing the disease
    e. you are at higher risk for developing the disease

18. What is neuropathy?
    a. sensory nerve damage
    b. the study of the brain
    c. nervous system surgery
    d. the study of kidney nerves
    e. the pathway of nerve transmissions

19. What signs might you see if someone is experiencing low blood glucose?
    a. the person is out of breath after a 1.5 mile run
    b. the person becomes emotional
    c. the person gets confused and may lose consciousness
    d. the person is not hungry
    e. the person can't do more than 10 curl-ups

20. How do you know if you have type 2 diabetes?
    a. you are more thirsty than normal and have blurry vision
    b. you feel really energetic but not very hungry
    c. a friend tells you that you have diabetes
    d. you are energetic and able to work out vigorously
    e. you are not thirsty after working out

REFERENCES

American Diabetes Association. (n.d.). *Gestational diabetes.* Available at http://www.diabetes.org/gestational-diabetes.jsp.

American Diabetes Association. (2007). Diagnosis and classification of diabetes mellitus. *Diabetes Care, 30,* 42-47.

American Podiatric Medical Association. (2007). *Facts on diabetes and the foot.* Available at http://www.apma.org/faqsdiab.html.

Canadian Diabetes Association. (2003). *Insulin: Things you should know.* Available at http://www.diabetes.ca/section_about/insulin3.asp.

Canadian Diabetes Association. (2004). Projection of prevalence & cost of diabetes in Canada: 2000–2016. *Canadian Journal of Diabetes, 28*(2).

Canadian Diabetes Association. (2006a). *About diabetes: Complications.* Available at http://www.diabetes.ca/section_about/complicationsIndex.asp.

Canadian Diabetes Association. (2006b). *About diabetes: Diabetes & shiftwork.* Available at http://www.diabetes.ca/section_about/shiftwork.asp.

Canadian Diabetes Association. (2007a). *About diabetic ketoacidosis.* Available at http://www.diabetes.ca/ilt/diabetes_answers/what_is_type_1_diabetes/about_diabetic_ketoacidosis.aspx.

Canadian Diabetes Association. (2007b). *Are you at risk?* Available at http://www.diabetes.ca/section_about/atrisk.asp.

Canadian Diabetes Association. (2007c). *Diabetes facts.* Available at http://www.diabetes.ca/section_about/thefacts.asp.

Dean H. (1998). NIDDM among youth in First Nation children in Canada. *Clinical Pediatrics, 37,* 89-96.

Diabetes Division, Health Canada. (1999). Diabetes in Canada—National statistics and opportunities for improved surveillance, prevention, and control. Ottawa: Health Canada.

Diabetes UK. (2006). *Diabetes and the police officer: Guidance for the recruitment and employment of police officers with diabetes.* Available at http://www.diabetes.org.uk/Documents/Reports/police_Guidance_FINAL.pdf.

First Nations and Inuit Regional Health Survey National Steering Committee. (1999). *First Nations and Inuit Regional Health Survey: National Report.* Ottawa: Health Canada.

Foster, A., & Edmonds, M. (2001). An overview of foot disease in patients with diabetes. *Nursing Standard, 16*(12), 45-52.

Health Canada. (2000). *Diabetes among Aboriginal (First Nations, Inuit and Métis) people in Canada: The evidence.* Ottawa: Author.

Health Canada. (2002). *Diabetes in Canada,* 2nd ed. Center for Chronic Disease Prevention and Control Population and Public Health Branch. Available at http://www.phac-aspc.gc.ca/publicat/dic-dac2/pdf/dic-dac2_en.pdf.

Health Canada. (2003). *Responding to the challenge of diabetes in Canada.* Catalogue no. H39-4/21-2003E. Ottawa: Author.

Institute for Clinical Evaluative Sciences. (2003). *ICES practice atlas: Diabetes in Ontario.* Available at http://www.ices.on.ca/webpage.cfm?site_id=1&org_id=32&morg_id=0&gsec_id=1510&item_id=1510&category_id=32.

Janghorbani, M., Jones, R.B., Murray, K.J., & Allison, S.P. (2001). Incidence of the risk factors for diabetic retinopathy in diabetic clinic attenders. *Ophthalmic Epidemiology, 8*(5), 309-325.

Lipscombe, L., & Hux, J. (2007). Trends in diabetes prevalence, incidence and mortality in Ontario, Canada 1995–2005: A population-based study. *Lancet, 369*(9563), 750-756.

Murphy, K., Gorber, S.C., & O'Dwyer, A. (2005). Population health impact of disease in Canada (PHI). Health state descriptions for Canadians: Diabetes. Catalogue no. 82-619-MIE2005002. Ottawa: Statistics Canada.

Pacaud, D. (2002). Hypoglycemia: The Achilles heel of the treatment of children with type 1 diabetes. *Canadian Journal of Diabetes, 26*(3), 215-222.

Public Health Agency of Canada. (2005). *The integrated pan-Canadian healthy living strategy.* Available at http://www.phac-aspc.gc.ca/hl-vs-strat/pdf/hls_e.pdf.

Public Health Agency of Canada. (2006). *National diabetes surveillance system.* Available at http://www.phac-aspc.gc.ca/ccdpc-cpcmc/ndss-snsd/english/index_e.html.

Public Health Agency of Canada. (2006, August). *Diabetes in Canada.* Available at http://www.phac-aspc.gc.ca/publicat/dic-dac99/d07_e.html.

Stone, C.A., McLachlan, K.A., Halliday, J.L., Wein, P., & Tippett, C. (2000). Gestational diabetes in Victoria in 1996: Incidence, risk factors and outcomes. *Medical Journal of Australia, 177*(9), 486-491.

Tjepkema, M., & Shields, M. (2004). *Nutrition: Findings from the Canadian Community Health Survey.* Issue no. 1. *Measured obesity: Adult obesity in Canada.* Ottawa: Statistics Canada.

US Department of Health and Human Services. (2001). *Diet and exercise dramatically delay type 2 diabetes.* Available at http://www.hhs.gov/news/press/2001pres/20010808a.html.

Zambanini, A., Newson, R.B., Maisey, M., & Feher, M.D. (1999). Injection related anxiety in insulin treated diabetes. *Diabetes Research in Clinical Practice, 46*(3), 239-246.

CHAPTER 11

Cardiovascular Disease

CHAPTER OBJECTIVES

After completing this chapter, you should be able to:

- Comment on the impact of cardiovascular disease on Canadian society.
- Understand the basic anatomy of the heart and the etiology of various cardiovascular diseases.
- Describe four common types of cardiovascular disease (arteriosclerosis, coronary heart disease, stroke, and hypertension).
- Describe the controllable and uncontrollable risk factors associated with cardiovascular diseases.
- List some of the symptoms of heart attacks and strokes.
- Make appropriate health decisions regarding your heart.

The term *cardiovascular disease* applies to any disease that affects the heart or blood vessels. Although a great deal of research and media attention has focused on diseases such as AIDS, hepatitis B, and cancer, cardiovascular disease has long been the number one cause of death in Canada, even with a small drop in rates from 1995 to 2002 (Public Health Agency of Canada, 2002; Sharratt & Sharratt, 1994). Cardiovascular disease accounted for 38 percent of all deaths in Canada in 1995 (Statistics Canada, 1997), accounting for 79,389 deaths. The figure for 1997 was only down to 37 percent (Statistics Canada, 1999). By 2002, 74,626 Canadian deaths (32 percent of all male deaths and 34 percent of all female deaths) were attributed to cardiovascular disease (Public Health Agency of Canada, 2002; Statistics Canada, 2004). Let's first take a look at the proportion of deaths attributable to the leading risk factors worldwide. The highest risk factor by far is high blood pressure (see figure 11.1).

FIGURE 11.1 Deaths Attributable to Leading Risk Factors Worldwide (2000)

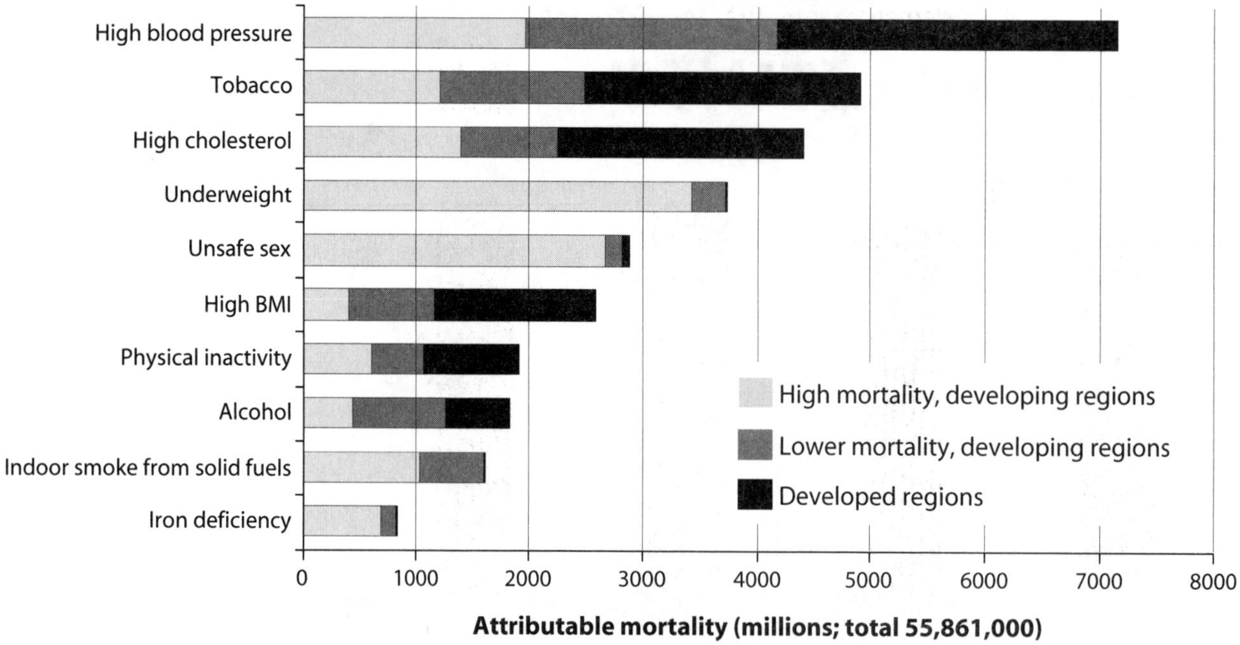

Source: Adapted from World Health Organization, Global Strategy on Diet, Physical Activity and Health, "Disease Burden and Deaths Attributable to Selected Leading Risk Factors," http://www.who.int/entity/dietphysicalactivity/publications/facts/en/.

CARDIOVASCULAR DISEASE: A CANADIAN CONCERN

The Heart and Stroke Foundation of Canada recently revealed that for the first time in 30 years, women have caught up to men when it comes to deaths from cardiovascular disease (Heart and Stroke Foundation of Canada, 2007c). In 1973, there were 23 percent fewer female deaths than male deaths from heart disease and stroke (34,924 female deaths versus 45,404 male deaths). By 2003, the number of male deaths had decreased by 19 percent, to 37,004, while the number of female deaths increased by 5 percent to 36,823. For the first time, the number of deaths from heart disease and stroke combined is virtually the same for women as for men. See figure 11.2.

Of all cardiovascular deaths, 54 percent are due to coronary artery disease, 20 percent to stroke, 15 percent to other forms of heart disease (malfunctioning of the electrical system of the heart, viral heart infections, and heart muscle diseases), and the remaining 10 percent to vascular problems, which includes arteriosclerosis, atherosclerosis, and high blood pressure (Heart and Stroke Foundation of Ontario, 2001).

Considerable research has identified the major risk factors for heart disease. It is important to manage the risks that you can influence, especially if you have other risk factors that are beyond your control.

Risk factors that you *cannot* control include age and gender (55 and over for women, 45 and over for men), ethnic descent (African, South Asian, and First Nations populations are at higher risk), and family history, which includes heart attacks or strokes before age 65, and angina.

FIGURE 11.2 **Number of Deaths from Heart Disease and Stroke**

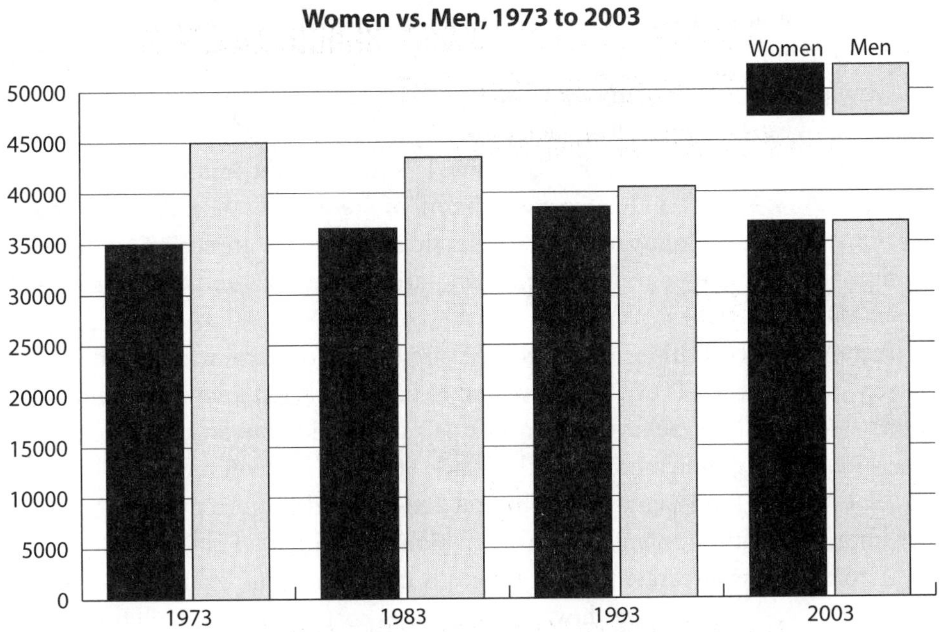

Source: Statistics Canada. (2007). Number of deaths from heart disease and stroke: Women vs. men (1973 to 2003). Based on data from Statistics Canada. (2004). *Mortality, summary list of causes.*

Risk factors that you *can* control or manage include high blood cholesterol, high blood pressure (hypertension), lack of exercise, being overweight, smoking, drinking too much alcohol, stress, lack of fruit and vegetables in your diet, and diabetes (Heart and Stroke Foundation of Canada, 2001a).

ON THE JOB

In the spring of 2002, "O" Division of the RCMP had cholesterol readings done for their officers. Statistics revealed that almost 50 percent of the officers tested had high cholesterol readings (Seguin, 2007). There are serious implications to this finding. Combined with any other risk factors, high cholesterol could be life threatening. Shift work, the lack of available nutritious foods on night shifts, and, for some officers, limited involvement in exercise programs, especially for those who are in isolated locations, can be a deadly combination. As an officer, you need to be aware of the risks associated with the career that you have chosen.

Cardiovascular Disease: Not Just a Disease of Old Age

Canadians run a high risk of developing cardiovascular diseases. We know that 8 out of 10 people have at least one risk factor associated with cardiovascular disease, and 1 in 10 have three or more risk factors (Heart and Stroke Foundation of Canada, 2003).

Young people carry a high level of risk factors. Nearly two-fifths of teenaged girls are physically inactive. Nearly one-quarter of adults in their 20s are overweight. One in five young women in their later teens (18 and 19 years) and one in four young men smoke cigarettes daily.

We know that women tend to be more physically inactive and have higher blood pressure. More men smoke, consume less than the recommended amounts of fruits and vegetables, and are overweight. All of these risks can lead to cardiovascular disease. Many cardiac rehabilitative exercise therapists are seeing an increasing numbers of patients in attendance who are between 25 and 50 years of age (Pepe, 2007).

Income and education also affect the prevalence of cardiovascular diseases. Those with higher levels of education tend to have increased knowledge and skills to undertake healthier behaviours. Individuals who live in poverty, however, must cope with meeting basic needs and their lack of income may limit their ability to purchase healthy foods, engage in physical activity, and acquire medications that may improve health problems such as high blood pressure and diabetes.

Cardiovascular diseases are the most costly contributors to health costs in Canada. Of total costs in 1998, cardiovascular diseases cost nearly $18.5 billion or 11.6 percent of the total cost of illnesses (Heart and Stroke Foundation of Canada, 2003).

Cardiovascular disease is not restricted to elderly people. It is the number two killer for ages 25–64 years, the number three killer for ages 0–14 years, and the number five killer for ages 15–24 years (Heart and Stroke Foundation of Canada, 2007a). Chronic diseases such as cardiovascular disease (accounting for 37 percent of all deaths) and cancer are now the leading causes of death and disability in Canada (MacLean, 2001). Eighty-five percent of Canadians over 65 have at least one modifiable risk factor for cardiovascular disease, and almost two-thirds of Canadians overall have at least one risk factor for cardiovascular disease. Two-thirds of Canadians lead sedentary lifestyles and over half are above a healthy weight (Mills, 2001). Hospitalization costs related to cardiovascular disease are over $4 billion annually (Heart and Stroke Foundation of Canada, 2003).

Of special note is a condition called bacterial endocarditis. This is an infection of the heart's inner lining (endocardium) or the heart valves. This can damage or destroy heart valves as bacteria enter the bloodstream and attack the heart. Some surgical procedures (such as tonsillectomies and gastrointestinal tract surgery) and respiratory procedures (such as professional teeth cleaning) cause brief bacteremia that enters the bloodstream and attacks the heart (American Heart Association, 2007).

Some medications (such as arthritic medication) and stimulants (such as caffeinated beverages) that individuals consume can cause the heart to race and may trigger heart attacks.

Cardiovascular Disease: Not Just a Man's Disease

The gap between men and women in the number of deaths from heart disease and stroke has narrowed significantly. In 2003, the number of deaths from heart disease and stroke was nearly equal for men and women (37,004 male deaths versus 36,823 female deaths) (Heart and Stroke Foundation of Canada, 2007c). And in 2004, more women died from stroke than did men (8,667 women versus 5,959 men) (Heart and Stroke Foundation of Canada, 2007c). The Heart and Stroke Foundation of Canada (2007c) has recently reported that women are 16 percent more likely than men to die within 30 days of a heart attack and 11 percent more likely than men to die within 30 days of a stroke.

Older women face the greatest danger, because the risk of falling victim to cardiovascular disease quadruples after menopause (Health Touch, 1998). At menopause, the ovaries slowly stop producing the hormone estrogen, which is heart-protective. There may be an increase in LDL or "bad" cholesterol and triglyceride levels, and a decrease in HDL or "good" cholesterol. Blood pressure also starts creeping up. Reduced estrogen may lead to an increase in body fat above the waist, which negatively affects the way blood clots and the way the body handles sugars (a precursor condition to diabetes).

In 2005, 16 percent of women and 22 percent of men in Canada aged 15 years and older were smokers. The good news regarding this statistic is that it is the lowest level in more than four decades of monitoring smoking rates (Statistics Canada, 2006). However, with smoking and the use of oral contraceptives combined, there is increased risk for blood clots and stroke in women (Stampfer, 2003).

Another frightening statistic is that 53 percent of Canadian women aged 18 and over are overweight or obese (Tjepkema, 2005). Obesity increases the risk of high blood pressure, diabetes, high blood cholesterol, heart disease, and stroke.

PERSONAL PERSPECTIVE

In the fall of 1999, a female graduate of that year at our college suffered a mild stroke. She was 21 years old. The doctors determined that smoking, social drinking, and taking birth control pills contributed to her stroke. With a strong will, she has struggled with regaining her speech and the use of her arm and foot. We all need to understand that what we consume can directly affect our bodies. Statistics indicate that women smokers who use birth control pills are 10–20 times more likely to have heart attacks or strokes than non-smoking women (Heart and Stroke Foundation of Ontario, 2006c).

Here are some sites to assist you if you are a smoker and interested in quitting. They are resources for self-help:

- One Step at a Time: Canadian Cancer Society .... www.cancer.ca
- Get on Track: Ontario Lung Association .... www.lung.ca
- Canadian Health Network .... www.canadian-health-network.ca
- Physicians for a Smoke-Free Canada .... www.smoke-free.ca
- QuitNet .... www.quitnet.org
- Quit Smoking Support .... www.quitsmokingsupport.com
- Quit 4 Life: Health Canada www.quit4life.com

With over 49 percent of women aged 12 and over inactive, women are doubling their risk of developing heart disease, doubling the risk of dying from cardiovascular disease, and increasing the risk of hypertension. If a woman becomes hypertensive, it increases the risk of cardiovascular disease by 3.5 times over a woman with normal blood pressure (Corrao, 1990). Combine any of these with diabetes, and the risk of developing cardiovascular disease becomes eight times greater than that for women without diabetes (Laakso et al., 1995).

Cardiovascular Disease and Children

In Canada rates of obesity among children and youth aged 2 to 17 years are increasing. In 1978–79, just 3 percent of children and youth were obese. By 2004, 8 percent, or an estimated 500,000, were obese (Shields, 2005). An additional 18 percent of Canadian children and youth are overweight. This means more than one-quarter (26 percent) of children are carrying too much weight. Excessive weight gain during adolescence and young adulthood may be one of the most important determinants of future development of heart disease and stroke (Connelly, 2005).

ANATOMY OF THE HEART

Located between your lungs, slightly to the left, and behind your sternum, is your heart. It weighs between 200 and 425 grams and is about the size of your fist. The average heart beats approximately 100,000 times a day, distributing about 7,200 litres (1,900 gallons) of blood. In your lifetime, it will beat approximately 2.5 billion times.

Your heart is designed to circulate blood. It pumps oxygen-rich blood to the rest of your body through a complex network of arteries, arterioles, and capillaries; deoxygenated (oxygen-poor) blood is carried back to the heart through the veins to send to the lungs to pick up oxygen and remove carbon dioxide.

HOW THE HEART FUNCTIONS

Your heart is a pump with four chambers. The two upper chambers are referred to as the left and right atria, and the lower ones are the left and right ventricles. Separating the left and right sides of the heart is a wall of muscle called the septum. There are four valves that separate each chamber and prevent the blood from coming back when the heart is at rest. Refer to figure 11.3.

The right two chambers of your heart (right atrium and ventricle) pump the deoxygenated blood to the lungs and exchange the waste (carbon dioxide) for oxygen. The blood then returns to the left chambers of the heart (left atrium and ventricle). The left ventricle is the largest and strongest chamber. Its job is to push blood through the aortic valve and into the superior and inferior vena cava, which distribute the blood to the rest of the body.

An electrical impulse starting the heartbeat and causing the atria to contract begins in a group of cells called the sinus node (SA node). It is called the pacemaker of the heart. This electric impulse spreads across into the lower part of the heart, stimulating the atrio-ventricular node (AV node), which causes the ventricles to contract and send blood pumping out with great force.

FIGURE 11.3 **Diagram of the Heart**

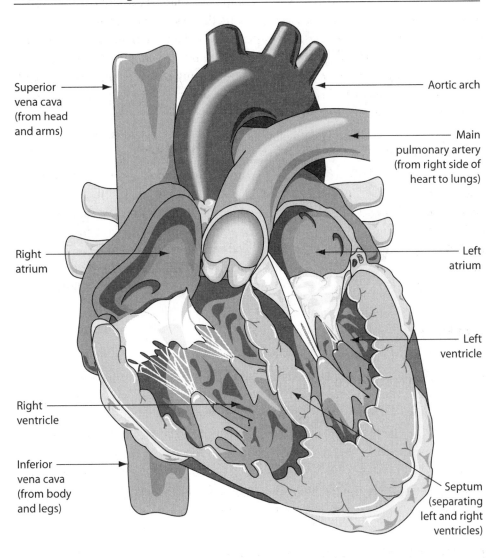

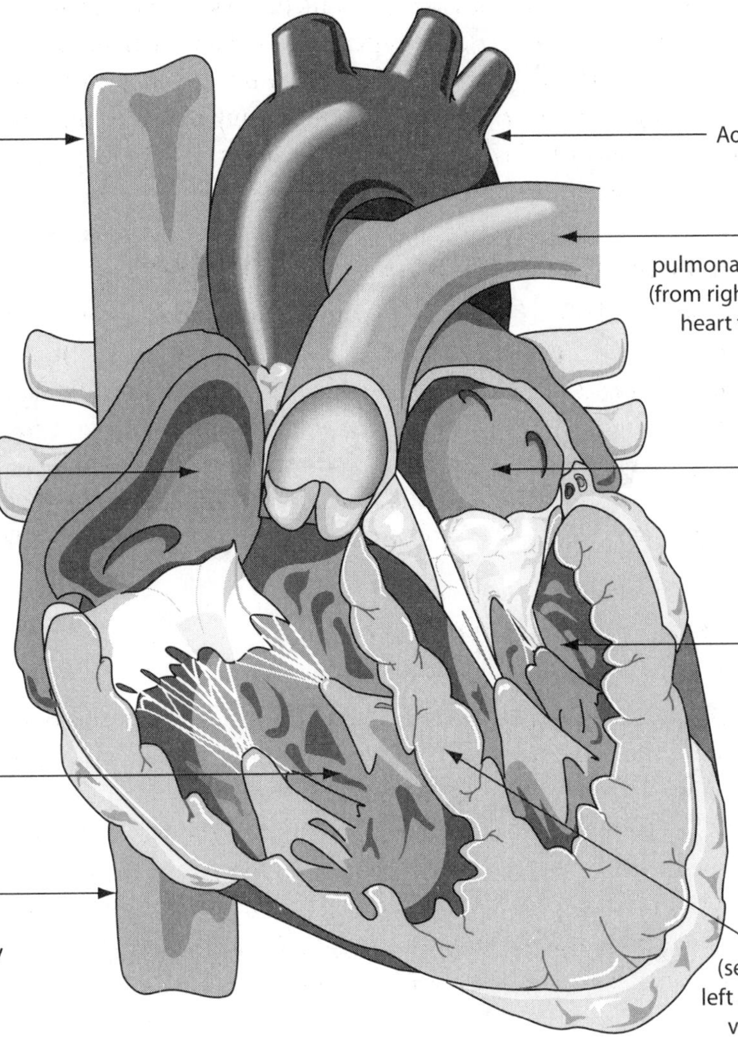

TYPES OF CARDIOVASCULAR DISEASE

The remainder of this chapter examines four common types of cardiovascular disease: arteriosclerosis, coronary heart disease, stroke, and hypertension.

Arteriosclerosis

Arteriosclerosis is not a single disease but a group of diseases characterized by a narrowing or hardening of the arteries. In these diseases, blood flow to vital organs is restricted by a progressive blockage of the arteries.

Atherosclerosis is a common type of arteriosclerosis, a slow, progressive disease that may start in childhood, in which arterial blockage results from fatty deposits collecting in the arteries. The deposits are typically composed of cholesterol, cellular debris, fibrin (a clotting material in the blood), and calcium. Atherosclerosis is not restricted to one area of the body, although some areas may experience a greater degree of blockage than others. This buildup of deposits in the arteries is called

arteriosclerosis
a blanket term for a group of diseases characterized by a narrowing or hardening of the arteries

atherosclerosis
a common type of arteriosclerosis; a slow, progressive disease in which arterial blockage results from fatty deposits collecting in the arteries

FIGURE 11.4 Atherosclerosis: Cross-Sectional View of an Artery

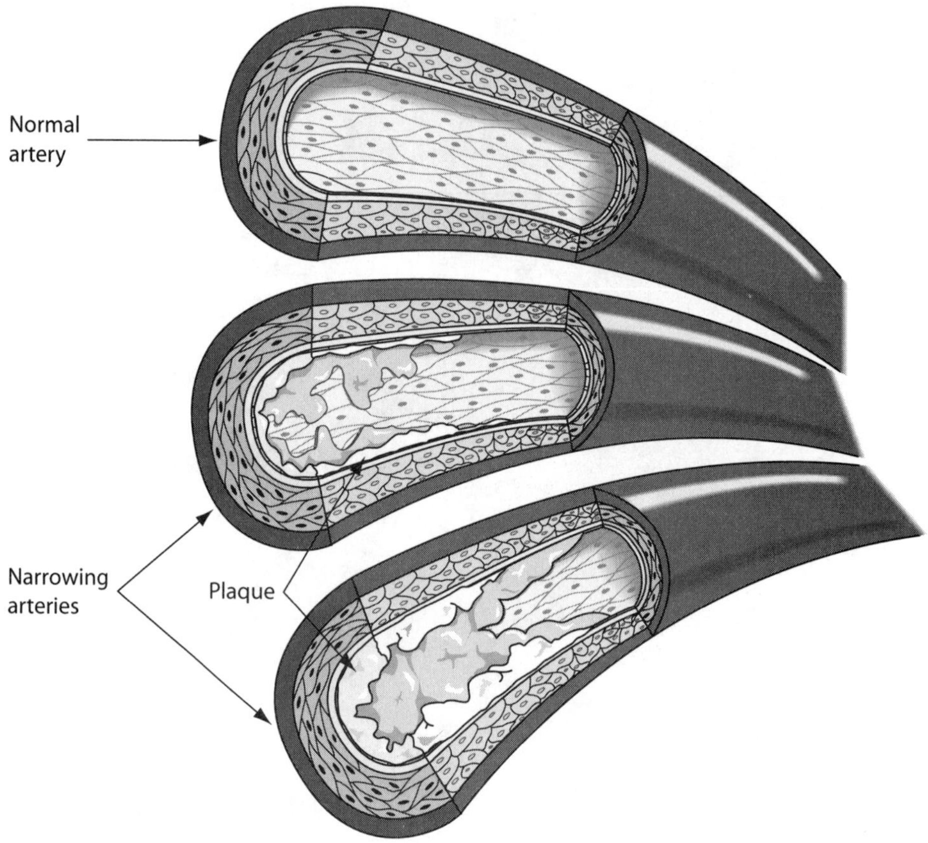

plaque (see figure 11.4). There are two types of plaque. Hard plaque causes the artery walls to thicken and harden. Soft plaque is more likely to break apart from the walls and enter the bloodstream, which can cause a blood clot that can partially or totally block the flow of blood in an artery. If this happens, the tissue past the blockage is deprived of blood and oxygen, and it may either die or suffer severe damage.

The causes of atherosclerosis are complicated. It is believed that the inner lining of the arteries becomes damaged and the body reacts by laying down the fatty deposits. Over time, the blood vessels become progressively thicker. High blood pressure, cholesterol, triglycerides in the blood, and smoking can contribute to the development of plaque.

Symptoms may not be apparent until the disease is far enough advanced to block a large part of the vessel. In the arteries of the heart (coronary arteries) it will cause angina (chest pain), which can lead to coronary artery disease. In the brain or carotid arteries (the two large arteries on either side of the head that carry blood to the head), it can cause a stroke.

coronary heart disease a type of coronary artery disease in which fatty deposits block one or more coronary arteries (arteries supplying the heart)

Coronary Heart Disease

Coronary heart disease, a type of coronary artery disease, occurs when fatty deposits block one or more coronary arteries (arteries supplying the heart). When the blockage becomes severe enough to cause ischemia (restricted blood flow), insuf-

FIGURE 11.5 Diagram of Myocardial Infarction (Heart Attack)

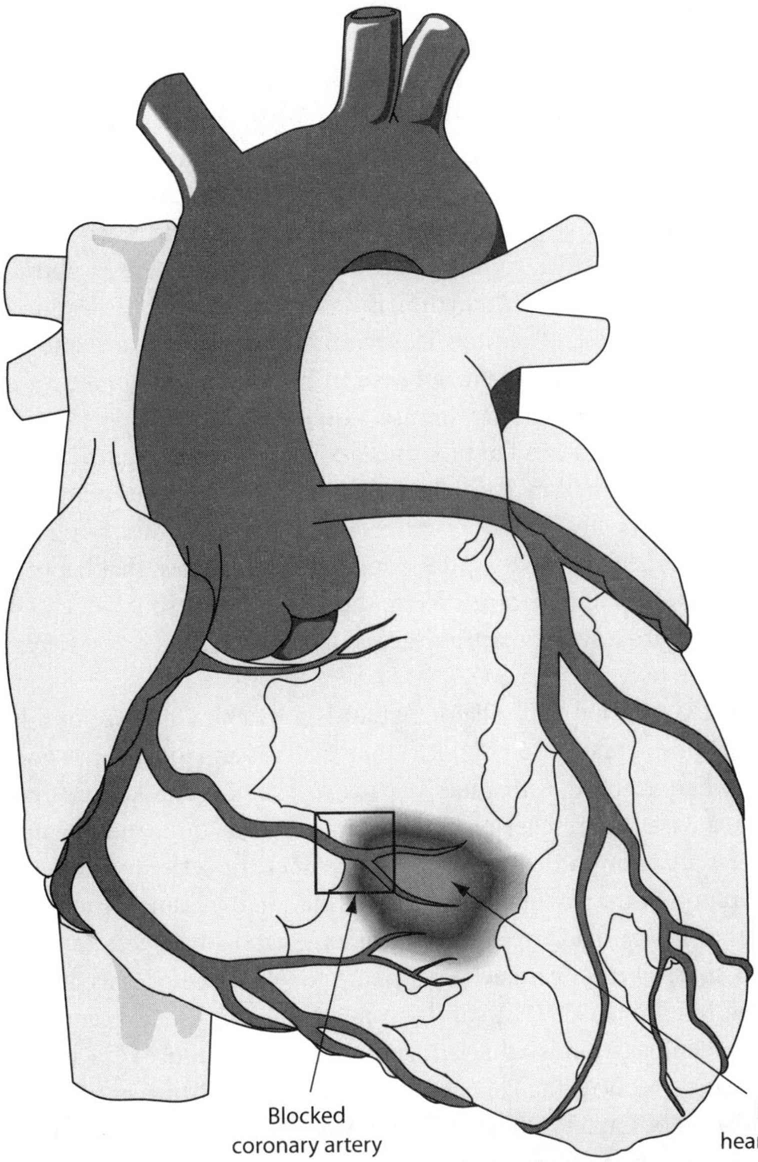

ficient oxygen reaches the heart and the person may experience severe chest pains called **angina pectoris**. Angina can be infrequent or constant, depending on the severity of the restriction.

In the most extreme cases, no oxygen can get past the blockage. When this happens, a heart attack (**myocardial infarction**) occurs (see figure 11.5). The cells past the blockage become damaged or die. The number of damaged and dead cells determines the seriousness of the attack—the greater the damage, the smaller the chance of recovery. Damage to the heart muscle may cause the heart to quiver rapidly (ventricular fibrillation), preventing the heart from delivering oxygenated blood to other organs and tissues, especially the brain. Permanent brain damage can occur within five minutes if the heart does not resume pumping blood to the brain. Myocardial infarction can also lead to **cardiac arrest** (the heart stops pumping).

angina pectoris
severe chest pains associated with advanced cases of coronary heart disease

myocardial infarction
a heart attack

cardiac arrest
cessation of the heart's pumping action

If emergency medical personnel reach a heart attack victim in time, they can administer medication to limit the damage and open up the coronary artery. If left untreated, the dead or damaged areas of the heart muscle are replaced by scar tissue, which weakens the pumping action of the heart and can lead to heart failure and other complications. The heart may go into arrhythmia (irregular heartbeat or rhythm), called ventricular fibrillation. Survival rates are highest for those victims able to receive clot-busting medication within an hour of a heart attack.

Sudden cardiac arrest is a major cause of death in Canada. Each year, more than 45,000 Canadians suffer from a sudden cardiac arrest (Heart and Stroke Foundation of Manitoba, 2007). Arrhythmias such as ventricular fibrillation cause most sudden cardiac arrests. The time between the onset of cardiac arrest and the performance of defibrillation is the major determinant for success in the resuscitation attempt. While cardiopulmonary resuscitation (CPR) can support circulation and ventilation for a short period of time, it is unlikely to convert ventricular fibrillation to a normal heart rhythm. Early defibrillation is the intervention that is most likely to save lives. If the heart is not restarted within a few minutes, brain damage and death will occur. Of those who suffer a sudden cardiac arrest that happens out of the hospital, fewer than 5 percent survive the trip to the hospital, due to delays in recognizing the cardiac emergency and access to the appropriate care (Heart and Stroke Foundation of Manitoba, 2007).

An automated external defibrillator (AED) is a machine the size of a laptop computer (but approximately 13 cm thick) that analyzes and looks for a shockable heart rhythm when attached, with adhesive pads, to a victim. The AED analyzes the heart rhythm, advises the rescuer of the need for defibrillation, and prompts the rescuer to press a button to deliver a controlled shock, or series of shocks, as required. Restoration of the rhythm requires defibrillation to be administered within a few minutes of the cardiac arrest. The use of external defibrillators can increase the chance of survival from cardiac arrest by up to 74 percent (Heart and Stroke Foundation of Manitoba, 2007). A survival rate of as high as 90 percent has been reported when defibrillation is achieved within the first minute of collapse. Every minute that passes reduces the chances of survival by 7–10 percent (Heart and Stroke Foundation of Canada, 2001b; St. John Ambulance, 2000). After more than 12 minutes of ventricular fibrillation (irregular, rapid, and chaotic firing of the ventricles), the survival rate is less than 5 percent (Larsen et al., 1993).

Administering CPR before emergency personnel arrive also increases the victim's likelihood of survival, and for this reason everyone should know CPR. CPR is the process of externally supporting the circulation and respiration of a person who has had a cardiac arrest. Artificial respiration and chest compression substitute for normal breathing and circulation until advanced life support measures can be taken. The flow of oxygen to the brain can be sustained and the amount of permanent damage can be reduced.

A heart attack victim may also undergo bypass surgery to provide new blood supply.

The common symptoms of a heart attack can include the following:

- a prolonged heavy squeezing pressure or squeezing pain in the centre of the chest, sometimes spreading to the shoulders, arms, neck, jaw, or throat; in women, pain may be a vague chest discomfort

- shortness of breath, paleness, sweating, or weakness
- nausea, vomiting, or indigestion
- a feeling of extreme anxiety and fear, or denial that anything is wrong.

Signs may be mild or severe. Until the 1980s, it was believed that male and female heart attack victims experienced the same symptoms. We know today that this is not always so. For example, women are more likely to experience unique symptoms such as vague chest discomfort, indigestion, back pain, and fatigue. As well, some heart attack tests and treatments may not work as well for women as for men.

Research on treating heart attacks has progressed a great deal in the past 30 years. There are now treatments to open blocked arteries while a heart attack is in progress or soon after. One particularly successful process, called reperfusion, uses drugs to restore blood flow to the heart muscle. Once the blocked arteries are opened, the heart attack usually stops. If treatment occurs early enough, damage to the heart muscle is minimized, and the pumping ability of the undamaged tissue is not as greatly impaired, which means that the heart attack survivor is able to enjoy a higher quality of life. Survival rates are highest for those victims who receive clot-busting medication within an hour of a heart attack.

THE FRAMINGHAM HEART STUDY

The objective of the Framingham Heart Study was to identify the common factors or characteristics that contribute to cardiovascular disease by following its development over a long period of time in a large group of participants who had not yet developed overt symptoms of cardiovascular disease or suffered a heart attack or stroke. Researchers recruited men and women between the ages of 30 and 62 from the town of Framingham, Massachusetts, and began the first round of extensive physical examinations and lifestyle interviews, which they would later analyze for common patterns related to the development of cardiovascular disease. Since 1948, the subjects have continued to return to the study every two years for a detailed medical history, physical examination, and laboratory tests. In fact, the third generation of these families is now being recruited and examined to understand how genetic factors relate to cardiovascular disease. This study, which has being going on for nearly six decades, is viewed as pioneering research throughout the world. For more information about the study, go to www.nhlbi.nih.gov/about/framingham.

UNCONTROLLABLE RISK FACTORS FOR CORONARY HEART DISEASE

The major uncontrollable risk factors for heart disease are the following:

- *Family history of coronary heart disease* Having a family history of cardiovascular disease appears to increase the risk significantly.
- *Ethnicity* South Asians, First Nations/Aboriginal peoples, Inuit, and blacks are at greater risk for hypertension and thus are at higher risk for

cardiovascular disease than are whites. These groups also have a worse chance of surviving heart attacks. (Heart and Stroke Foundation of Canada, 2003).

- *Gender* Men have a greater risk of suffering cardiovascular disease in their younger years. Women catch up to men quickly after reaching menopause because the protection of hormones is removed. Some women increase their risk before menopause if they smoke and take oral contraceptives.

CONTROLLABLE RISK FACTORS FOR CORONARY HEART DISEASE

Many police services now offer educational programs to help officers assess their risk of developing coronary heart disease and to modify risky behaviours. Smoking-cessation programs, cholesterol assessments, blood pressure clinics, and the fitness pin award offered by the Police Fitness Personnel of Ontario are some of the initiatives that have been undertaken.

Here are some of the risk factors for coronary heart disease that you can control:

- *Smoking* Smoking poses the greatest risk for heart disease. Smokers increase their risk for cardiovascular disease by 70 percent. Exposure to second-hand smoke may increase the risk of cardiovascular disease by 30 percent (Breslow, 1997). Although we do not fully understand how cigarettes damage the heart, there are two possible explanations. One is that carbon monoxide in cigarette smoke may cause a deficiency of oxygen in the body, causing the heart to work harder. The other centres on the nicotine and tar released in cigarette smoke, which cause damage to the blood vessel walls and allow cholesterol and plaque to build up. In addition, women who both smoke and use oral contraceptives have an increased risk of stroke (Heart and Stroke Foundation of Canada, 2003).
- *Physical inactivity* Individuals who do not participate in at least moderate physical activity increase their risk for cardiovascular disease. Exercise increases levels of "good" (HDL) cholesterol, improves serum lipids and blood pressure, helps people manage stress, and improves the efficiency of the heart, lungs, and muscles. Exercise also reduces body weight and improves diabetes. Individuals who are having difficulty becoming physically active should seek professional assistance (such as a certified personal trainer), and those who have been diagnosed with heart disease or who have identified risk factors should seek professionally trained personnel who are familiar with these issues (such as a certified exercise physiologist).
- *High blood cholesterol* Abnormally elevated cholesterol, low-density lipoproteins (LDL), and triglycerides, and low levels of high-density lipoproteins (HDL) are increased risk factors for developing vascular diseases, particularly for coronary artery disease. We know that elevated levels of total serum cholesterol and low-density lipoprotein cholesterol are important risk factors for strokes, including carotid artery disease (Heart and Stroke Foundation of Canada, 2003).
- *High blood pressure* Defined as blood pressure greater than 140/90. High blood pressure is a major risk factor for strokes, coronary artery disease, peripheral vascular disease, and congestive heart failure. A great deal of research indicates that lowering blood pressure can reduce the incidence of

stroke, myocardial infarction, ischemic heart disease, vascular disease, renal (kidney) disease, heart failure, and overall death rate. We know that those who are overweight, physically inactive, drink heavily, and consume excessive salt have a higher risk of developing high blood pressure. There is also a higher risk of metabolic cardiovascular risk factors, which include insulin resistance, obesity, hyperuricemia (an excess of uric acid in the blood, often producing gout), and dyslipidemia (an abnormal concentration of lipids or lipidproteins in the blood) (Heart and Stroke Foundation of Canada, 2003). A startling statistic is that 42 percent of us with high blood pressure don't even know that we have it (Heart and Stroke Foundation of Canada, 2007b).

- *Diabetes* People with diabetes tend to have elevated blood fat levels and increased atherosclerosis. Since overweight individuals have an increased risk for diabetes, it becomes more difficult to differentiate the effects on cardiovascular disease. Cardiovascular disease is in fact the leading cause of death in diabetics. Diabetes increases the risk of high blood pressure, strokes, and heart and vascular diseases, particularly in women. There are also added risks of peripheral vascular disease, eye problems, and kidney disease. After the age of 50, the percentage of men with diabetes is higher than the percentage of women (Heart and Stroke Foundation of Canada, 2003).
- *Obesity* Being overweight puts additional strain on your entire body. If you are more than 13.5 kg (30 pounds) overweight, you are at higher risk for heart disease and stroke (Heart and Stroke Foundation of Canada, 2001a). Your heart must work harder to push blood through extra capillaries that feed the excess fat. This pressure can damage the vessels. People who are overweight or obese are at risk of developing high blood pressure, high blood lipids, and diabetes, all of which put them at a high risk for cardiovascular or heart disease. Being overweight—either excess weight (defined by WHO as a body mass index (BMI) of 25.0–29.9) or obesity (BMI ≥ 30.0)—among individuals aged between 18 and 64 years is one of the most common factors that influence the development of high blood pressure and diabetes, which are two risk factors for cardiovascular diseases (Heart and Stroke Foundation of Canada, 2003, p. 27, 2003).
- *Stress* As discussed in chapter 13, people who have especially high stress levels are considered time bombs for a heart attack. When under stress, the body produces stress chemicals, which in turn increase blood pressure. Chronic hostility and hate are two key personality factors related to the greatest risk.
- *Inadequate consumption of fruits and vegetables* According to *Canada's Food Guide* (2007), 5 to 10 servings of fresh fruits and vegetables are recommended for daily intake. Fruits and vegetables are associated with reduced risk of cardiovascular diseases. They are important for intake of natural vitamins, antioxidants, and fibre. Potassium, which is present in many fruits and vegetables (for example, bananas, tomatoes, and sweet potatoes), has been shown to be protective, particularly against strokes (Heart and Stroke Foundation of Canada, 2003).

- *Poor dental hygiene* Periodontal disease (gum disease) is associated with heart disease, strokes, and diabetes. Good dental hygiene is important for reducing gum disease and the risk of heart disease. With increased risk of endocarditis, police officers who work 12-hour shifts need to be aware of how important it is to brush their teeth regularly and floss daily. This means taking a toothbrush to work. It is also important to avoid food that contains excessive amounts of sugar.

Stroke

Stroke—paralysis and a sudden loss of consciousness caused by an interruption of blood flow to the brain—is one of the leading causes of death in Canada. Between 40,000 and 50,000 people suffer a stroke in Canada each year, and one out of every four dies (Heart and Stroke Foundation of Ontario, 1996). Of the survivors, only a third make a full recovery.

A stroke can occur when a blood clot travels to the brain and interrupts the blood supply (and thus the oxygen supply) to the brain. As a result, brain cells die and the parts of the body they control can stop functioning. This is called a thrombotic or thromboembolic stroke and it occurs in about 80 percent of the stroke population (Heart and Stroke Foundation of Ontario, 2006b).

A stroke may also occur when very high blood pressure causes a weakened blood vessel near the brain to break. This is called a hemorrhagic stroke and accounts for 20 percent of strokes (Heart and Stroke Foundation of Ontario, 2006e). **Subarachnoid hemorrhage** is uncontrolled bleeding on the surface of the brain, in an area between the brain and the skull. **Intracerebral hemorrhage** occurs when an artery deep within the brain ruptures. Both can be caused by structural problems with the blood vessels in the brain. An **aneurysm** is a weakened area in the blood vessel wall that fills with blood and bulges. As a result of high blood pressure or trauma, the vessel can rupture and cause uncontrolled bleeding in the brain. An **arteriovenous malformation** (AVM) is a malformation of the blood vessels, usually present at birth, that becomes weak and risks hemorrhaging.

A **transient ischemic attack** (TIA) occurs when the blood supply to the brain is temporarily interfered with. About 15,000 Canadians each year suffer a TIA. People who have had a TIA are five times more likely than the general population to have a full-blown stroke within two years (Heart and Stroke Foundation, 2006a). These attacks can last for seconds or hours and can happen for a variety of reasons. They do not cause permanent neurological damage and are not necessarily a warning sign of an impending stroke.

A stroke damages the brain and causes a sudden loss of brain function. Since your brain is divided into a number of sections, there are different effects for each.

The effects of left hemisphere strokes include:

- weakness or paralysis on the right side of the body
- trouble reading, talking, thinking, or doing math
- behaviour that is more slow and cautious than usual
- trouble learning or remembering new information
- requiring frequent instructions and feedback to finish tasks.

stroke
paralysis and a sudden loss of consciousness caused by an interruption of blood flow to the brain; a thrombotic or thromboembolic stroke occurs when blood flow is interrupted by a blood clot that travels to the brain; a hemorrhagic stroke occurs when very high blood pressure causes a weakened blood vessel near the brain to break

subarachnoid hemorrhage
hemorrhage that occurs when a blood vessel on the surface of the brain bleeds into the space between the brain and the skull

intracerebral hemorrhage
bleeding in the brain resulting from the rupture of a blood vessel

aneurysm
a weak or thin area in a blood vessel that causes it to expand and fill with blood; aneurysms may occur as a result of a disease, an injury, or a congenital abnormality in the vessel

arteriovenous malformation
a malformation of the blood vessels of the brain, usually present at birth; an arteriovenous malformation can increase the risk of stroke

transient ischemic attack
a temporary interference with the blood supply to the brain

The effects of right hemisphere strokes include:

- weakness or paralysis on the left side of the body
- vision problems
- problems with depth perception, up and down, front and back
- inability to pick up objects, button up a shirt, or tie a shoe
- inability to understand a map
- short-term memory loss
- forgetting or ignoring objects or people on your left side
- having difficulty with judgment, including acting impulsively or not realizing your own limitations.

Brain stem strokes (at the base of brain), which are uncommon, include the following problems:

- difficulty with breathing and heart function
- body temperature control problems
- difficulties with balance and coordination
- weakness or paralysis of your arms and legs on both sides of the body
- difficulty with chewing, swallowing, and speaking
- vision problems.

Strokes in the cerebellum are also less common, but they have more severe effects, including:

- ataxia (inability to walk with coordination and balance)
- dizziness
- headache
- nausea and vomiting.

Even if these symptoms seem to quickly disappear, one should seek medical attention immediately. More than 40 percent of potential stroke patients who receive medical treatment within the critical three-hour time window will significantly reduce the risk or degree of long-term impairment. Since 1998, mortality rates for patients 30 days after a stroke have decreased 4.5 percent in Ontario (Heart and Stroke Foundation of Canada, 2007c).

THE RISK FACTORS FOR STROKE

Risk factors for stroke that you can control include the following:

- *High blood pressure* High blood pressure affects one in five Canadians and is the number one risk factor for stroke. Blood pressure that is consistently more than 140/90 is considered high, but if you are diabetic, 130/80 is high (Heart and Stroke Foundation of Canada, 2007b). With high blood pressure there is an increased risk of burst blood vessels, resulting in a stroke.
- *Smoking* Smoking, whether primary or second-hand, can contribute to plaque buildup in your arteries and increase the risk of blood clots, doubling the risk of an ischemic stroke (Heart and Stroke Foundation, 2006c).

- *High blood cholesterol* Increased levels of LDL cholesterol build up plaque on your arteries causing atherosclerosis, which can lead to a blockage in the brain.
- *Obesity* Those who carry extra weight are more at risk to suffer from high blood pressure, which places a great strain on the blood vessels of the brain.
- *Physical inactivity* Those who do not stay physically active increase their risk of unhealthy weight, high blood pressure, high cholesterol, and higher stress levels.
- *Excessive alcohol consumption* Those who drink too much alcohol can increase their blood pressure, which can lead to a stroke. A recent meta-analysis published in the *Journal of the American Medical Association* concluded that heavy alcohol consumption increases the relative risk of stroke, while light or moderate alcohol consumption may be protective against total and ischemic stroke (Reynolds et al., 2003).
- *Stress* Stress releases hormones that increase blood pressure and blood cholesterol, which leads to atherosclerosis.
- *Heart disease–atrial fibrillation* Atrial fibrillation affects approximately 200,000 to 250,000 Canadians. It is estimated that up to 15 percent of all strokes are due to atrial fibrillation. Caused by high blood pressure, atrial fibrillation can cause blood clots to form, leading to strokes (Heart and Stroke Foundation of Canada, 2006d).

Risk factors for stroke that you can't control include the following:

- *Age* Although strokes can occur at any age, most strokes occur in persons over 65.
- *Family history of stroke* Those with a parent or sibling who had a stroke before age 65 are at increased risk of having a stroke.
- *Ethnicity* First Nations people and those of African or South Asian descent are more likely to have high blood pressure and diabetes, putting them at higher risk for strokes.
- *Gender* Until menopause, women have lower risk of stroke than men. After that, women take the lead.
- *Prior stroke or TIA* If you've had a previous stroke or a TIA, your risk is greater for another stroke.
- *Socioeconomic status* Lower socioeconomic levels increase the risk of poorer nutritional intake.

Recommendations to Prevent Strokes

The Heart and Stroke Foundation (Coordinated Stroke Strategy, 2005) makes the following recommendations:

- Consider taking medication if you have conditions including cardiovascular disease, diabetes, truncal obesity (high amounts of abdominal fat), or abnormally high LDL cholesterol levels; if you have a strong family history of these conditions; if you are a smoker; or if you lead a sedentary lifestyle.
- Lead a healthier lifestyle, including regular physical activity (at least 30 minutes of moderate-intensity activity daily) and appropriate nutrition

(enrich your diet with fruits, vegetables, whole grains, nuts, and omega-3 fatty acids).

- Reduce your intake of sugars if you are diabetic.
- Make an effort to limit or quit smoking.
- Reduce consumption of alcohol. Follow the Canadian low-risk drinking guidelines (two or fewer standard drinks per day, with consumption not exceeding 14 standard drinks per week for men and nine standard drinks per week for non-pregnant women).
- Avoid medication that increases blood pressure, which may put you at risk for stroke.
- Those with symptoms may consider surgical intervention (such as carotid stenting, which is the opening of the carotid arteries to allow better blood flow to the brain).

Turn to **assignment 11.1**, "First Aid for Heart Attack and Stroke Victims" (in the appendix). Using your first aid text and Internet sites, research how you as a law enforcement officer should be prepared to deal with heart attacks and strokes.

Hypertension

hypertension
high blood pressure—the term *essential hypertension* is used for cases in which the cause is unknown

Hypertension (high blood pressure) is estimated to be the leading risk for death in the world (World Health Organization, 2002). Known as the silent killer, this health risk can be prevented by following an appropriate lifestyle that is relatively easy to manage. Hypertension affects about 25 percent of the adult population in Canada, and with the current lifestyles we lead, over 90 percent are at risk of developing hypertension (Wolf-Maier et al., 2003; Vasan et al., 2002). It has been documented that 40 percent of hypertensive adults in Canada are unaware they have hypertension. Of those that are aware, only about two-thirds are being treated pharmacologically and about 13 percent are being treated and controlled (Joffres et al., 2001). Unfortunately, it is predicted that the prevalence of hypertension will rise with an aging sedentary population that has poor dietary habits and increasing obesity (Impending Global Pandemic, 1999). High blood pressure can double or even triple your risk of heart disease and stroke, and increase your risk of kidney disease.

THE DASH EATING PLAN

The DASH Eating Plan, supported through the National Heart, Lung and Blood Institute (NHLBI), was developed as an eating plan that is low in sodium, saturated fat, cholesterol, and total fat. It emphasizes fruits, vegetables, whole grain products, fish, poultry, nuts, and fat-free or low-fat milk and milk products that are rich in potassium, magnesium, and calcium, along with protein and fibre. It is a diet that limits the consumption of red meats, sweets, added sugars, and sugar-containing beverages. This diet's emphasis is to lower blood pressure and decrease the risks of cardiovascular disease and diabetes. It also stresses losing weight, regular exercise, and limiting consumption of alcohol. For more information about this plan, visit www.nhlbi.nih.gov/health/public/heart/hbp/dash/new_dash.pdf.

Approximately 11 percent of the Canadian adult population (3.6 million) has high normal blood pressure (130–139/85–89 mmHg). In 2006, a trial was conducted to "prevent" hypertension in overweight adults with high normal blood pressure with the use of pharmacotherapy (Julius et al., 2006). In the participants treated with a placebo, a startling 40.4 percent developed hypertension within two years and 63.0 percent within four years. This very high risk is confirmed by the Framingham study, where 37.3 percent of those aged 35–64 and 49.5 percent of those above age 65 with high normal blood pressure developed hypertension within four years (Vasan et al., 2001).

The focus of the Canadian Hypertension Education Program (CHEP) is to encourage adults to regularly monitor their blood pressure, reassess blood pressure in those with high normal values, educate on preventable lifestyles, and educate to reduce dietary sodium (World Health Organization, 2002; Hooper et al., 2002). In 2006, CHEP recommended the DASH type of diet ("Lowering Your Blood Pressure with DASH") for the prevention and management of hypertension (Touyz et al., 2004; Khan, 2006). For 2007, additional evidence has become available on the antihypertensive effectiveness of soluble fibre, whole grains, and protein from plant sources (Appel et al., 2005; He et al., 2005; Rasmussen et al., 2006). This recommendation emphasizes fruits, vegetables, low-fat dairy products, dietary and soluble fibre, and whole grains and protein from plant sources, which will reduce saturated fat and cholesterol.

There are two forms of high blood pressure: essential (or primary) and secondary. Essential hypertension is a common condition that accounts for 95 percent of hypertension. Risk factors for this type of hypertension include the following:

- family history of hypertension
- gender (men are more likely to have hypertension, but women's risk increases significantly after menopause)
- age (more often in people over 35)
- ethnicity (the risk is higher for South Asians, First Nations/Aboriginal peoples, Inuit, and blacks than whites)
- obesity (if you are 20 percent or more above your ideal body weight)
- smoking
- sensitivity to sodium (high salt or sodium in your diet)
- heavy alcohol consumption
- use of oral contraceptives
- physical inactivity

Secondary hypertension, which accounts for 5 percent of hypertension cases, is caused by specific abnormalities in one of the organs or systems of the body. Specifically, causes of secondary hypertension include:

- the narrowing of the renal arteries, which causes renal hypertension in the kidneys
- tumours of the adrenal glands (glands that sit right on top of the kidneys), which can cause other conditions, such as hyperaldosteronism, Cushing's syndrome, and pheochromocytoma

- coarction of the aorta (a rare hereditary disorder characterized by the narrowing of the aorta above the renal arteries, causing lack of sufficient blood flow to the kidneys and influencing the release of a number of hormones to boost blood pressure to the kidneys)
- pregnancy and pre-eclampsia (commonly called toxemia), which is an increase in blood pressure that can lead to kidney damage, convulsion, and coma in the mother, as well as eye or brain damage in the fetus
- metabolic syndrome and obesity

ABOUT BLOOD PRESSURE

Blood pressure is measured in two parts and is expressed as a fraction—for example, 120/80 or 120 over 80. The first number refers to systolic pressure, or the pressure that is applied to the walls of the arteries when the heart contracts. The second value is diastolic pressure or the pressure on the arterial walls during the heart's relaxation phase. This is the phase where the heart refills with blood. The higher your systolic or diastolic pressure, and the length of time during which it stays high, the more damage to your blood vessels will occur. Strokes and heart attacks are caused by damaged blood vessels.

Normal blood pressure varies for different individuals based on their weight, age, gender, ethnicity, and physical condition. Table 11.1 classifies blood pressure to give you a clearer idea of what your blood pressure means.

For most people, blood pressure should be less than 140/90. It is now recommended that people with diabetes or kidney disease have blood pressure less than 130/80. Blood pressure less than 120/80 is very good unless it causes dizziness (CHEP, 2007).

TABLE 11.1 Classification of Hypertension

(Pre-hypertension) 120–139/80–89

Category	Systolic	Diastolic
Optimal	< 120	< 80
Normal	< 130	< 85
High-normal	130–139	85–89
Grade 1 (mild hypertension)	140–159	90–99
Grade 2 (moderate hypertension)	160–179	100–109
Grade 3 (severe hypertension)	≥ 180	≥ 110
Isolated systolic hypertension (ISH)	≥ 140	< 90
The category pertains to the highest-risk blood pressure		

Source: Chalmers J., et al. (1999). *Journal of Hypertension*, *17*, 151-185.

A physician will diagnose you with hypertension under the following conditions (CHEP, 2007):

- if your blood pressure is extremely high (above 200/120)
- if your blood pressure is higher than 160/100 over three visits
- if your blood pressure is higher than 140/90 over five visits
- if you have diabetes or kidney disease and blood pressure higher than 130/80
- if your blood pressure is higher than 135/85 when measured over a week at home, twice a day, in the morning and evening (go to a doctor to confirm).

It is important to have regular checkups with your doctor to ensure that your blood pressure is normal and your general health is good. If you have high blood pressure, you will not be able to perform a BFOR test (see chapter 16) without medical clearance. Since the test is a means of screening for law enforcement recruits, you should be aware of your blood pressure. If you are unsure, consult your instructor or doctor. Some people experience "white coat syndrome"—elevated blood pressure that is caused by anxiety about the tester who is taking your blood pressure or anxiety over the result of the test. For those people, it is important to understand what blood pressure is and to have their blood pressure tested repeatedly. Some individuals who are being tested for a BFOR will bring documentation from a doctor who has diagnosed the syndrome as proof that they have been cleared by their physician for testing.

PREVENTION OF CARDIOVASCULAR DISEASES

Generally, you can help prevent these diseases if you do the following:

- Exercise. Be physically active for 30 to 60 minutes every day of the week—five times a week you need to work at an intensity of 70 to 85 percent (see chapter 6 for more information).
- Choose foods such as fruits, vegetables, and whole grains and those lower in saturated and trans fats and salt, and limit fast foods and prepared foods (see chapter 8).
- If you are overweight, losing about 5 kg may help you get within a healthy range (see chapter 9).

APPENDIX: CARDIOVASCULAR DISEASE GLOSSARY

If you research cardiovascular diseases, you may come upon terminology that is new. Here is a glossary to help you understand these terms more clearly.

acute myocardial infarction
The formation of a blood clot in one or more of the blood vessels to the heart, causing damage to the heart muscle from a lack of blood flow; sometimes called a heart attack.

angina pectoris
A symptomatic manifestation of ischemic heart disease, describing a severe squeezing or pressure-like thoracic pain brought on by exertion or stress

angioplasty
The dilatation of a blood vessel by means of a balloon catheter where the balloon is inflated to flatten plaque against the artery wall.

arrhythmia
An irregular heartbeat. There are two types: those that are too slow (bradycardia) and those that are too fast (tachycardia).

cardiovascular diseases
All diseases of the circulatory system including acute myocardial infarction, ischemic heart disease, valvular heart disease, peripheral vascular disease, arrhythmias, high blood pressure, and stroke.

carotid endarterectomy
The excision of thickened atheromatous (fatty deposit) areas of the innermost layer of the carotid artery.

cerebrovascular disease
Diseases of one or more blood vessels of the brain that can result in a stroke.

cholesterol
A soft waxy substance found among the lipids (fats) in the blood and in every one of our body's cells. Too much cholesterol in the blood can lead to heart disease.

congenital heart disease
A class of cardiac disease caused by abnormal development of the heart prior to birth.

congestive heart failure
The inability of the heart to maintain adequate pumping function.

coronary artery disease
see ischemic heart disease.

diabetes mellitus
A condition associated with an elevation of blood glucose levels.

elevated serum cholesterol
Serum cholesterol level in the blood greater than or equal to 5.2 mmol/litre.

endocarditis
An infection of the heart or vascular system, most often superimposed on pre-existing valvular heart disease.

high blood pressure
Diastolic blood pressure equal to or greater than 90 or systolic blood pressure equal to or greater than 140.

hypercholesterolemia
High levels of cholesterol in the blood.

ischemic heart disease
Any condition in which the heart muscle is damaged or works inefficiently because of an absence or relative deficiency of its blood supply; most often caused by atherosclerosis, it includes angina pectoris, acute myocardial infarction, chronic ischemic heart disease, and sudden death.

myocardial infarction
Another name for a heart attack, which refers to the blockage of blood flow to the heart muscle.

obesity
According to the World Health Organiz ation, having a body mass index of 30 or more.

pacemaker
An electronic device that sends tiny electrical signals through a wire (called an electrode catheter) to the heart. These electrical signals cause the heart muscle to contract and generate a heartbeat. Pacemakers are most commonly used to maintain an adequate heart rate in patients suffering from bradycardia, although they also have other uses.

stenosis
Refers to the area of narrowing or blockage in the coronary artery caused by atherosclerosis.

thrombolysis
The process whereby a blood clot is broken up or dissolved.

transient ischemic attack
Attack that occurs when the blood supply to the brain is temporarily blocked by a blood clot. The attack usually lasts 10 minutes or less and does not cause permanent neurological damage.

triglycerides
A form of lipid, essentially chains of fatty acids, that provide much of the energy that the body's cells need in order to function. High levels are associated with increased risk of coronary artery disease.

ventricular fibrillation (VF)
A chaotic, extremely rapid, and highly irregular heart arrhythmia originating in the ventricles. Ventricular fibrillation causes immediate loss of consciousness and is fatal unless stopped (usually by using a defibrillator). VF is the most common cause of sudden death.

ventricular tachycardia (VT)
Disturbance of the heart's rhythm, causing the ventricles to beat rapidly and inefficiently.

OTHER POINTS OF INTEREST

Further information on cardiovascular disease is available from the Heart and Stroke Foundation of Canada's website (www.heartandstroke.ca) and through the Ontario Heart and Stroke Foundation's local offices. The following topics might be of special interest to you or your family:

- blood clots
- aneurysms
- congestive heart failure
- congenital heart defects
- stress testing
- surgical procedures (including intra-uterine surgery to correct heart defects before birth)
- drug therapy
- pacemakers

KEY TERMS

arteriosclerosis

atherosclerosis

coronary heart disease

angina pectoris

myocardial infarction

cardiac arrest

stroke

subarachnoid hemorrhage

intracerebral hemorrhage

aneurysm

ateriovenous malformation

transient ischemic attack

hypertension

EXERCISES

Review

1. What is arteriosclerosis?

2. What is coronary heart disease?

3. What are some possible signs of a heart attack?

4. How does hypertension affect the heart and arteries?

5. What special concerns surround women and cardiovascular disease?

6. Drawing on what you have learned so far, list five ways that people can lower their risk of cardiovascular disease. Include explanations of how these lower the risk.

7. What causes strokes?

8. What are the typical symptoms of an impending stroke?

9. Why is hypertension known as the silent killer?

10. Why is it important to learn CPR and AED?

Multiple Choice

1. The condition where the artery walls become thickened, hard, and non-elastic is
   a. arteriosclerosis
   b. atherosclerosis
   c. coronary embolism
   d. coronary thrombosis
   e. high blood pressure

2. Which of the following are considered controllable risk factors for heart disease?
   a. family history of heart disease, stress, obesity
   b. gender, high blood pressure, obesity
   c. inactivity, gender, high blood pressure
   d. high cholesterol levels, stress, inactivity
   e. diabetes, family history of heart disease, obesity

3. Which of the following is considered a primary risk factor for heart disease that you can change?
   a. diabetes
   b. inactivity
   c. high blood lipids
   d. gender
   e. smoking

4. A myocardial infarction is caused by
   a. high blood pressure
   b. diabetes
   c. a clot in the brain
   d. weakness in the heart muscle
   e. a blockage in one of the coronary arteries

5. What is the *main* benefit of good blood supply and circulation in the coronary arteries?
   a. it strengthens heart valves by moving more blood through the heart
   b. it nourishes the heart and reduces the risk of a heart attack
   c. it helps to prevent blood pooling in the lower limbs
   d. it increases blood pressure in the heart

6. Which of the following lifestyle practices may help control or prevent hypertension?
   a. maintaining a healthy body weight
   b. exercising regularly
   c. not drinking alcohol, or doing so only in moderation
   d. practising stress management
   e. all of the above

7. A stroke is caused by
   a. a blood clot in the coronary arteries
   b. a severe headache
   c. a blood clot in the brain
   d. a blood clot in the leg
   e. hardening of the arteries

8. Arteriosclerosis is a term for
   a. chest pain
   b. myocardial infarction
   c. angina
   d. hardening of the arteries
   e. blood clot

9. High blood pressure is, most directly, a measure of
   a. potential pain
   b. heart stress
   c. pressure within blood vessels
   d. cholesterol levels
   e. advanced aging

10. AED stands for
    a. arterial external defibrillator
    b. automated energy device
    c. arterial emergency dialysis
    d. automated external defibrillator
    e. atrial emergency device

11. The leading cause of death in Canada is
    a. cancer
    b. HIV/AIDS
    c. cardiovascular disease
    d. high blood pressure
    e. motor vehicle accidents

12. The two upper chambers of the heart are called the
    a. atria
    b. ventricles
    c. aortic valves
    d. sinoatrial nodes
    e. aortic branches

13. The two lower chambers of the heart are called the
    a. atria
    b. ventricles
    c. aortic valves
    d. sinoatrial nodes
    e. aortic branches

14. The general term for the thickening and hardening of arteries is
    a. atherosclerosis
    b. arteriosclerosis
    c. plaque formation
    d. myocardial infarction
    e. carotid plaque

15. The upper limit of high normal blood pressure is
    a. 120/80
    b. 160/110
    c. 140/90
    d. 139/89
    e. 150/100

16. The reduction in oxygen flow to the heart causing chest pain is known as
    a. ischemia
    b. angina pectoris
    c. arrhythmia
    d. myocardial infarction
    e. atrial fibrillation

17. An irregular heartbeat is called
    a. tachycardia
    b. fibrillation
    c. arrhythmia
    d. bradycardia
    e. atrial flutter

18. Which of the following risk factors for cardiovascular disease is uncontrollable?
    a. heredity
    b. smoking
    c. physical inactivity
    d. drinking
    e. consuming large quantities of fat

19. Which of the following risk factors for cardiovascular disease is controllable?
    a. gender
    b. age
    c. high cholesterol level
    d. family history
    e. ethnicity

20. A mild form of a stroke, leaving only temporary symptoms, is called a(n)
    a. embolism
    b. thrombosis
    c. subarachnoid hematoma
    d. transient ischemic attack
    e. atrial flutter

21. Premenopausal women may have lower rates of heart attacks compared with men due to
    a. pregnancy
    b. the ability to cope with stress
    c. hormone replacement therapy
    d. eating better
    e. estrogen

22. Normal blood pressure is considered to be
    a. 120/90
    b. 120/80
    c. 130/90
    d. 130/80
    e. 110/60

23. Hypertension is known as the silent killer because
    a. people don't know how to take their blood pressure
    b. people don't pay attention to the symptoms
    c. people are unaware that they have high blood pressure
    d. people don't understand what their blood pressure means
    e. people ignore their symptoms in order to do things they want to do

REFERENCES

American Heart Association. (2007). *Bacterial endocarditis.* Available at http://www.americanheart.org/presenter.jhtml?identifier=4436.

Appel, L.J., Sacks, F.M., Carey, V.J., et al. (2005). Effects of protein, monounsaturated fat, and carbohydrate intake on blood pressure and serum lipids: Results of the OmniHeart randomized trial. *Journal of the American Medical Association, 204,* 2455-2564.

Breslow, J.L. (1997). Cardiovascular disease burden increases, NIH funding decreases. *Nature Medicine, 3,* 6000-6009.

Campbell, N.R.C., Onysko, J., Johansen, H., & Gao, R.-N. (2006). Changes in cardiovascular deaths and hospitalization in Canada. *Canadian Journal of Cardiology, 22,* 425-427.

Canadian Centre for Health Information. (1989). Cardiovascular disease in Canada. *Health Reports, 1,* 1-22.

Canadian Hypertension Education Program (CHEP). (2007). Recommendations. Available at http://www.hypertension.ca/chep/en/default.asp.

Chockalingam, A., & Balaguer-Vintró, I. (Eds.). (1999). *Impending global pandemic of cardiovascular disease.* Barcelona, Spain: Prous Science.

Coordinated Stroke Strategy. (2005). Working to provide Ontario citizens with the best possible stroke care. *Heart and Stroke Foundation of Canada Professional Education.* Available at http://www.strokestrategyseo.ca/pdf_docs/Prevention % 20Workshop % 20Overview % 20July % 2005.pdf.

Connelly, C. (2005). *Interventions Related to Obesity: A state of the evidence review.* 2003. Ottawa: Report commissioned by the Heart and Stroke Foundation of Canada.

Corrao, J.M., Becker, R.C., Ockene, L.S., & Hamilton, G.A., et al. (1990). Coronary heart disease risk factors in women. *Cardiology, 77,* 8-12.

He., J., Gu, D., Wu, X., Chen, J., Duan, X., & Whelton, P.K. (2005). Effect of soybean protein on blood pressure: A randomized controlled trial. *Annals of Internal Medicine, 143:* 1-9.

Health Touch. (1998). *Heart Disease, Women & Nutrition.* Available at http://www.healthtouch.com/bin/EContent_HT/hdShowLfts.asp?lftname=DCC003&cid=HTHLTH.

Heart and Stroke Foundation of Canada. (2001a). *Risk factors.* Available at http://ww2.heartandstroke.ca.

Heart and Stroke Foundation of Canada. (2001b). *Types of Attacks.* Available at http://ww2.heartandstroke.ca.

Heart and Stroke Foundation of Canada. (2003, May). *The growing burden of heart disease and stroke in Canada.* Ottawa: Author.

Heart and Stroke Foundation of Canada. (2006a). *Mini strokes: What you need to know!* Available at http://ww2.heartandstroke.ca/Page.asp?PageID=1965&ArticleID=5005&Src=stroke&From=SubCategory.

Heart and Stroke Foundation of Canada. (2006b). *Ischemic stroke & TIA (mini-stroke).* Available at http://ww2.heartandstroke.ca/Page.asp?PageID=1965&ArticleID=5068&Src=stroke&From=SubCategory.

Heart and Stroke Foundation of Canada. (2006c). *Smoking, heart disease and stroke.* Available at http://ww2.heartandstroke.ca/Page.asp?PageID=1965&ArticleID=4989&Src=stroke&From=SubCategory.

Heart and Stroke Foundation of Canada. (2006d). *Heart disease-atrial fibrillation.* Available at http://ww2.heartandstroke.ca/Page.asp?PageID=1965&ArticleID=4993&Src=stroke&From=SubCategory.

Heart and Stroke Foundation of Canada. (2006e). *Hemorrhagic stroke.* Available at http://ww2.heartandstroke.ca/Page.asp?PageID=1965&ArticleID=5069&Src=stroke&From=SubCategory.

Heart and Stroke Foundation of Canada. (2007a). *Health dictionary.* Available at http://ww2.heartandstroke.ca/Page.asp?PageID=1936.

Heart and Stroke Foundation of Canada. (2007b). *High blood pressure.* Available at http://ww2.heartandstroke.ca/Page.asp?PageID=1965&ArticleID=4984&Src=stroke&From=SubCategory.

Heart and Stroke Foundation of Canada. (2007c). Report cards on health: 2007 Report on Canadians' health—Time to bridge the gender gap, says the Heart and Stroke Foundation. Available at http://ww2.heartandstroke.ca/Page.asp?PageID=1613&ContentID=24339&ContentTypeID=1.

Heart and Stroke Foundation of Manitoba. (January 2007). *Automated external defibrillators (AEDs)—Getting started.* Available at http://ww2.heartandstroke.ca/Page.asp?PageID=1613&ContentID=23077&ContentTypeID=1.

Heart and Stroke Foundation of Ontario. (1993). *Planned giving: A gift from your heart could save a life.* Toronto: Author.

Heart and Stroke Foundation of Ontario. (1996). *Stroke facts, heart and stroke healthline, disease and lifestyle information.* Toronto: Author.

Heart and Stroke Foundation of Ontario. (2001). *General info—Incidence of cardiovascular disease.* Available at http://ww1.heartandstroke.on.ca.

Hooper, L., Bartlett, C., Smith, G.D., & Ebrahim, S. (2002). Systematic review of the long term effect of advice to reduce dietary salt in adults. *British Medical Journal, 325,* 628-637.

Joffres, M.R., Hamet, P., MacLean, D.R., L'Italien, G.J., & Foder, G. (2001). Distribution of blood pressure and hypertension in Canada and the United States. *American Journal of Hypertension, 14,* 1099-1105.

Julius, S., Nesbit, S.D., Egan, B.M., et al. (2006). Feasibility of treating prehypertension with an angiotensin-receptor blocker. *New England Journal of Medicine,* 354, 1742-174.

Khan, N.A., McAlister, F.A., Rabkin, S.W., et al. (2006). The 2006 Canadian Hypertension Education Program recommendations for the management of hypertension: Part II—Therapy. *Canadian Journal of Cardiology, 22,* 583-593.

Laakso, M., Ronnemaa, T., Lehto, S., Puukka, P., Kallio, V., & Ryorala, K. (1995). Does NIDDM increase the risk for coronary heart disease similarly in both low- and high-risk populations? *Diabetologia, 38,* 487-493.

Larsen, M.P., Eisenberg, M.S., Cummins, R.O., & Hallstrom, A.P. (1993). Predicting survival from out-of-hospital cardiac arrest: A graphic model. *Annals of Emergency Medicine, 22,* 1642-1658.

Laurent, M., Belanger, A., Berthelot, J.M., & Carriere, Y. (2005). *Healthy today, healthy tomorrow? Findings from the National Population Health Survey.* Catalogue no. 82-618-MWE2005004. Ottawa: Statistics Canada.

Onysko, J., Maxwell, C., Elaisziw, M., Zhang, J., Johansen, H., & Campbell, N. (2006). Large increases in hypertension diagnosis and treatment in Canada following a health care professional education program. *Hypertension, 48,* 853-860.

Pepe, J. (2007, March 7). Certified exercise physiologist. Telephone conversation.

Pradhan, A.D. (2001). C-reactive protein, interleukin 6, and risk of developing type 2 diabetes mellitus. *Journal of the American Medical Association, 286,* 327-334.

Public Health Agency of Canada. (2002). *Economic burden of illness in Canada, 1998.* Available at http://www.hc-sc.gc.ca/ahc-asc/media/nr-cp/2002/2002_ebic-femc_e.html.

Rasmussen, B.M., Vessby, B., Uusitupa, M., et al. (2006). Effects of dietary saturated, monounsaturated, and n-3 fatty acids on blood pressure in healthy subjects. *American Journal of Clinical Nutrition, 83,* 221-226.

Reynolds, K., Lewis, L.B., et al. (2003). Alcohol consumption and stroke: A meta-analysis. *Journal of the American Medical Association, 289*, 579-588.

Seguin, R. (2007, March 7). RCMP "O" Division Fitness and Lifestyle Coordinator. Telephone conversation.

Sharratt, M.T., & Sharratt, J.K. (1994). Potential health benefits of active living for persons living with chronic conditions. In H.A. Quinney, L. Gauvin, & T. Wall (Eds.), *Toward active living* (pp. 42-43). Champaign, IL: Human Kinetics.

Shields, M. (2005). *Nutrition: Findings from the Canadian Community Health Survey—Overweight Canadian children and adolescents* Catalogue no. 82-620-MWE2005001. Ottawa: Statistics Canada.

St. John Ambulance. (2000). Automated external defibrillation—AED. *First aid: First on the scene.* Ottawa: St. John Ambulance.

Stampfer M.J., et al. (2003). Primary prevention of coronary heart disease in women through diet and lifestyles. *NEJM, 343*, 16-22.

Statistics Canada. (1997). *Causes of death 1995.* Catalogue no. 84-208-XPB. Ottawa: Author.

Statistics Canada. (1999). *Causes of death in Canada, 1997.* Catalogue no. 84F0208XPB. Ottawa: Author.

Statistics Canada. (2003). *Causes of death 2001.* Catalogue no. 84-208-XIE. Ottawa: Author.

Statistics Canada. (2004). *Causes of death 2002.* Catalogue no. 84F0503XPB. Ottawa: Author.

Statistics Canada. (2006). *Canadian tobacco use monitoring survey (CTUMS).* Available at http://www.hc-sc.gc.ca/hl-vs/tobac-tabac/research-recherche/stat/ctums-esutc/2006/index_e.html.

Tjepkema, M. (2005). Measured obesity. Adult obesity in Canada: Measured height and weight. *Nutrition: Findings from the Canadian Community Health Survey.* Issue no. 1. Catalogue no. 82-620-MWE2005001. Ottawa: Statistics Canada.

Touyz, R.M., Campbell, N., Logan, A., et al. (2004). The 2004 Canadian recommendations for the management of hypertension: Part III — Lifestyle modifications to prevent and control hypertension. *Canadian Journal of Cardiology, 20*, 55-59.

Vasan, R.S., Beiser, A., Seshadri, S., et al. (2002). Residual lifetime risk for developing hypertension in middle-aged women and men. *Journal of the American Medical Association, 287*, 1003-1010.

Vasan, R.S., Larson, M.G., Leip, E.P., Kannel, W.B., & Levy, D. (2001). Assessment of frequency of progression to hypertension in non-hypertensive participants in the Framingham Heart Study: A cohort study. *Lancet, 358*, 1682-1686.

Wolf-Maier, K., Cooper, R.S., Banegas, J.R., et al. (2003). Hypertension prevalence and blood pressure in 6 European countries, Canada and the United States. *Journal of the American Medical Association, 289*, 363-369.

World Health Organization. (2002). *The world health report 2002.* Geneva: Author.

CHAPTER 12

Back Pain

CHAPTER OBJECTIVES

After completing this chapter, you should be able to:

- Describe the prevalence of back pain and back injuries in policing.
- Describe the functions of the spine.
- Describe the causes of back pain, and identify the special risks to a healthy back posed by policing.
- Describe how arthritis, osteoporosis, and repetitive strain injuries have a potential impact on a person involved in law enforcement.
- Describe how a healthy back may be maintained.
- Describe how back injuries are treated.

Back pain, most of which occurs in the lower back, is one of the most common health complaints among Canadian adults. Almost everyone experiences some type of back pain during the course of their lives. In most cases the pain subsides within a couple of days or weeks. However, for some it may occur repeatedly and in some cases it may never go away. For some people it has a major impact on their ability to do regular chores around the house and perform simple daily tasks. More than 70 percent of back problems begin during routine daily activities. Accidents and other forms of trauma account for only 30 percent of back problems (Canadian Physiotherapy Association, 2006). Next to the common cold, low-back pain is the most common reason for missing work. On average, 90 percent of people with acute low-back pain will recover within four weeks (Canadian Physiotherapy Association, 2006).

Low-back pain is a disease of inactivity. More than 80 percent of low-back pain problems are caused by inadequate muscular development. Low-back pain usually makes its first appearance between the ages of 30 and 50, at a point in life when people are spending more time on family and job-related activities and are less physically active (National Institute for Neurological Disorders and Stroke, 2003). Routine activities such as housework, taking out the garbage and blue boxes, gardening, or reaching for an object may trigger an episode of acute back pain, which may last for hours, days, or even years.

In this chapter we will look at the causes of low-back pain, including the special risks faced by law enforcement officers. We will also look at preventing and managing back pain.

Researchers in Canada conducted a survey in the late 1990s of a random sample of 1,002 members of the Royal Canadian Mounted Police (RCMP) to determine if back problems were more common in this group than the general public (Brown et al., 1998). Researchers found that the general public reported a one-year prevalence rate between 25 and 62 percent, while the RCMP had a one-year prevalence rate between 44 and 62 percent (Brown et al., 1998). The researchers concluded that the prevalence of back problems in the sample of RCMP officers was similar to that of the general public, and that police officers did not have a higher risk of back problems due to certain aspects of their job such as wearing a seatbelt or riding in a patrol vehicle all day (Brown et al., 1998). However, a later study found that there was a small effect of wearing boots on posture and the biomechanical load on the spine. In this study, researchers also found that the duty belt did not have any significant effect on an officer's flexibility and range of motion, but it did increase the metabolic cost of wearing the equipment, which could tire constables by the end of the day and predispose them to low-back pain precipitation (Kumar & Narayan, 2001). Another study found that exposure to wearing heavy body armour, combined with exposure to vehicle vibration for over two hours per day, did increase the risk of low-back pain (Burton et al., 1996), while yet another found that officers who drove and sat in the same vehicle were at greater risk than those whose daily tasks were varied, such as those who spent part of their day walking (Gyi & Porter, 1998).

Wearing a vest and firearms or carrying an overloaded backpack may lead to poor posture, overstretching of the soft tissue of the neck and back, and excessive strain on muscles and joints. Over time, the physical strain of carrying heavy loads may lead to the following problems:

- Harmful strain and fatigue in the muscles and soft tissues of the back from overuse. Constantly carrying the weight on one side may cause the spine to develop an adaptive curve, and leaning forward too much may affect the natural curve of the lower back and increase the curve of the upper back and shoulders.
- Spinal compression and/or improper alignment, which may hamper the proper functioning of the discs between the vertebrae that provide shock absorption, which in turn leaves the back more vulnerable to injury.
- Stress to or compression of the shoulders and arms, which in turn causes the nerves to be compressed, resulting in tingling, numbness, or weakness in the arms or hands.

THE SPINE

vertebrae
the bones of the spine (singular: vertebra)

To understand back pain, you first need to know something about the spine. The spine has 33 bones, called **vertebrae**. These extend from the base of the skull to the end of the trunk (see figure 12.1). The spine is naturally curved, which ensures proper balance and weight bearing. The spine has the following functions (Fahey, Insel, & Walton, 1997):

FIGURE 12.1 **The Spine**

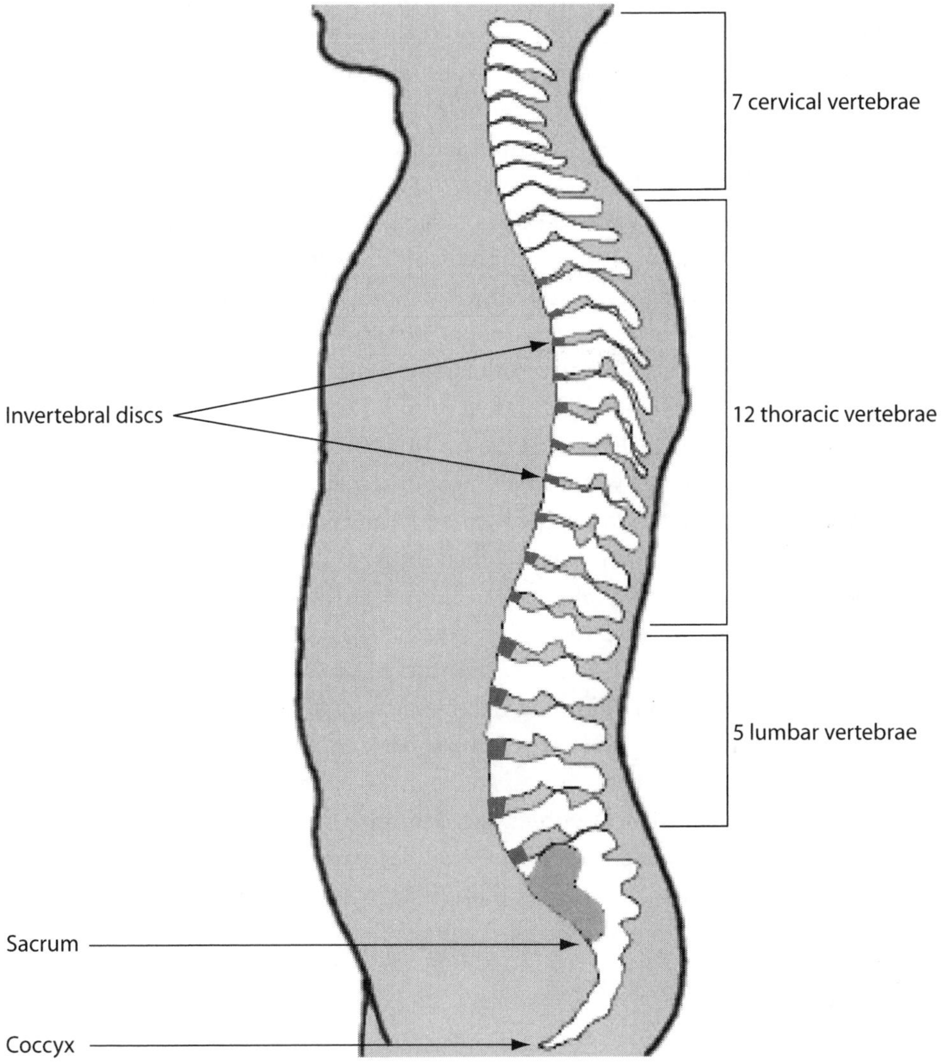

- It provides structural support for the body, especially the thorax (chest).
- It surrounds and protects the spinal cord (a column of nervous tissue that acts as a continuation of the brain and connects the brain to the rest of the nervous system).
- It serves as an attachment site for a large number of muscles, tendons, and ligaments. (Tendons are strong, fibrous structures that attach muscles to bones. Ligaments are also strong and fibrous, and link two bones together at a joint.)
- It allows movement of the neck and back in all directions.

Each vertebra is made up of a large bone, called the body, and a bony ring. The vertebrae link together to form a "tunnel" that protects the nerves and spinal cord. The lumbar vertebrae are under constant pressure from the weight of the upper body. The wear and tear of this pressure over a period of time may contribute to the development of low-back pain. The vertebrae are separated by flexible, gelatinous, shock-absorbing pads called **intervertebral discs**, which are approximately

intervertebral discs flexible, gelatinous, shock-absorbing pads that separate the vertebrae

90 percent water in young people but only about 70 percent water in older people (we lose the water as we age) (Greenberg & Dintiman, 1997). As a result, in older people the spine is more vulnerable to injury. The discs act as shock absorbers between the vertebrae in the spine. As we age or experience disc degeneration (typically age 40 onward), the normal gelatin-like centre of the discs degenerates and the spaces between the vertebrae narrow. This puts additional stress on the vertebrae, which causes further wearing and may cause pressure on the spinal cord or nerve endings. Degeneration of the intervertebral discs, which is often called **degenerative disc disease (DDD)** of the spine, is a common disorder of the lower spine. Disc degeneration may lead to disorders such as spinal stenosis (narrowing of the spinal canal that houses the spinal cord and nerve roots and may affect the lumbar or cervical nerves), spondylolisthesis (forward slippage of a disc and vertebra), and retrolisthesis (backward slippage of a disc and vertebra). Disc degeneration in the neck is referred to as cervical disc disease, in the mid-back it is referred to as thoracic disc disease, and in the lumbar spine area it is referred to as lumbago. Age, repetitive strain, and possibly genetics cause disc wear and tear. Since there is little blood supply to the discs, they cannot repair themselves if injured.

degenerative disc disease (DDD)
degeneration of the intervertebral disc

One common injury is a "slipped" or herniated disc, which occurs when sudden pressure causes the disc to rupture and its gelatinous interior to protrude through the outer coat of the disc. (See figures 12.2 and 12.3.) The protruding material may put pressure on adjoining nerves, causing considerable low-back pain, which radiates into the legs. However, most back problems involve the muscles, tendons, or ligaments, not the bones. As we grow older, the discs become flatter, and if stressed or weakened, the outer part (annulus) may bulge or tear. The location of the pain is dependent on where the disc is pressing on the nerve. In the lumbar region it is called sciatica, a condition we will discuss later in the chapter.

OSTEOPOROSIS

Another problem that is occurring in our aging population is an increase in back injuries as a result of osteoporosis. **Osteoporosis** is a condition common in older people, in whom bones become increasingly soft and porous, thinner, and more brittle, making them susceptible to risk of fracture, particularly of the hip, spine, and wrist. Seventy percent of hip fractures are osteoporosis-related. Hip fractures result in death in up to 20 percent of cases, and disability in 50 percent of those who survive. Osteoporosis is known as the "silent thief" because bone loss occurs without symptoms. Approximately 1.4 million Canadians suffer from osteoporosis (Osteoporosis Canada, 2007). As we age, the discs begin to lose their gelatinous mass, resulting in compression of the vertebrae. One of the signs of osteoporosis is a substantial decrease in height and a stooped appearance (see figure 12.4). Increased pressure on the adjoining nerves and vertebrae causes the vertebrae to crack. Women are at a greater risk for osteoporosis due to a greater loss of calcium and lower bone density. This risk increases at menopause when protective hormones are reduced. Osteoporosis may be prevented by taking calcium supplements and hormone replacements and by doing weight-bearing exercises. Research indicates that calcium loss may begin as early as 25–30 years old; the onset of calcium loss may depend on hormone imbalance, so those who do not have as much of the

osteoporosis
a condition common in older people, in whom bones become increasingly soft and porous, thinner, and more brittle, making them susceptible to risk of fracture, particularly of the hip, spine, and wrist

FIGURE 12.2 Process of Herniation of an Intervertebral Disc: Side View

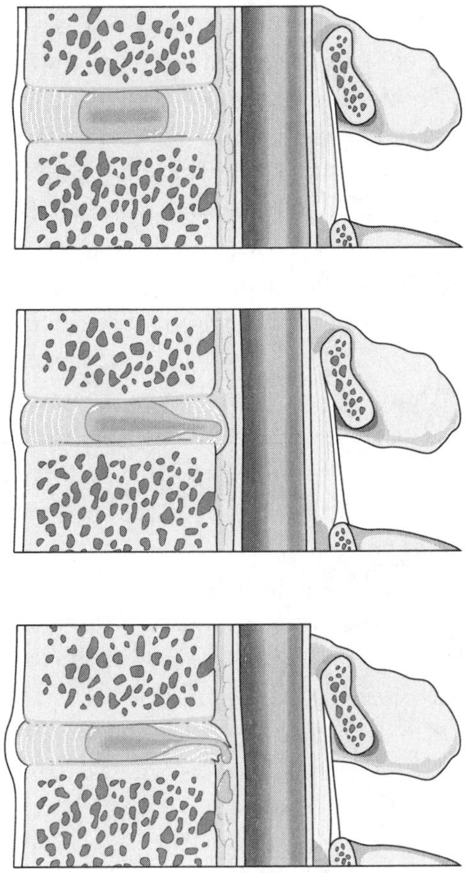

FIGURE 12.3 Herniation and Rupture of an Intervertebral Disc: Top View

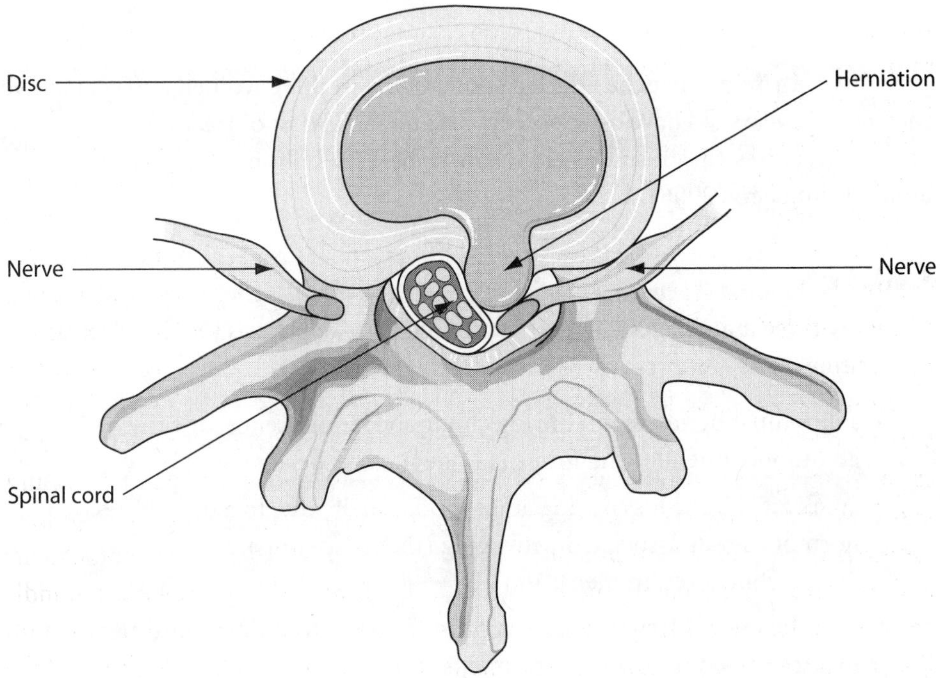

FIGURE 12.4 **Osteoporosis and Its Effects on the Spine**

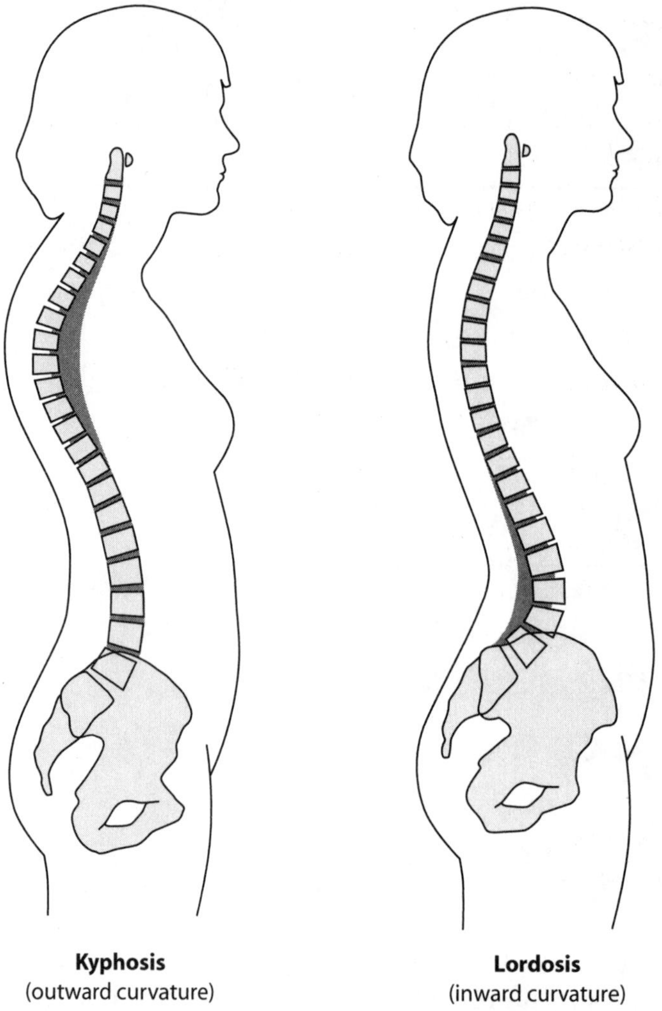

protective hormones may be affected sooner. One in three women and one in five men over 50 years old have osteoporosis. The financial cost of treating osteoporosis and the fractures that result is estimated to be $1.9 billion each year in Canada alone (Henneberg, 2006).

Causes

There are three main factors that are attributed to osteoporosis (National Institutes of Health, 2003):

- suboptimal bone growth during childhood, adolescence, or early adulthood, not allowing for peak bone mass to be achieved;
- accelerated bone loss during adulthood, usually due to a drop in sex hormone levels associated with aging (that is, menopause in women, low testosterone levels in men); and
- bone loss secondary to disease conditions including eating disorders, medications, and medical treatments.

Risk Factors

The risk factors for osteoporosis include (National Institutes of Health, 2003):

- *Gender* Women are at higher risk.
- *Fracture history* Personal history of fracture after age 50 or a family history of fractures increases the risk.
- *Race* Asian and Caucasian women are at greater risk.
- *Body frame and weight* Women who have a small frame or who are below 127 pounds are at greater risk.
- *Age* Risk increases with age.
- *Menopause* Women can lose more than 20 percent of their bone mass in the first five to seven years following menopause.
- *Low testosterone in men* Testosterone levels decrease with age.
- *Absence of or abnormal menstruation* Delayed menarche, no menstruation, or an abnormal menstrual cycle can increase the risk.
- *Certain medications and conditions* Medications and conditions that affect vitamin D and calcium absorption increase the risk.
- *Lack of physical activity* Inadequate weight-bearing activity increases the risk.
- *Lifestyle factors* Cigarette smoking and excessive alcohol use increase the risk.

Diagnosis of Osteoporosis

Four major risk factors for fractures are age (over 65 years), low bone mineral density, fragility fractures after age 40, and family history of osteoporosis. Some of the minor risk factors include excessive caffeine and alcohol use, smoking, low calcium intake, early menopause (before age 45), and weight less than 57 kg (Mills, 2006). Osteoporosis Canada has recommended that everyone over the age of 65, and those who are over 50 and have at least one major risk factor or two minor risk factors, should have a DXA bone densitometer test, which assesses density of the hip, spine, and forearm on a yearly basis (Mills, 2006). The bone densitometry allows accurate and precise skeletal assessment, and enables detection of osteoporosis prior to actual fractures. It can determine if there is any onset of fractures in the spine and limbs. With information about a patient's risk factors and the results of a bone densitometer test, a physician can determine diagnosis of mineral loss in the bone.

THE CAUSES OF BACK PAIN

Although some people have a weak back for genetic reasons, inadequate muscular development is the major cause of back pain. The strength of a muscle is directly related to the amount of work it does. Strength increases the more the muscle is made to work against an opposing force. If the muscle is not worked enough, it loses strength. In physically inactive people, the large muscle groups are not worked enough and therefore lack sufficient strength. For the back, insufficient muscle strength means that correct body alignment is compromised.

The back is supported and its movement is controlled by 140 muscles. Typically, a muscle, ligament, or tendon strain or sprain causes nearby muscles to spasm (involuntarily contract) in an attempt to support the back. It is estimated that 70 percent of back problems are due to improper alignment of the spine and pelvic girdle (hip bones) caused by inflexible and weak muscles (Greenberg & Dintiman, 1997). Poor flexibility and weak muscles in the back, pelvis, and thighs may increase the curve of the lower back and cause the pelvis to tilt too far forward. Good flexibility in these areas, along with good muscle strength and good posture, helps prevent abnormal pressure on sensitive spinal nerves.

Poor abdominal muscle group development is another common cause of low-back pain. If the abdominal muscles are weak, they cannot exert enough pressure to keep the pelvis in place, and it tilts forward. This in turn causes the vertebrae in the lower back to become slightly displaced and press against one another, producing an ache in the lower back.

The hamstring muscles are another muscle group implicated in low-back pain. This group consists of three large muscles, located at the back of each thigh, which are associated with movement at the hip and knee joints. The difficulty most people face in trying to touch their toes with their fingertips without bending their knees is largely due to the hamstrings' inability to stretch far enough. This inability stems from an inflexibility or shortening of the hamstrings caused by physical inactivity or long periods of sitting. Hamstrings' inflexibility or shortening may cause pain in the hamstrings themselves and "referred" pain in the lower back.

Factors that may compound low-back pain include physical injury, hard sneezing or coughing, improper lifting or bending, long hours of sitting or standing, sitting slumped in overstuffed chairs or car seats, anxiety, depression, obesity, and diseases such as arthritis. Vertebral joints may be affected by degenerative arthritis, causing inflammation within the joint. Although back pain may result from sudden, traumatic injuries, in most cases people cannot identify a specific injury as the starting point of their condition.

RISK FACTORS

Although we know that anyone can be subjected to back pain, there are a number of factors that increase your risk. Several of these factors are not under your control:

- growing older
- having a family history of back pain
- being a man; statistically, more men work in physically demanding careers that increase their risk of injury
- having children; two or more full-term pregnancies triple a woman's risk of osteoporosis and potential collapse of the vertebrae
- having a congenital birth defect
- having a degenerative disease of the spine, such as osteoporosis or arthritis

Factors that you can control include the following:

- A lack of exercise.

FIGURE 12.5 **Improper and Proper Techniques for Lifting Heavy Objects**

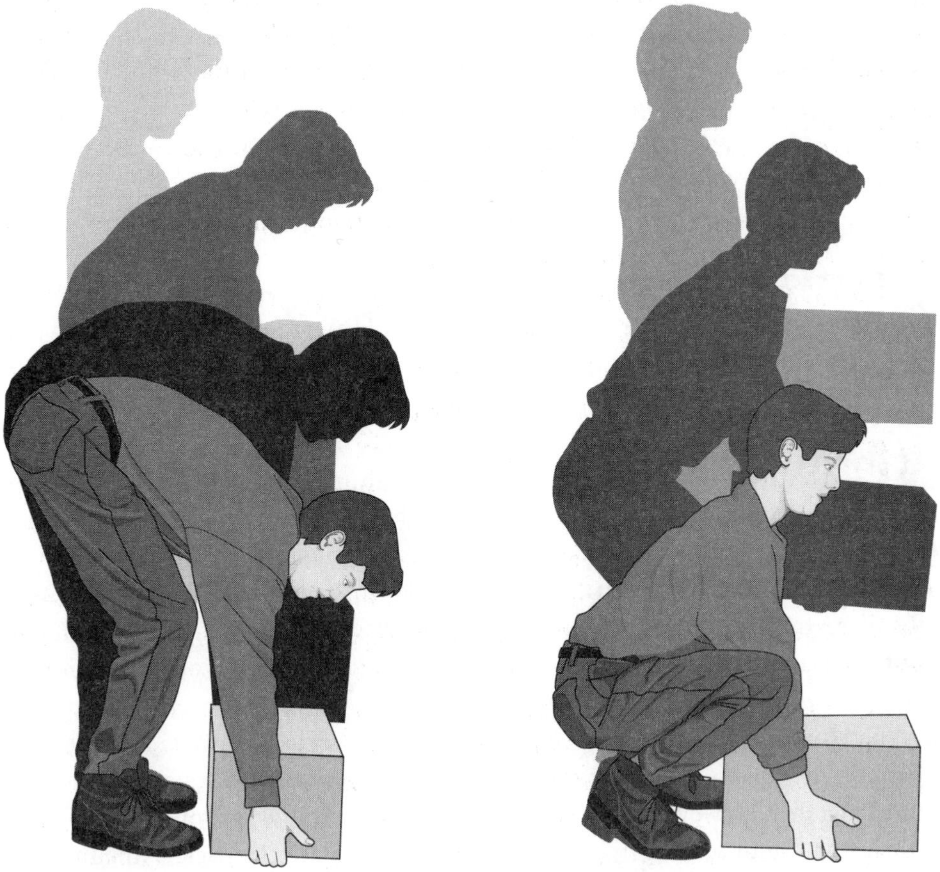

- Sitting for long periods of time, lifting or pulling heavy objects without using proper form (see figure 12.5), bending or twisting frequently, heavy physical exertion, repetitive motions, and exposure to constant vibration such as driving.
- Smoking. You are twice as likely to have low-back pain if you smoke or are exposed to second-hand smoke. Lorentzon et al. (2007) have shown that adolescent smokers have significant loss in bone mass density resulting in a lower peak bone mass, mainly as a consequence of reduced cortical thickness (the density of the outer layer of the bone).
- Being overweight. Weighing more than 20 percent over your ideal body weight increases your risk of back problems. However, Zhao (2006) feels that lowering weight to reduce back problems may increase the risk of osteoporosis.
- Having poor posture.
- Having an illness or disease that causes chronic coughing.
- Having a mental health problem, such as severe anxiety or depression.
- Suffering from a significant amount of stress.

There are also several activities that can increase your risk of back pain and injury:

- running or jogging without the proper equipment or on uneven surfaces
- skiing and snowboarding
- sledding, snowmobiling, or tobogganing
- sports like gymnastics, trampolining, and wrestling, which require forceful twisting
- contact sports like football or rugby
- work-related activities that require repeated lifting, bending, or twisting of the back

Arthritis

arthritis
a group of conditions in which there is a degeneration of the joint following trauma to the joint (as a result of an infection or aging)

fibromyalgia
chronic disorder characterized by widespread musculoskeletal pain, fatigue, and multiple "tender points," particularly in the neck, spine, shoulders, and hips

Arthritis is a group of conditions that affect the joints of the body. It comprises more than 100 conditions, including lupus, fibromyalgia, gout, and scleroderma. The most common type of arthritis in Canada is osteoarthritis (see figure 12.6), affecting 3 million Canadians, or 1 in 10 (Murphy et al., 2006). It is a degenerative joint disease, and occurs following trauma to the joint (as a result of an infection or aging). Osteoarthritis is also sometimes confused with or may be associated with degenerative disc disease, a gradual deterioration of the discs between the vertebrae of the spine. This is because osteoarthritis and degenerated discs are commonly found together. However, they are separate conditions. Rheumatoid and psoriatic arthritis are autoimmune diseases (that is, the body attacks itself). Rheumatoid arthritis is the second most common type of arthritis, affecting 300,000 Canadians, or 1 in 100 (Murphy et al., 2006). It is an autoimmune disorder in which the immune system attacks healthy joints, resulting in damage to cartilage, bone, tendons, and ligaments. Twice as many women as men get rheumatoid arthritis and it most commonly appears between the ages of 25 and 50. Septic arthritis is caused by joint infection. Gouty arthritis occurs when uric acid deposits build up in the joints, causing joint inflammation. **Fibromyalgia** is a chronic disorder characterized by widespread musculoskeletal pain, fatigue, and multiple "tender points," particularly in the neck, spine, shoulders, and hips. Additional symptoms may include sleep disturbances, morning stiffness, and anxiety (National Institute for Neurological Disorders and Stroke, 2003).

Long-term disability accounted for almost 80 percent of the economic costs of arthritis in 1998, at nearly $3.5 billion, and the 35–64 year age group incurred 70 percent of these costs. Two-thirds of those with arthritis are women, and nearly 60 percent are under the age of 65. Epidemiologists predict there will be about 100,000 new cases of arthritis each year over the next 30 years. It is estimated that by 2026, more than 6 million Canadians over the age of 15 will have arthritis. Musculoskeletal diseases (arthritis and osteoporosis) cost Canadians $16.4 billion every year—the second highest cost of disease after heart disease. Of this total, $2.6 billion is in direct costs such as physician and hospital care and drugs, and $13.7 billion is in indirect costs, including premature disability and death. The economic burden of all musculoskeletal conditions in Canada accounted for 10.3 percent of the total economic burden of all illnesses (Canadian Institutes of Health Research, 2005).

FIGURE 12.6 **Progression of Osteoarthritis**

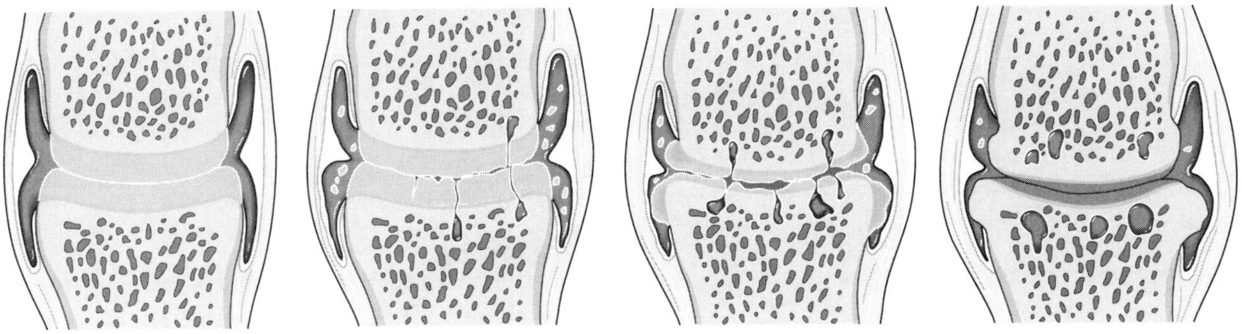

Healthy knee joint deteriorating as a result of osteoarthritis →

All arthritis causes pain. Chronic pain and reduced mobility and function are the most common outcomes of long-term arthritis. Osteoarthritis is typically worse at night or following rest. Rheumatoid arthritis, on the other hand, is usually worse in the mornings. Warm showers or baths seem to relieve the symptoms, but many who experience this pain are less likely to use the affected joint.

Treatment revolves around the history of the pain, such as when it started, how many joints are affected, how long the pain lasts, what aggravates the inflammation, and what helps to relieve the pain. Physical examinations and X-rays confirm the state of the condition, and blood tests confirm the diagnosis. There are medications that you may discuss with your doctor regarding treatment. Early diagnosis of arthritis may help prevent irreversible joint damage (see figure 12.7).

Repetitive Strain Injury

Repetitive strain injury (RSI) is also associated with back pain. RSI arises when soft tissue is subjected to repeated trauma (such as typing or using a computer mouse) without the chance to recover from each trauma. In the upper body it results in injuries such as carpal tunnel syndrome or tennis elbow. Repetitive activity damages tendons, affects circulation, and causes biomechanical stresses on soft tissue by not allowing enough recovery time between movements. Symptoms include pain, numbness, and tingling in the affected body parts (Tjepkema, 2003). Repetitive strain injuries take a toll not only physically but mentally. An RSI may affect work with functional and activity limitations, and may cause sleep disturbances. In 2001, 10 percent of Canadians aged 20 or older reported having an RSI serious enough to have limited their usual activities at some point in the previous 12 months (Tjepkema, 2003). Most RSIs affect the upper body—specifically, 25 percent of cases occur in the neck and shoulders, 23 percent in the wrists or hands, 19 percent in the upper or lower back, 16 percent in the elbows or lower arms, and 17 percent in a lower extremity or unspecified body part.

repetitive strain injury (RSI)

an injury that arises when soft tissue is subjected to repeated trauma (such as may be caused by typing or using a computer mouse) without the chance to recover from each trauma

There are two broad groupings of repetitive strain injuries: tendon-related disorders and peripheral nerve entrapment disorders. Tendon-related disorders, which involve the inflammation of the tendon and sheath or injuries to them, include tendonitis (inflammation of the tendon), tenosynovitis (inflammation of the tendon sheath), epicondylitis (golfer's or tennis elbow), and rotator cuff tendonitis. Peripheral nerve entrapment disorders involve compression of a nerve. The most

FIGURE 12.7 **Effect of Arthritis on the Hip Joint**

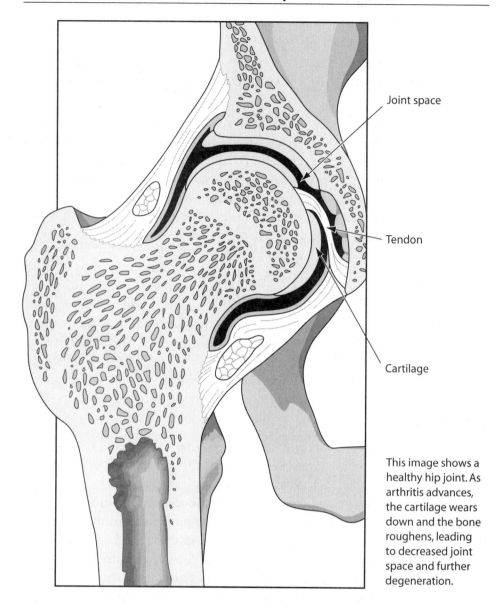

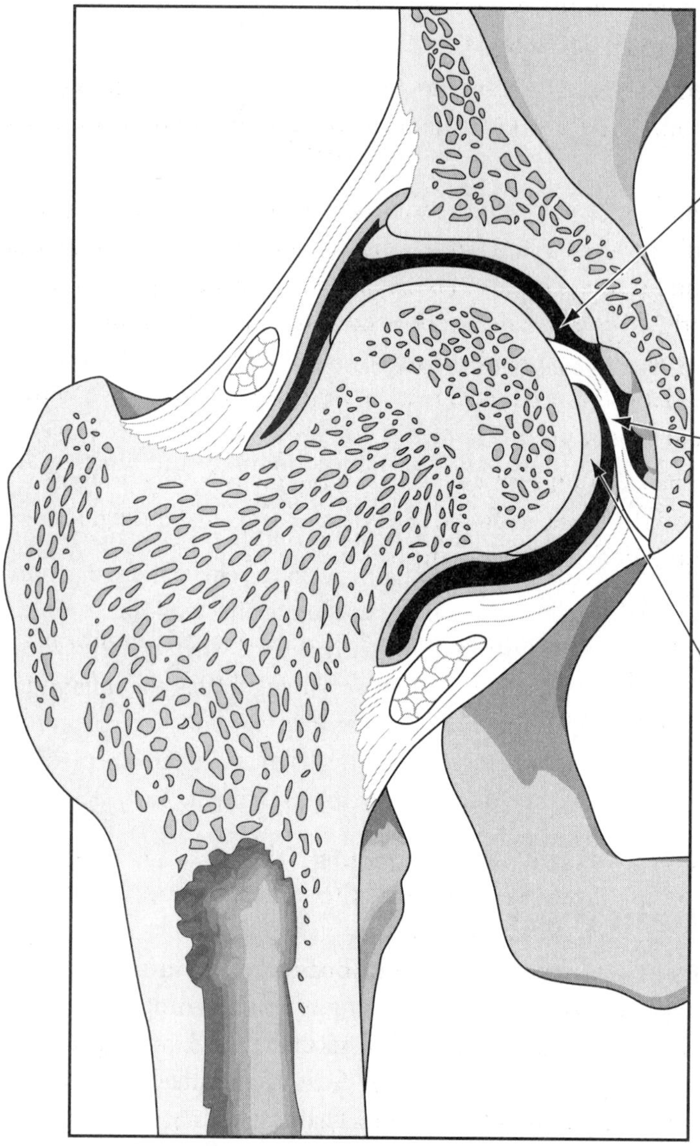

This image shows a healthy hip joint. As arthritis advances, the cartilage wears down and the bone roughens, leading to decreased joint space and further degeneration.

common is carpal tunnel syndrome (compression of the medial nerve), and the second most common is cubital tunnel syndrome (compression of the ulnar nerve) (Tjepkema, 2003).

Many workers have jobs in which they have little or no control over how the job is done or the rate at which the job must be completed. Often these jobs involve rapid, repetitive tasks. Law enforcement officers, for example, are often required to perform repetitive tasks that adversely affect their back and shoulder muscles and tendons. Altercations and repetitive movements such as use of force or firearms training may cause inflammation. With the introduction of computers into vehicles and poor ergonomic conditions (such as the location of the computer, inability to move the display, vest and belt hampering movement to face the display, etc.) many officers are complaining about shoulder and wrist pain. Ranney (1995) identifies several features of law enforcement that are conducive to RSI and back problems generally:

- Law enforcement may require officers to perform the same task for a long time without a chance to rest or exercise a different set of muscles. Sitting in a cruiser for hours is an example.
- Law enforcement may require substantial muscular force—for example, when an officer must restrain a person or remove him or her from a volatile situation.
- Law enforcement may require officers to maintain an awkward posture that is difficult to hold for even a short time. For example, officers are sometimes required to stand for long periods in boots that provide inadequate foot support. Similarly, cruiser seat design does not address the needs of different body types. If a seat has been damaged by excessive use and has not been repaired, officers are forced to sit in a position that does not allow them to maintain proper posture, which puts additional strain on the back.
- The equipment belt that uniformed officers wear weighs 5–9 kg or more and puts strain on the lower back whether one is sitting or standing. In addition, the equipment attached to the belt may cause an officer to sit in an awkward position.
- Officers who work outdoors in winter face a higher risk of back injuries. If they have to respond quickly to an altercation or other incident, their cold, stiff muscles and joints are more likely to suffer damage.

Sciatica

Sciatica, or sciatic neuritis, is a common back condition. The sciatic nerve exits the spinal column between the lowest vertebrae and the sacrum (see figure 12.1 on p. 245). This nerve supplies sensation to the back of the thighs and buttocks, knee flexors, and foot muscles. When it is compressed, inflamed, or irritated anywhere along its length, pain may result. Sciatica may result in wasting of the muscles of the lower leg. It may result from poor posture, disc degeneration, a bulging disc, or pregnancy where the fetus is pushing on the nerves. Symptoms range from a sensation of "pins and needles" or numbness to a burning feeling in the leg or foot region. The pain from a bulging disc is usually worse when you're active, and feels better when you're resting. Coughing, sneezing, sitting, driving, and bending forward may make the pain worse because these movements put more pressure on the nerve.

sciatica
pain anywhere along the sciatic nerve as the result of compression, inflammation, or irritation; generally, the pain travels from the back of the thigh to the back of the calf, and also may extend upwards, to the hip

This problem is especially hard on officers who must sit in their cruisers for long periods of time. With extended sitting in a vehicle, many people feel their legs burn or go numb, making it very difficult to get out of the cruiser quickly and respond to emergencies.

PREVENTING BACK PAIN

Physical conditioning is the key to avoiding back injury. In addition to getting regular aerobic exercise, officers need to develop strong back and stomach muscles, which are necessary to support the spine. Prevention is the key to a healthy back. Law enforcement personnel need to learn the proper ways to stand, bend, lift, sit, rest, and sleep. They must regularly perform exercises that stretch and strengthen the major muscles affecting the back, and be as active as possible. Flexibility is a key factor to back health. Without it, many individuals suffer back strain.

Exercises for a Healthy Back

Flexion and extension exercises will help you maintain a healthy back and are also used to recover from low-back injuries.

FLEXION EXERCISES

- *Cat back* Kneel on the floor, resting on your hands and knees. Allow your spine to sag slightly. Then arch your back like a cat as high as possible. Try to hold this position for a few seconds. Performing this exercise is often easier if you lower your head as you arch your back.
- *Pelvic tilt* Lie on your back with knees bent and feet flat on the floor. Press the small of your back against the floor and tighten your stomach and buttock muscles. Do not push with your feet. Performing this exercise correctly should cause the lower part of your pelvis to rotate forward and flatten your back against the floor. Hold for six seconds, and then relax the muscles for six seconds. Repeat six times. When learning this exercise, it is often helpful to put a hand in the hollow of your back so that you can feel the small of your back pressing down toward the floor.

EXTENSION EXERCISES

When used to alleviate low-back pain, these exercises should be repeated at two-hour intervals six to eight times a day. For prevention, these exercises may be done daily.

- *Lower-back relaxing* Lie on the floor on your stomach, arms at your sides and head turned to one side. Now try to relax the muscles in your lower back. Hold for a few minutes.
- *Upper-back lift (modified)* Lie on your stomach with your chin resting on the floor. Put your elbows under your shoulders on your chest and support your body on your forearms. Keep your neck in a straight line. If you notice a reduction in pain, hold this position for up to five minutes. If the pain increases, discontinue immediately. If this exercise helps, move on to the next one.
- *Upper-back lift* Lie on your stomach with your chin resting on the floor. Put your hands under your shoulders with forearms flat on the floor. Straighten (extend) your elbows as you tighten your back muscles to lift your body up without triggering pain. Keep the pelvis, hips, and legs completely relaxed. Try to extend your back as much as possible, but do not push with your arms. Hold this position for two seconds and then return to the starting position. Repeat 10 times.

Exercises to Avoid

A number of exercises that were popular in the 1960s and 1970s and are still recommended by some people put too much strain on the spine and should be avoided. Here are a few examples:

- standing toe touch while keeping the legs straight
- standing hamstring stretch where the legs are straight (which puts excessive strain on the knees and lower back)
- prone arch—lying on your stomach and trying to bring your head to your feet
- yoga plough—lying on your back and trying to put your feet up behind your head (which strains the neck and back)
- sit-ups, especially where you put your hands behind your head and pull on your neck to assist the sit-up (which may pull your vertebrae out of alignment)

If you are involved in a fitness program and believe an exercise you are asked to do may harm your back, speak to the instructor and ask for an alternative. Do not do anything that causes pain. Protecting your back is more important than adhering strictly to a fitness program, and you are the person most aware of your body's limitations.

Tips for a Healthy Back

In addition to exercising, you may take many steps in everyday life to help your back. The following tips will help you keep your back healthy and prevent low-back pain. Remember, your back is meant to give you a lifetime's worth of support, and it is essential that you look after it. To keep it healthy, you need to strengthen it and keep it flexible.

- When lifting an object, bend at the knees and hips rather than keeping your legs straight and bending at the waist. Your feet should be shoulder-width apart. Lift gradually, keeping your arms straight and pushing up with your leg muscles. Ensure that the object is close to your body when you are lifting and carrying it. Do not twist; if you have to turn while holding the object, first pick it up and then move your feet rather than twisting at the waist.
- When standing, make sure most of your weight is on the balls of your feet and not on your heels. Your feet should be shoulder-width apart, your knees should be slightly bent, and your arms should fall naturally to your sides. Periodically, you should shift your weight from one foot to the other.
- It is important to keep your body aligned. When you stand up against a wall, the back of your head, shoulders, and bottom should touch the wall.
- When sitting, keep your knees slightly higher than your hips. Sit upright rather than with your shoulders forward by placing your feet on a footrest (books, pillows, or a cardboard box may be used as a substitute). If you use a back support, make sure it fits you.
- Do not sit in the same position for a long period of time. Get up and move around. This will reduce the strain on your back muscles and ligaments and help improve circulation to reduce muscle fatigue and discomfort.
- Leaning against a solid support when you are sitting such as sitting on a chair rather than a bench with no back helps to reduce fatigue.

- When sitting at a desk or in front of a computer, place your chair as close as possible to the desk or computer so that you are sitting in an upright position. If your back flattens when you sit, try putting a lumbar roll (the low-back pillow that is often sold in drugstores) behind your lower back. Your feet should be flat on the floor and your knees higher than your hips.
- Once a day, lie on your back with your feet up on a couch at a 90° angle. This straightens the lower back. Doing the pelvic tilt on the floor will also reduce the strain on your lower back.
- When sleeping, try to lie on your side with your knees and hips bent. If you lie on your back, place a pillow under your knees. Do not lie on your stomach because this hyperextends the back. Your mattress should be firm enough to support your spine in its neutral position. It should not sag. Consider adding a layer of foam for extra support.
- When walking, keep your toes pointed straight ahead. Keep your back flat, your head up, and your chin in.
- To warm up for an activity, swing any tool you will be using (such as an adze, rake, shovel, axe, or golf club) lazily back and forth around your head and shoulders in different positions, gradually working up to a full range of motion. Gradually, work your way up to the effort required to do the activity.

Proper Sitting in a Vehicle

It is essential to sit properly, especially when driving. Since law enforcement officers may spend a great deal of time in vehicles, it is important that you look after your back. Officers complain of low-back pain and general backaches as the result of sitting in cruisers that are damaged and uncomfortable. Whether you are on the job or enjoying a drive, here are some guidelines to assist you in sitting correctly (Mack, 2002):

1. When adjusting your seat, begin by sitting with your bottom as far back in the seat as possible. Make sure that your lower back is pressing firmly against the back of the seat. Then move your seat forward until your right foot is on the floorboards behind the pedal with your knee slightly bent (this will ensure maximum pressure when you are braking in an emergency).
2. Your backrest should be near the upright position to place less pressure on the lower back. Your chest should be at least 20–25 cm from the centre of the steering wheel. Your wrists should be able to reach over the wheel when stopped, and your elbows should be slightly bent when your arms are placed in the normal driving position. Shorter individuals may require seat cushions and pedal extenders to accomplish this. When driving, officers are encouraged to sit back with their torsos at an approximate 100° angle or more (Kumar & Narayan, 2001).
3. Your head restraint is important for preventing whiplash. The middle of the back of your head should come in full contact with the restraint.
4. Your rearview mirror should be positioned so that you can see the two rear pillars as well as the roofline and bottom of the rear window. Your

side mirrors should be positioned so that you can see the adjacent lane rather than the side of the vehicle.

5. Seatbelt position is very important. The lap portion should be pulled down snugly over the hipbones to prevent the belt from riding up in a crash (which could cause internal injuries). The shoulder belt should be high enough to ensure that the belt does not fall off your shoulder (to prevent hitting the steering wheel or windshield).
6. When getting into the vehicle, first sit on the seat, and then rotate your legs in as one unit to prevent abnormal twisting of the spine. When exiting the vehicle, make sure to rotate your legs as one unit to the door, place your feet on the ground, and then stand up. If you have spent a long time in the vehicle, this will prevent excessive twisting of the spine, which has lost mobility from sitting in one position.
7. Redistribution of the components in your duty belt can help you sit properly. Kumar & Narayan's (2001) study proposed that the minimal amount of equipment be attached to an officer's duty belt. It suggested that the baton be moved to a pocket on the thigh and the radio to a pocket on the chest in a designed uniform. Many police services are now issuing phones to their officers, and even BlackBerry devices in order to supply a lightweight phone and computer in a single piece of equipment. The magazine of bullets, handcuffs, and pepper spray should all be placed on the front of the duty belt to ensure that the back is fully supported by the backrest.
8. During normal policing when emergencies are not expected, officers should consciously and periodically change their postures, move around, or change physical activity. It is recommended that every 50 minutes of continuous work of one type should be followed by a 10-minute period of another activity (Kumar & Narayan, 2001).
9. When sitting in a vehicle, do not keep your legs fully extended. Your knees should be bent to prevent back strain and shortening of the hamstring muscles. Push the front seat of your vehicle forward so that your knees will be higher than your hips. This will reduce the strain on your back and shoulder muscles.

NUTRITIONAL CONSIDERATIONS FOR A HEALTHIER BACK

When an excess amount of protein, refined carbohydrates, and fats are consumed over a period of time, the body becomes more acidic. Since the body prefers alkaline minerals, calcium in particular is removed from bones and transported to the rest of the body to neutralize the acidic environment. Some goes into the kidneys and is excreted out. In addition, phosphorus competes with calcium for absorption in the intestines. The more phosphorus there is, the less calcium will be absorbed, and as we age, this becomes a concern.

TABLE 12.1 Daily Calcium Requirements

Age	Daily calcium requirement (mg)*
0–6 months	210
7–12 months	270
1–3 years	500
4–8 years	800
9–18 years	1300
19–50 years	1000
51+ years	1200

* Applicable to males and females, including during pregancy.

Source: Adapted from Dietary Reference Intakes Tables at http://www.hc-sc.gc.ca/fn-an/nutrition/reference/table/ref_elements_tbl_e.html.

How Much Calcium Do You Need?

Calcium requirements are age-related. As we get older, we require more calcium in our diet since we lose our ability to absorb calcium. We need to maximize our intake in order to continue to have calcium-dense bones. Table 12.1 outlines calcium requirements by age.

How to Maximize Your Calcium Intake Through Diet

By consulting a reliable food chart, such as the one found on the *Canada's Food Guide* Web page (see www.hc-sc.gc.ca/fn-an/food-guide-aliment/index_e.html), you can calculate your daily calcium intake. Osteoporosis Canada (www.osteoporosis.ca) has a calculator that can help you find out whether you're getting the recommended levels.

Foods Containing Easily Absorbed Calcium

Excellent sources of calcium include milk, cheese, and yogurt. Skim milk has the same amount of calcium as whole milk, with less fat and cholesterol. The calcium in soy beverages is absorbed at the rate of 75 percent of milk. Some soy beverages and orange juices are fortified with calcium (check their labels). There are also vegetables and fish (canned salmon and sardines), and meat alternatives such as lentils and beans that are rich in calcium. If you cannot consume or do not like dairy products, it is important that you make sure you are eating alternative calcium-rich choices. If you are unsure, consult a dietitian.

Foods That Cause Calcium Loss Through Urination

Over 90 percent of sodium comes from food rather than table salt. Since salt acts as a diuretic, you should read labels to ensure that sodium levels are kept to a minimum in your foods, especially if you eat a lot of canned or packaged foods. Caffeine is also a diuretic. If you consume more than four cups of coffee a day, you should drink one glass of milk for every cup of caffeine-containing beverage, or avoid caffeinated beverages altogether.

Vitamin D and Calcium

Vitamin D is also involved with bone health. It helps with the maintenance of serum calcium (the amount of calcium found in the bloodstream) and phosphate concentrations in the body (Institute of Medicine, 1997). It improves muscle strength, reduces fracture rates, and reduces rates of falling (Bischoff-Ferrari et al., 2004a, 2004b, 2005). In some cases it plays a role in the prevention of certain cancers and protection against autoimmune diseases (Garland et al., 2006).

Many people (particularly those over 50) do not get enough vitamin D from food sources alone. Health Canada recommends that everyone over the age of 50 take a 10 g (400 IU) supplement of vitamin D (Health Canada, 2007) every day.

TREATING BACK INJURIES

Although prevention is the key to keeping your back healthy, almost everyone will experience low-back pain at some point. Treatment usually involves the following:

- one to three days of bed rest on a firm mattress supported by plywood
- moderate application of heat and cold; a prolonged bath may relax a strained back, but make sure the water is not too hot (a warm bath with epsom salts relaxes muscles)
- gentle massage until muscle spasms are eliminated or significantly reduced
- after recovery, daily exercises to strengthen the back and abdominal muscles

In the longer term, you are encouraged to do the following:

- Exercise aerobically for 30 minutes three or four times a week, working towards 30 minutes every day.
- Reduce abdominal fat by changing your dietary habits. Abdominal fat puts strain on the lower back.
- Continue your daily back and abdominal exercises.

For patients with a new episode of low-back pain, prompt access to physiotherapy is cost- and time-effective. More than 70 percent of patients require only a single clinic visit, and less than 5 percent need to be referred to a specialist (Pinnington, Miller, & Stanley, 2004).

Surgery is rarely needed to correct low-back problems, but be sure to consult a physician for diagnosis and treatment in all cases of back pain. Do not take your back's health lightly.

KEY TERMS

vertebrae

intervertebral discs

degenerative disc disease (DDD)

osteoporosis

arthritis

fibromyalgia

repetitive strain injury (RSI)

sciatica

EXERCISES

Review

1. Describe the functions of the spine.

2. Summarize the causes of low-back pain.

3. What is a herniated disc? What are some of the causes of this type of injury?

4. What is arthritis and what impact does it have on your joints?

5. What is an RSI? What are some of the symptoms associated with RSI?

6. What is osteoporosis, and what can you do to prevent the disease?

7. What special risks to a healthy back do law enforcement officers' duties create?

8. Describe some techniques for preventing low-back pain.

9. How are back injuries treated?

Multiple Choice and True or False

1. The solution for reducing muscular imbalances is to ________________ tight back muscles and ________________ weak abdominal muscles.
   a. strengthen, stretch
   b. strengthen, rest
   c. stretch, strengthen
   d. shorten, strengthen
   e. rest, exercise

2. Which of the following is true of posture?
   a. a rigid posture is desirable
   b. muscle weakness does not influence posture
   c. alignment of one body part may affect another
   d. good posture requires additional muscular effort
   e. poor posture has not been linked to any health problems

3. The most common health complaint in people under the age of 50 is
   a. headache
   b. neckache
   c. backache
   d. leg problems
   e. foot problems

4. Which of the following is recommended for lifting a heavy load?
   a. lift with the leg muscles
   b. push or pull an object instead of carrying it
   c. carry the load in one arm to keep the other arm free
   d. let the arm muscles do most of the work
   e. bend over the object with a straight back and lift up with your arms

5. What is *least* likely to lead to back problems?
   a. lack of coordination
   b. lack of strength
   c. poor flexibility
   d. poor coordination
   e. protruding abdomen

6. When directing traffic, what standing position should you avoid?
   a. back arched
   b. knees locked
   c. knees bent
   d. one foot forward
   e. back straight

7. The most common cause of low-back pain is
   a. a slipped disc
   b. a herniated disc
   c. weak back muscles and strong stomach muscles
   d. weak stomach muscles
   e. weak stomach muscles and lack of back flexibility

8. Which of the following factors can contribute to low-back pain or increase the risk for low-back pain?
   a. being between the ages of 50 and 64
   b. depression, apathy, inattentiveness, boredom, emotional upsets, and lack of focus when doing your job
   c. strong abdominal muscles, which pull the back out of place
   d. all of the above put an individual at higher risk for low-back pain
   e. there are no known factors that contribute to back pain

9. Pain that radiates down the back of the leg is known as
   a. osteoarthritis
   b. sciatica
   c. osteoporosis
   d. fibromyalgia
   e. repetitive strain injury

10. Back flexibility and strengthening exercises should be done daily to maintain a healthy back.
    a. True
    b. False

11. When lifting the 80-lb. (36-kg) bag in the PARE test, it is best to keep your knees straight and lift primarily with your arms to prevent back strain.
    a. True
    b. False

12. Sharp muscle pain in the back is an indication that you should stop the activity you are engaged in.
    a. True
    b. False

REFERENCES

Bischoff-Ferrari, H.B., Dawson-Hughes, B., Willett, W.C., Staehelin, H.B., Bazemore, M.G., Zee, R.Y., & Wong, J.B. (2004a). Effect of vitamin D on falls: A meta-analysis. *Journal of the American Medical Association, 291*, 1999-2006.

Bischoff-Ferrari, H.A., Dietrich, T., Orav, J., Hu, F.B., Zhang, Y., Karlson, E.W., & Dawson-Hughes, B. (2004b). Higher 25-hydroxyvitamin D concentrations are associated with better lower-extremity function in both active and inactive persons aged 60 years. *American Journal of Clinical Nutrition, 80*, 752-758.

Bischoff-Ferrari, H.A., Willett, W.C., Wong, J.B., Giovannucci, E., Dietrich, T., & Dawson-Hughes, B. (2005). Fracture prevention with vitamin D supplementation: A meta-analysis of randomized control trials. *Journal of the American Medical Association, 295*, 2257-2264.

Brown, J.J., Wells, G.A., Trottier, A.J., Bonneau, J., & Ferris, B. (1998). Back pain in a large Canadian police force. *Spine, 23*, 821-827.

Burton, A.K., Tillotson, K.M., Symonds, T.L., Burke, C., & Mathewson, T. (1996). Occupational risk factors for the first-onset and subsequent course of low back trouble: A study of serving police officers. *Spine, 21*(22), 2612-2620.

Canadian Institutes of Health research. (2005). *Health research—Investing in Canada's future 2004–2005.* Available at http://www.irsc.gc.ca/e/28892.html.

Canadian Physiotherapy Association. (2006). *Back pain "Oh, my aching back!"* Available at http://www.physiotherapy.ca/PublicUploads/222460BackPainInfo.pdf.

Fahey, T.D., Insel, P.M., & Walton, T.R. (1997). *Fit and well: Core concepts and labs in physical fitness and wellness* (2nd ed.). Mountain View, CA: Mayfield.

Garland, C.F., Garland, F.C., Gorham, E.D., Lipkin, M., Newmark, H., Mohr, S.B., & Holick, M.F. (2006). The role of vitamin D in cancer prevention. *American Journal of Public Health, 96*, 252-261.

Greenberg, J.S., & Dintiman, G.B. (1997). *Wellness: Creating a life of health and fitness.* Needham Heights, MA: Allyn and Bacon.

Gyi, D.E., & Porter, J.M. (1998). Musculoskeletal problems and driving in police officers. *Occupational Medicine (London), 48*(3), 153-160.

Health Canada. (2007). *Vitamin D for people over 50: Background.* Available at http://www.hc-sc.gc.ca/fn-an/food-guide-aliment/context/evid-fond/vita_d_e.html.

Henneberg, E. (2006). Canadian research contributions are front and centre. IOF World Congress on Osteoporosis, Toronto 2006. *Osteoporosis Update, 10*(3).

Institute of Medicine (IOM). (1997). *Dietary reference intakes for calcium, phosphorus, magnesium, vitamin D and fluoride.* Washington, DC: National Academy Press.

Kumar, S., & Narayan, Y. (2001). Low back pain among RCMP officers: An investigation into vehicles, duty belts and boots. *Canadian Police Research Centre (CPRC) Technical Report*, September, 1999. TR-01-99.

Lorentzon, M., Mellstrom, D., Haug, E., & Ohlsson, C. (2007). Smoking is associated with lower peak bone mineral density mainly as a result of reduced cortical thickness in young adult men: *Journal of Clinical Endocrinology & Metabolism, 92*(2), 428-429.

Mack, T. (2002, February–March). Health news: Just sit right here. *Leisureways.* Oakville, ON: Formula.

Mills, K. (2006). *Standards for bone mineral density testing.* Available at http://www.osteoporosis.ca/english/Mediapercent20Room/Background/Densitormetrypercent20Standards/default.asp?s=1.

Murphy, K.A., Spence, S.T., McIntosh, C.N., & Connor Gorber, S.K. for the Population Health Impact of Disease in Canada (PHI). (2006). Health state descriptions for Canadians: Musculoskeletal diseases. Statistics Canada, catalogue no. 82-619-MIE2006003. Ottawa: Statistics Canada.

National Institute for Neurological Disorders and Stroke. (2003). *Low-back pain fact sheet.* Available at http://www.ninds.nih.gov/disorders/backpain/detail_backpain.htm.

National Institutes of Health. (2003). *What is osteoporosis?* Available at http://www.niams.nih.gov/bone/hi/FF_Osteoporosis.pdf.

Osteoporosis Canada. (2002). *10 top things you need to know about osteoporosis.* Available at http://www.osteoporosis.ca/english/News/2002/Top%2010%20About%20Osteoporosis/default.asp?s=1.

Osteoporosis Canada. (2007). *What is osteoporosis?* Available at http://www.osteoporosis.ca/english/about%20osteoporosis/default.asp?s=1.

Pinnington, M.A., Miller, J., & Stanley, I. (2004). An evaluation of prompt access to physiotherapy in the management of low back pain in primary care. *Family Practice, 21*(4), 372-380.

Ranney, D. (1995). *Pain at work and what to do about it.* Waterloo, ON: Department of Kinesiology, University of Waterloo.

Tjepkema, M. (2003). Repetitive strain injury. *Ministry of Industry: Health Report, 14*(4). Statistics Canada, catalogue no. 0040282-003-XIE.

Zhao, L.J. (2006). Interventions decreasing obesity risk tend to be beneficial for decreasing risk to osteoporosis: A challenge to the current dogma. *Osteoporos International, 17* (Suppl. 2): S37 (Abstract P152SU).

CHAPTER 13

Stress

CHAPTER OBJECTIVES

After completing this chapter, you should be able to:

- Explain the differences among neutral, good, and bad stress.
- Describe the health effects of stress.
- Describe the kinds of stress that law enforcement personnel face.
- Explain what a critical incident is, how it can cause stress for law enforcement personnel, and how the stress should be handled.
- Explain what post-traumatic stress disorder is, how to recognize someone suffering from it, and what you can do to help an individual.
- Describe the characteristics of type A, type B, and type C personalities.
- Implement stress management techniques.

Many officers view stress as a normal part of their career. Others, who have been on the service for 10 to 20 years, report feeling considerably more pressure than when they began their career. Their stress levels continue to increase as there are increased levels of violent crime as well as greater public scrutiny and adverse publicity, perceived or not. There is increased risk of contracting air- and blood-borne diseases such as tuberculosis and HIV/AIDS. Added to these stressors are the issues of having to deal with cultural diversity and the imperative of "political correctness."

CHANGING ROLES OF LAW ENFORCEMENT AND ITS IMPACT ON OFFICERS

In the past 10 years, community policing has come to the forefront of policing. Working directly with the community can provide job satisfaction and provide overall departmental efficiency. However, the transition to community policing has caused apprehension on the part of officers who must implement this fundamental shift in policing philosophy on a day-to-day basis. At times, the stress to perform to both service and community standards can be overwhelming.

Everyone lives with stress. Stress is neither positive nor negative. How you handle or react to what you perceive as stress is what determines its effect on your life. In this chapter we will examine what stress is; its causes, effects, and symptoms;

and how it can be managed. The World Health Organization (2003) has described stress as "a global epidemic" (p. 7). Stress is described as an equal opportunity destroyer, affecting people in all demographics. More specifically, we will look at stress in law enforcement, with a special focus on critical incidents and post-traumatic stress disorder. We will also look at strategies for managing stress.

DEFINING STRESS

stress
a "non-specific response of the body to any demands made upon it" (Dr. Hans Selye)

Dr. Hans Selye (1974) was the first to define **stress**, which in his words is the "non-specific response of the body to any demands made upon it." Shafer (1996) explains stress as the arousal of the mind and body in response to demands made on them. Experts in the field of psychoneuroimmunology (PNI) suggest that as much as 85 percent of all disease and illness—from the common cold to cancer—can be linked to stress (Kiecolt-Glaser, 1999; Seaward, 2005).

THE TYPES OF STRESS

There are three types of stress:

1. *Neutral stress (neustress)* With this kind of stress the mind and body are aroused but the stress is neither harmful nor helpful (Morse & Furst, 1979). An example is observing that traffic is slowing down in front of you.
2. *Good stress (eustress)* This kind of stress is caused by the factors that initiate emotional and psychological growth. Eustress provides pleasure, adds meaning to life, and fosters an attitude that tries to find positive solutions to problems. It encourages optimal performance. An example is competing with classmates to win a race.
3. *Bad stress (distress)* This kind of stress results in negative responses. Unchecked negative stress can interfere with the physiological and psychological functioning of the body and may ultimately give rise to a hypokinetic disease or disability (Selye, 1974). Examples are being faced with a physical challenge you can't do (such as performing a timed run in a certain time) or not having enough money to pay for next month's rent.

Turn to **assignment 13.1** (in the appendix) to fill out the Life Experience Survey and answer the questions.

THE STRESS RESPONSE

general adaptation syndrome (GAS)
the body's reaction to stress

Hans Selye concluded that the body reacts to good and bad stress in the same way. He labelled the stress response—the body's reaction to stress—the **general adaptation syndrome (GAS)**. It includes three stages: the fight-or-flight response, the stage of resistance, and the stage of exhaustion (Selye, 1956).

The *fight-or-flight response* (or alarm stage) is the stage when the body prepares itself to cope with a stressor. The response is a warning signal that a stressor is present (whether real or imagined). This is really a primitive survival mechanism that today is not triggered often. As the body prepares for fight or flight, powerful stress hormones and steroids are pumped into the bloodstream, senses become more acute, muscles tense, digestion ceases, breathing and blood pressure rates increase, and there is an urge to go to the washroom. If the stressor is only imagined, over time we suffer the ill effects of chronic arousal, leading to excessive wear and tear on the body. So, we need to avoid those triggers that illicit the stress response.

In the *stage of resistance*, the body actively resists and attempts to cope with the stressor. If you are able to channel that energy, your body returns to normal. However, being aroused for too long and too often may lead to fatigue. Headaches, forgetfulness, constipation, diarrhea, asthma, anxiety attacks, and high blood pressure are all signs of prolonged arousal.

The *stage of exhaustion* can result in illness and ultimately death. During this phase, the body is subjected to repeated stress response breakdowns. If you are healthy enough, you will be successful in resisting stress. However, if the body can't cope, disease and malfunction of organ systems will result. For example, chronic high blood pressure can lead to kidney and heart disease, which can result in premature death.

The Effects of Stress

Most people look after their cars better than their bodies. While they may watch what they put in their gas tanks, they have little regard for what they eat. Under stress, most people tend to lose their appetite; they eat less, eat irregularly, and eat poorer-quality food. This usually means a decrease in energy intake to levels too low to sustain normal activities, let alone cope with stressful situations.

Stress combined with poor eating habits can wear your body down. Stress can have a short- or long-term effect on your body. When your body responds negatively to stress, such responses often manifest as **psychosomatic symptoms** (physical symptoms resulting from mental conflict). Let's look at some of the short- and long-term effects of stress and their physical consequences.

psychosomatic symptoms
physical symptoms resulting from mental conflict

SHORT-TERM EFFECTS OF STRESS

Short-term effects are seen soon after stress is experienced and can be corrected with proper stress management. The effects are as follows:

- less energy and more fatigue (a result of lower blood sugar levels)
- paleness
- slowing down of bodily functions such as digestion and wound healing (a result of loss of important minerals and reduced absorption of nutrients from food)
- higher blood pressure and heart rate
- loss of appetite and decreased taste for food
- depression
- more susceptibility to infections

Under these conditions, some people resort to artificial means to regain normal function. They consume over-the-counter stimulants or caffeine to remain alert and large doses of vitamins to replace depleted resources. They also resort to concoctions such as condensed-liquid vitamins and "power bars." But these simply put additional stress on the body. Caffeine, for example, increases irritability, interferes with sleep, and, by destroying stomach enzymes, weakens the stomach lining. If left untreated, these short-term effects will slowly or quickly wear away at your physical and mental health, with serious ramifications.

LONG-TERM EFFECTS OF STRESS

The possible long-term effects of stress include the following:

- nervous stomach and stomach aches
- constipation or diarrhea
- ulcers
- inflammation of the digestive system
- indigestion
- headaches
- high blood pressure
- allergic reactions such as asthma, eczema, and hives
- an inability to function under normal circumstances, including loss of concentration and an inability to focus

Chronic Exposure to Stress

Without proper stress management, constant or chronic exposure to stress—sometimes bottled up over several years—can lead to long-term or continual effects, such as

- elevation of heart rate and blood pressure
- weakening of the immune system
- inflammation of the stomach lining
- allergic reactions such as hives, hay fever, asthma, and congested breathing
- muscle-tension and migraine headaches
- muscle stiffness, aches, cramps, and backaches
- hypokinetic diseases (diseases brought on by partial or complete lack of physical activity and, in this case, stress, including cardiovascular diseases, digestive diseases, diabetes, excessive fat, and lower-back pain)

Emotional Effects of Chronic Stress

Chronic stress can also have emotional consequences, such as

- depression, leading to an inability to function normally at work and at home
- cynicism and suspiciousness
- emotional detachment from various aspects of daily life
- excessive aggressiveness (which may trigger an increase in citizen complaints)
- marital or family problems
- alcoholism and other substance abuse
- suicide

STRESSORS

A **stressor** is any physical, psychological, or environmental event or condition that initiates the stress response. However, what is stressful for one person may not be stressful for another. Also, what is stressful for someone at a certain time may not be stressful for that same person at another time.

stressor
any physical, psychological, or environmental event or condition that initiates the stress response

Stressors in Daily Life

Some common stressors in daily life include:

- changes and transitions (marriage, separation, divorce, death of a loved one, moving, job change or loss, going to school away from home or for the first time in a number of years)
- relationships (continued conflicts, lack of support)
- lifestyle (inconsistent with values, too committed to a particular lifestyle)
- money problems (inflation, credit card debt, financial losses)
- loss of self-esteem (falling behind academically and professionally, failing to meet others' expectations)
- fatigue or illness (poor diet, lack of sleep, lack of exercise)
- attempting to juggle family, academic, and career demands

Stressors in Law Enforcement

Finn (1997) identified five main categories of stress in law enforcement:

1. *Problems in the officer's personal life* can increase stress levels. The divorce rate for officers is five times that of the general population. Some officers' significant others must assume the role of both parents, rearrange their agendas to fit duty schedules (especially in specialized units), or simply learn to function independently. This can sometimes result in a breakdown in communication. Family may be affected by passive coolness or angry attacks from the stress of an officer's exposure to conflict, which leads them to feel alienated or frightened. An officer's children may react to concerns over their parents' safety with nightmares, regressive behaviour, a lack of emotion, anxiety, and aggressive and inappropriate outbursts.
2. *Pressure of law enforcement work* is produced by real threats and dangers, such as entering a dark and unfamiliar building, responding to a weapons call, pursuing lawbreakers at high speeds, or responding to a prison inmate disturbance. It also revolves around keeping current with technology and the workload itself (a shortage of personnel can affect the workload of individuals). For those in isolated communities, the time spent away from family and boredom sometimes also cause stress.
3. *Organizational stress* is produced by elements inherent in the paramilitary character of public (and some private) policing and corrections work. Examples include constant adjustment to changing schedules, working at odd hours, and complying with detailed rules and procedures.

4. *The attitude of the general public and other police officers toward police work and officers* can impact issues around community policing and expectations of the officers. It also can arise when an officer's gender or race is not accepted by particular colleagues. Difficulties "fitting in," perceptions of bias, and social isolation can all lead to stress.
5. *Operational stress* is produced by the realities of modern policing, such as understaffing, constantly having to adopt a "Band-Aid" approach to problems, lack of equipment, and having to deal with criminals, derelicts, and people in distress. It also has to do with police bureaucracy and the feeling of not being supported by one's bosses. Other stress-creating situations include being lied to often, being required to put oneself in dangerous situations to protect the public, the seeming injustice of some of our laws, and the constant awareness that one may be held legally liable for one's actions. In addition there are issues around promotional opportunities, lack of support, and decisions made that only top-level police administrators have control over.

Stressors from Workplace Health and Safety Hazards

There are many occupational health and safety risks that police officers may encounter on a daily basis or at some point in their career. They are grouped into five categories (Parsons, 2004):

- *Physical hazards,* such as a criminal with a weapon (visible) or radiation (invisible). Ellis (1993) found that police officers were at the greatest risk of assault when arresting and transporting suspects and prisoners. One Canadian study indicated that police officers are at greatest risk of time loss due to violence (Boyd, 1995).
- *Chemical hazards,* including furnace fumes, car exhaust, or, in a situation like 9/11, clouds of carcinogens. There has been some research around exposure to radio frequency, the use of police traffic radar, and sunshine being linked to cancer, including testicular, cervical, colon, and skin cancer (including melanoma) (Van Netten et al., 2003).
- *Biological hazards,* including micro-organisms in the air or communicable diseases like HIV/AIDS, tuberculosis, and hepatitis A, B, or C.
- *Ergonomic hazards,* including injuries to the musculoskeletal system from uncomfortable working positions, heavy physical tasks, or altercations with and handcuffing of criminals. A study of RCMP officers found the main source of back problems to be seatbelt use and riding in a patrol car all day (Brown et al., 1998); however, other research found issue around vibrations (such as motorcycles), wearing body armour, and working on a computer terminal in a confined space (such as car computers) (Gyi & Porter, 1998).
- *Psychosocial hazards,* including difficulties with supervisors or fellow workers, sexual harassment, discrimination, or dealing with issues like suicide. One study found that after dealing with lying, cheating, and hostile people on the street, officers can start mistrusting friends and even family,

or develop a negative attitude toward their work (Kohan & O'Connor, 2002). Police suicides can result from the stressful nature of police work in terms of overload shift work and exposure to violent and life-threatening situations. Departmental politics, inadequate resources to do the job, and lack of support and recognition from management also increase the stressful nature of police work (Loo, 2003).

These are just some of the stressors that may affect your future work in law enforcement. Remember that some individuals perceive particular stressors as positive, while others perceive the same stressors as negative. As a result, the impact of particular stressors varies from person to person.

CRITICAL INCIDENTS

A **critical incident** is a situation faced by police and other emergency service personnel that causes them to experience unusually strong emotional reactions that have the potential to interfere with their ability to function at the scene (current stress) or later (residual stress). Critical incidents are sudden and unexpected; disrupt one's sense of control; disrupt beliefs and values, as well as assumptions about the world in which we live, the people in it, and the work we do; involve the perception of a life-damaging threat; and may involve emotional or physical loss. It cannot be predicted how a given person will react to a particular event on a particular day. For those who are used to being in control of their emotions and their surroundings, it may be surprising, embarrassing, frustrating, or overwhelming to discover that an incident can be so debilitating.

critical incident
a situation faced by police and other emergency service personnel that causes them to experience unusually strong emotional reactions that have the potential to interfere with their ability to function at the scene (current stress) or later (residual stress)

The intensity of such an experience takes time to subside. If vivid "flashback" experiences or nightmares haunt you, make you feel emotionally numb or overwhelmed, and you are losing sleep, it is possible that you are suffering from post-traumatic stress disorder (PTSD).

This trauma is stress run amok. Stress will deregulate the nervous system for a short period of time. Within days or weeks we go back to equilibrium as the nervous system calms down. When we are traumatized, there is a residual effect on our lives, relationships, and overall ability to function, including our ability to perform daily tasks.

Types of Critical Incidents

Law enforcement personnel are often faced with critical incidents related to life and death. The following are some examples and the kinds of feelings they cause:

- *Death/injury/shooting in the line of duty* The myth of invulnerability is shattered.
- *Suicide of a co-worker* Job and personal life pressures, and the pressure of balancing the two, come into focus. Colleagues also experience guilt over not being there to help.
- *Death of a child* The innocence represented by children can have a profound impact on officers, sometimes pushing them over the edge. The officers may feel that what they stand for is useless. Should an officer have a family of his or her own, "factors of identification" can add even more stress.

- *Prolonged but failed rescue attempt* If the officer has come to know the victim, the officer may exhibit a great deal of stress arising out of a deep sense of personal failure.
- *Mass-casualty incidents* Incidents involving carnage or mass fatalities (such as the attack on New York City's World Trade Center in September 2001, the crash of a Swissair plane off the coast of Nova Scotia in 1998, the Oklahoma City bombing in 1995, and the Hurricane Katrina disaster in 2005), coupled with staff and resource shortages and mass confusion, can override an officer's ability to cope.
- *Officer's safety is unusually jeopardized* Daily exposure to potential danger, combined with a specific situation in which an officer becomes unusually vulnerable and lacks control, can trigger a stress reaction.
- *Responding officer knows the victim* Arriving on the scene and discovering that you know the victim can trigger a critical stress reaction of the "If only I had driven faster" variety.
- *Officer responding to an abused individual* Officers must respond to incidents involving serious physical assault, including sexual assault, incest, molestation, and gang assaults that go beyond comprehension of human decency.

Factors Affecting Responses to Critical Incidents

Some officers are better able than others to cope with the stress of critical incidents. The following are some factors that affect coping (Connor & Butterfield, 2003):

- *Nature of the event* Has the officer witnessed this type of incident before? How severe is the incident?
- *Degree of warning* Was the officer dispatched to the scene with an appropriate warning, or did the officer happen upon the scene?
- *Ego strength/coping style* Does the officer cope with tragic situations more easily than others do by accepting those situations as fate?
- *Prior mastery of the experience* How many times has the officer been exposed to a similar situation?
- *Proximity* How close does the officer feel to the person or incident (for example, if a child is involved, is she or he the same age as the officer's child)?
- *The amount of stress in the officer's life at the time* Is there already a great deal of stress in the officer's life, either at work or at home? If so, the incident may have a stronger impact.
- *The nature and degree of social support available to an officer after a critical incident* The more support an officer receives, the better are his or her chances of coping with the stress of a critical incident. The reactions of those supporting the officer may or may not be appropriate, and thus may further affect the individual.

Symptoms of Stress Arising out of Critical Incidents

Critical incidents can be overwhelming. We have to remember that the personnel who respond to them are human. Each officer will respond differently, and what may be easy to cope with one day is impossible to cope with the next. Most people are resilient enough to move through the incident, while others will never be the same. We have to be sensitive to the pressures faced by people who confront extreme situations every day. Recognizing the symptoms of stress can allow us to help them. Developing symptoms is never a sign of weakness. Symptoms should be taken seriously.

For some, these symptoms can be overwhelming to every part of their being. For others, the effects will take weeks, months, and possibly years to be totally felt. These overwhelming responses to stress can result in **post-traumatic stress disorder (PTSD)**. This disorder changes the way the body responds to stress, probably as a result of chemical imbalances that increase the levels of stress hormones and alter the reaction of the nervous system. Trauma victims have recurring images of the critical incident and respond in a distressful way to similar situations.

post-traumatic stress disorder (PTSD)
disorder that changes the way the body responds to stress, probably as a result of chemical imbalances that increase the levels of stress hormones and alter the reaction of the nervous system

The symptoms of stress exhibited after a critical incident can be divided into four kinds: physical, cognitive, emotional, and behavioural (American Psychiatric Association, 2000, pp. 429-484).

1. *Physical symptoms*
   - aches, pains, muscle tension, trembling, and poor coordination
   - jumpiness and being startled by sudden sounds or movements
   - cold sweats, dry mouth, pale skin, and difficulty focusing the eyes
   - feeling out of breath, hyperventilating until the fingers and toes cramp or go numb
   - upset stomach, vomiting, diarrhea, constipation, and frequent urination
   - chronic fatigue and pain—every movement requires a great deal of effort
   - a distant, haunted, faraway stare
   - substance abuse
   - sexual dysfunction
   - insomnia
2. *Cognitive symptoms*
   - difficulty making decisions
   - confusion
   - detachment and withdrawal
   - disorientation
   - poor concentration and loss of interest in activities
   - memory loss, especially with respect to recent events or the trauma itself
   - inability to perform multiple tasks
   - flashbacks (visual or auditory)

- daydreams, nightmares, and bad dreams
- avoidance of reminders of the event
- contemplation of suicide
- compulsive behaviour patterns
- attention deficit hyperactivity disorder (ADHD) symptoms

3. *Emotional symptoms*
   - grief, including spontaneous crying
   - numbness
   - guilt
   - feelings of hopelessness and being overwhelmed
   - depression, extended periods of sadness
   - anxiety, fear, and edginess
   - panic attacks
   - self-doubt
   - irritability, anger, and resentment
   - hyper-startled responses
   - feeling detached from reality
   - vigilant to the point of being paranoid
   - intrusive thoughts
   - flashbacks or nightmares
   - sudden floods of emotions or images related to the initial event
   - a loss of previously sustained beliefs
4. *Behavioural symptoms*
   - decreased job performance and increased absenteeism
   - detachment and increased isolation from friends, colleagues, and family
   - increased premature departure from work or social gatherings
   - outbursts of laughter or tears
   - changes in normal humour patterns
   - excessive talkativeness or silence
   - low morale
   - hostile tone of voice
   - hypervigilance, jumpiness, or an extreme sense of being "on guard"
   - substance abuse
   - acting like an adolescent and taking up reckless, sometimes life-threatening hobbies
   - avoidance of situations that resemble the initial event
   - obsession with death

Twice as many police officers die by their own hand as do in the line of duty. Suicide among police officers is at a rate of almost twice that of the general population. Officers going through a divorce are five times more likely to commit suicide, and if they are in serious trouble on the job, suspended, or facing termination, they are seven times more likely to commit suicide (Goldfarb, 1999).

Helping a Colleague Cope with Critical Incidents

The police subculture holds on to many myths that can lessen an officer's ability to cope with the aftermath of a critical incident. An officer's recovery can be hampered by beliefs such as "If you can't deal with it, you need to find a new line of work" and "Officers should keep their problems to themselves." Attempting to deny their reactions to stress can cause officers to suffer in silence and not seek help, and in some instances to disrupt their lives and the lives of their families. It is important that officers cope with their stress and come to terms with stressful incidents. It is also important for colleagues to help officers cope with the stress of critical incidents.

The process of debriefing officers has advanced in the last 15 years. Debriefing involves the provision of assistance by a qualified mental health professional to officers who have been involved in a traumatic incident. Although many police services take officers who have been involved in traumatic incidents off duty to deal with the situation, depending on staffing issues, the process may be delayed for up to 72 hours. The process is intended to help alleviate the trauma felt by the officers and to help speed up the recovery process. The process does not deal with blame or cause of the incident but rather with the emotional and psychological consequences of the incident, such as guilt, sadness, or anger. It does not substitute for therapy.

Whether debriefing is done in an individual or platoon setting, it is important that supervisors ensure that this is done in a timely fashion (Everly & Mitchell, 2000). This is what we know about debriefing (Fullerton et al., 2006):

- People with high levels of disaster exposure are 3.1 times more likely to attend a debriefing than those with low levels of exposure.
- Females are 2.7 times more likely to attend a debriefing than males.
- Those with previous disaster experience are 2.7 times more likely to attend a debriefing than those without prior experience.
- Older subjects are more likely than young subjects to talk about the critical incident with their spouse/significant other, a co-worker, or another person.
- People with higher education are more likely than those with lower education to talk about the critical incident with their spouse/significant other, co-worker, or another person.

In addition to debriefing, awareness of the initial psychological and physiological responses to traumatic events may also be reassuring when adverse responses occur. Such education can more readily identify individuals who are at risk and provide earlier intervention (Ghahramanlou & Boradbeck, 2000; Figley, 1995).

Here are some ways you can help others who are suffering the effects of stress after a critical incident:

1. *Manage the situation*
   - Maintain a calm and reassuring presence.
   - Remove the officer from the scene as soon as possible.
   - Facilitate the officer's understanding of the situation. Encourage him or her to talk. Let the officer tell and retell the story. Asking, "Are you okay with this?" is better than saying nothing.
   - Encourage the officer to talk about his or her feelings. Acknowledge that reactions of grief and fear are normal. Let the person know that you are there and that you care.
   - Normalize the officer's reactions as much as possible. Reassure the officer that his or her symptoms are normal.
2. *Mobilize support*
   - Assess the social, familial, and community resources and supports available. Help the officer notify family members that he or she is safe. Encourage family and friends to listen to his or her story. Encourage family and friends to share their feelings.
   - Give the officer plenty of fluids (but no alcohol or coffee).
   - Encourage the officer to engage in physical activity as soon as he or she is able.
   - Provide phone numbers or help the officer access employee assistance programs, chaplain services, and family counselling.
   - If the officer experiences chest pain, hyperventilates, has an elevated heart rate, or exhibits other serious physical symptoms, have him or her seek immediate medical attention.
3. *Follow up*
   - Keep the officer informed about the facts surrounding the incident and any ongoing investigations.
   - Check back with the officer to see how he or she is coping and whether available resources and supports are being used. Encourage others to check as well.
   - Offer to support the officer at court hearings, community meetings, meetings with insurance companies—any event that directly relates to the trauma.
   - If necessary, initiate referrals for outside agencies or participation in counselling (including family) and psychotherapy.
   - Post-traumatic stress disorder may actually alter the way the brain functions. Serotonin, a chemical in the brain, is drastically affected by stress. Encouraging the officer to seek medical intervention may be necessary.

Research (Brown, 2003) indicates that officers should be followed up on for at least two years following a critical incident, since often the individual does not recognize the symptoms of stress. For many, the symptoms generally subside and normal function gradually returns. For some, symptoms may appear to be gone, but they surface again in another stressful situation.

Do *not* do the following:

- Second-guess the officer.
- Say, "I understand how you feel." (You may think you do, but to a victim, his or her pain is unique.)
- Say, "Everything is going to be fine." Acknowledge that things may never be the same but they will get better over time.
- Try to protect the officer by withholding information (but use your judgment in this regard, and seek legal advice if necessary).
- Say things like "It could have been worse," "You can always get another (pet, house, car)," "It's best if you just stay busy," and "You need to get on with your life."
- Say, "When this happened to me ..." Even if you had an identical experience, the victim's need to talk about his or her own trauma is probably greater than the need to listen to other people's experience.
- Give too much advice.
- Make promises and not come through.

Some officers will find that moving on to another career is appropriate, but law enforcement is as much of a calling as medicine or the clergy, as suggested by the large number of students who have known since they were five or six years old that all they ever wanted to be was a police officer. Make sure you have exhausted all methods of support before letting someone—possibly yourself—make such a monumental decision.

If you are helping a child through a critical incident, here are some additional points to consider:

- Answer questions honestly but without frightening details.
- Don't be afraid to admit that you don't have all the answers.
- Allow the child to express her or his feelings so you have a starting point for talking about the situation.

ADDITIONAL STRESS IN YOUR TEENS INTO ADULTHOOD

As you prepare for your career in law enforcement, you too may be faced with additional stress while you gain experience through education, volunteering, and life experiences. Teen stress is similar to adult stress in terms of signs and symptoms. However, adolescents have unique stressors that they face, such as the following:

- physical changes, including an increase in weight and height, menarche, and pubertal changes
- mental changes, including issues with independence, attraction toward the opposite sex, aggressive behaviour, and exposure to experimenting with new things (such as substance abuse)

- emotional issues, which include changing relationships with peers, responsibilities to their families, demands placed on them in school, financial issues, separation or divorce of parents, romantic relationships, and even getting along with siblings

BEHAVIOUR TYPES

Why do different people respond differently to stress? The theory of behaviour types offers some answers.

Type A Behaviour

First identified in the late 1950s by Drs. Meyer Friedman and Ray Rosenman (1994), type A behaviour is the term for behaviour in which a person is competitive, impatient, and a polyphasic thinker (thinks of two or more things at once). A type A personality also experiences an intense sense of urgency, is aggressive and frequently hostile, is intensely driven toward achievement but frequently lacks properly defined goals, and is unable to concentrate on work because distracting thoughts intrude.

Type A personalities are likely to be highly stressed. Recent research indicates that people who are hostile, cynical, and angry a great deal of the time face a higher risk of heart disease, atherosclerosis, and hypertension (Myrtek, 2001). They are very competitive and tend to be tense and agitated when it comes to work. They have poor impulse control and always need to be active. Type A personalities have a mixture of right- and left-brain dominance. They express their anger with outbursts and verbal comments and experience negative emotions. They like to have control over everything, so they tend to be leaders. In addition, they often react in a hostile manner when criticized and they tend to be risk takers.

Type B Behaviour

Type B behaviour is the term for behaviour in which a person takes things one at a time; concentrates effectively; is flexible, unaggressive, and patient; and does not get upset if daily tasks are not completed. A type B personality also takes life as it comes, living in the "here and now"; does not get extremely upset at failing to achieve a goal; usually sets more realistic goals than a type A person; makes time for activities such as exercise, hobbies, and seeing friends; and handles stressful situations more effectively. Type B personalities are intuitive, spontaneous, and patient. They are right-brained dominant and non-judgmental. They are open to criticism and use humour to make their point. When they are angry, their anger is directed at the problem, not the person. They support others, are adaptable and flexible, express positive feelings, and generally believe that everyone can get along.

Type C Behaviour

Some people who resemble type A personalities may actually use their type A behaviours to resist stress. These hardy people have been characterized as type C. They are able to channel their energies into creative endeavours or physical fitness without suffering the effects of high stress. Type C personalities take as much time as they need and want; they are future-oriented. They like to weigh pros and cons before making a decision. They tend to be left-brain dominant and more patient than type A personalities. They analyze and try to figure out what to expect. Type C personalities, however, can be more sensitive to criticism. Thus, they can be resentful and more likely to give the "silent treatment" to a person with whom they are angry. Overall, they have a higher risk of cancer, and have a tendency to be inflexible.

The type C personality has five unique traits ("the **five Cs**") (Kobasa, 1982) that can help them deal with stress effectively:

five Cs
the five unique traits of the type C personality: control, commitment, challenge, choices in lifestyle, and connectedness

1. *Control*—hardiness with a sense of control over life events and their outcomes and the ability to take daily annoyances in stride by thinking and planning
2. *Commitment*—a sense of purpose in life and the ability to set short- and long-term goals involving such things as community projects, religious values, and time with family and friends
3. *Challenge*—a great deal of confidence in one's ability to do one's work, perceiving life as a challenge and accepting setbacks as a part of life and an opportunity for growth
4. *Choices in lifestyle*—integration into daily life of lifestyle choices that enhance health and reduce stress (for example, exercise, proper nutrition, avoiding substance abuse, and use of relaxation techniques)
5. *Connectedness*—a positive social network

Go to **assignment 13.2** (in the appendix) and assess your behaviour type. Answer the questions after you have done the survey.

COPING WITH STRESS

Police officers tend to believe that the emotions and stress reactions arising from critical incidents must be hidden. But this way of coping with stress is unhealthy. Once we recognize that we are under stress, we find that the skills to cope with that stress are right at our fingertips. Many stress management programs now include cognitive aspects (for example, time management, social engineering), but few address the spiritual issues of stress: values, relationships, and even the purpose of life.

Here are some strategies for coping with stress:

1. Exercise—aerobic exercise is one of the keys to coping with stress. Aerobic exercise releases chemical compounds called endorphins that combat stress.
2. Make better nutritional decisions to keep your body healthy and fight infections.
   - Eat a balanced diet of fresh food including fruits, vegetables, and grains (as set out in *Canada's Food Guide to Healthy Eating*).
   - Drink plenty of water every day (at least eight glasses).
   - Avoid overeating.

- Decrease your intake of artificial sweeteners.
- Limit your salt intake to prevent hypertension.
- Limit your caffeine intake.

3. Avoid alcohol and drug abuse (including cigarette smoking).
4. Manage self-talk (how you perceive and express yourself).
   - Reframe your point of view and accentuate the positive.
   - Perceive adverse situations as opportunities rather than setbacks.
   - Stop blaming others.
   - See adverse situations as temporarily bearable.
   - Take things less seriously.
   - Feel okay no matter what.
5. Manage your actions.
   - Learn to say no and stick by it.
   - Be assertive.
   - Learn to listen to people.
   - Use more appropriate communication styles.
6. Use appropriate time-management skills.
   - Balance work and play; set aside time for recreational activities.
   - Set aside time for idleness each day (without guilt).
   - Set realistic goals.
7. Develop a support group.
   - Learn to ask for help. Call a friend.
   - Spend quality time with family and friends who have a positive outlook on life.
   - Develop satisfying relationships.
8. Control physical stress responses.
   - Use breathing exercises.
   - Use muscle relaxation exercises.
   - Use mental health exercises.
   - Use yoga.
9. Remember to take the time to laugh at yourself.
10. Resolve issues of anger and fear.
11. Engage in hobbies like drawing, writing, singing, or playing with pets.
12. Watch stress-relieving programs such as comedies or cartoons.

Relaxation Techniques

Let's look at how stress responses can be controlled by relaxation techniques. To benefit from these techniques, you must prepare by not drinking caffeinated beverages, eating, or smoking for at least an hour beforehand, and by not exercising for at least two hours beforehand.

BREATHING

Breathing is affected by the stress response. When you are stressed, your breathing becomes more rapid and shallow, and your heart rate increases. To elicit a relaxation response, you must slow down your breathing and learn to take deeper breaths. By breathing right, you will have more efficient oxygenation of the blood, which will trigger the parasympathetic "quieting response" (a sense of control over the body and its reactions to stressors).

Try the following breathing exercises:

1. Monitor your heart rate for 15 seconds and then multiply by 4 to obtain beats per minute.
2. Sit up straight with your back against a chair.
3. Put your left hand over your chest and your right hand over your abdomen.
4. Breathe normally. You will probably notice that your chest expands more than your abdomen.
5. Now practise a new way of breathing by holding in your breath and then slowly releasing the air. To do this most effectively, breathe through your nose. When you take a deep breath, you should feel your diaphragm push down and your abdomen expand outward (as you get oxygen into the lower third of the lungs).
6. Continue to breathe slowly for about five minutes while attempting to relax and slow your breathing down. At the end of the five minutes, you should feel relaxed and be able to resume normal activities.
7. Monitor your heart rate again. If you are more relaxed, your heart rate should be down. Diaphragmatic breathing is a skill that takes practice. Practise it several times each day.

MEDITATION

Meditation can involve focusing the mind, and thereby quieting the body, by sitting or lying down comfortably and quietly with eyes closed for 10–20 minutes once or twice a day. It does not involve thinking, though you will probably find that turning off thoughts is almost impossible. Try not to get caught up in your thoughts rather than fighting them while you meditate.

Meditation methods include the following:

- Mindful meditation is simply listening to internal thoughts and bodily processes, such as your breathing (Kabat-Zinn, 1991).
- Transcendental meditation involves entering a meditative state twice a day by closing your eyes and repeating a mantra (a sound without meaning).
- Zen meditation focuses on breathing.
- Benson's (1975) method of relaxation is a technique in which you focus on words or phrases associated with your beliefs. The idea is to turn to your inner self to find harmony.

AUTOGENIC FEEDBACK

Through passive suggestion, you practise focusing on the heaviness and relaxed state of your warm muscles. The following is an autogenic feedback exercise. Begin by lying or sitting in a comfortable position, and say each phrase to yourself slowly and distinctly several times. All four stages in this exercise can be completed in five minutes, or you can take as long as you want.

Stage 1

- "My legs feel heavy."
- "My arms feel heavy."
- "My shoulders feel heavy."
- "My head feels heavy."
- "I can no longer lift my limbs off the ground."

Stage 2

- "My legs feel warm."
- "My arms feel warm."
- "My shoulders feel warm."
- "My face feels warm."
- "My entire body feels warm and comfortable." (Some people imagine putting a blanket on to add to the sense of warmth.)

Stage 3

- "My heartbeat is slowing and I am becoming calm."

Stage 4

- "My breathing is slowing and I am relaxed."

PROGRESSIVE MUSCLE RELAXATION

This technique requires you to alternately tense and relax your muscles.

1. While lying on your back or sitting in a comfortable position, monitor your heart rate for 15 seconds and then multiply by 4 to obtain beats per minute. Concentrate on relaxing and slowing your breathing.
2. Do each of the following exercises twice. Hold for 10 seconds each time.
   a. Curl your toes and hold. Release.
   b. Pull your toes up toward your head and hold. Release. Then take a deep breath and slowly exhale.
   c. Tighten your calf muscles. Release.
   d. Tighten your thigh muscles. Release. Then take a deep breath and slowly exhale.
   e. Tighten your abdominal muscles. Release.
   f. Do a pelvic tilt (described in chapter 12). Release. Take a deep breath and slowly exhale.
   g. Tighten your back muscles to bring your shoulder blades together. Relax.

h. Make a fist with both hands. Release.
i. Tighten your shoulders. Release.
j. Gently tighten your neck muscles. Release.
k. Scrunch up your face by tightening your facial muscles. Release. Take a deep breath and slowly exhale.

3. Ensure that your muscles are relaxed. You may have to tense and relax them again.
4. Monitor your heart rate again to see whether it has gone down.

VISUALIZATION

Also called mental imagery, guided imagery, or guided daydreaming (Samuels & Samuels, 1975), this technique involves imagining yourself in a quiet and peaceful place, usually a natural setting. Known as Jacobson's method of relaxation, the objective of this method is to work on the peripheral nervous system to reduce the physiological symptoms of anxiety (Jacobson, 1938) by progressive relaxation of the body and the use of mental imagery to achieve relaxation. It can be done entirely on your own or with the help of instructors or recordings (such as tapes of ocean or bird sounds). In a recent cardiology study, Paul-Labrador et al. (2006) found that patients who used visualization improved their blood pressure and insulin-resistance components of metabolic syndrome, as well as cardiac autonomic nervous system tone (including heart rate, the heart's ability to contract, and tolerance to physical activity), thereby reducing the physiological response to stress and improving coronary heart disease (CHD) risk factors.

The following visualization exercise is based on memories of locations that have had special meaning for me. Feel free to visualize locations of your own once you have tried this exercise.

You will probably need someone to read these instructions to you the first time you try this exercise. I usually do this exercise immediately after doing the progressive muscle relaxation technique described above.

Find a quiet, comfortable spot in which to sit or lie down. Begin by monitoring your heart rate for 15 seconds.

> Take a deep breath and relax. Concentrate on how relaxed you are becoming and how comfortable you are. Close your eyes and concentrate on your breathing. Relax your back, arms, and legs. Concentrate on releasing the tension stored in your body. Feel your chest go up and down with your breathing. Relax and concentrate on your breathing.
>
> Now imagine that you are getting up from your spot to walk down a corridor toward a door. Open that door and walk through it to an escalator. Together let's go down the escalator: 1, 2, 3, 4, 5, 6, 7, 8, 9, 10. Now step off the escalator and go to the door.
>
> When you reach that door, imagine that you are taking off your shoes, picking up a towel lying beside the door, and then walking through the door. On the other side of the door is a beach and you can feel the warmth of the sun on your body and the white sand at your feet. Close the door behind you.
>
> As you walk toward the dark blue ocean on the right, you can feel the sun on your face and back. You are able to hear the waves and feel a slight breeze on your face. You can feel the cool sand underneath your feet. Above you, the sky is a clear

blue. Find a place to sit or lie down. Remember you have a towel to use if you need it. You will continue to feel the warmth of the sand and sun. You will hear the waves and the birds in the distance. You are relaxed and quiet. For the next several minutes, allow your mind to relax and continue to enjoy the beach. Enjoy the stillness, warmth, and quiet you are experiencing.

Next, imagine that you are getting up and walking to the water's edge. Dip your hand in the water and splash it on your face. You can now return to the door feeling refreshed and alert and at peace. Open the door and take one last look at the beach. Close the door. Lock the door with the key that's hanging by the door and put the key in your pocket.

You are now going back up the escalator to the first door. Together let's go back up the escalator: 10, 9, 8, 7, 6, 5, 4, 3, 2, 1. Step off the escalator. Open the door, walk down the corridor, and return to the spot where you began your journey. Take a moment to remember the peaceful time you spent at the beach.

Bring your attention back to the here and now.

Take a deep breath. Before you get up, see whether you were able to lower your heart rate. You should feel refreshed and alert.

OTHER RELAXATION TECHNIQUES

Hypnosis

Hypnosis acts as a stress reducer by getting the subject to concentrate on key words and images. It is a scientifically verified and effective technique that can promote accelerated human change. With hypnosis you can create desired changes in behaviour and encourage mental and physical well-being. People use it to lose weight, quit smoking, reduce physical pain, and deal with traumatic events.

Biofeedback

Biofeedback is a form of alternative medicine that assesses bodily processes such as blood pressure, heart rate, skin temperature, galvanic skin response (sweating), and muscle tension to raise a person's awareness and conscious control over physiological responses. It involves a physiological feedback monitor such as an electrocardiograph for monitoring heart activity. It allows you to learn appropriate relaxation responses (Choe et al., 2007).

Music

Music conjures up images and memories, and can be relaxing and renewing. The music you choose will depend on your own preferences, although quiet, slower music is more relaxing.

Yoga

Yoga is a discipline that seeks to unite the mind, body, and soul (Seaward, 2005). The practice of yoga combines breathing, stretching, and balance to achieve a spiritual focus.

T'ai Chi Ch'uan

Known as the softest martial art (Seaward, 2005), this discipline brings the body and mind together through the "chi," or life force, when you do a series of graceful martial arts movements. T'ai Chi Ch'uan attempts to achieve deep relaxation and as much "softness" in the musculature as possible. It is characterized by the leverage through the joints based on the relaxation of muscles to enhance and increase breathing, body heat, the lymph system, and peristalsis, working toward a homeostasis state (returning your internal circulation back to a healthier and balanced state). This discipline can help you keep calm and steady under pressure. Many communities offer programs.

Massage

Massage stimulates blood flow and improves muscle tone. It relaxes the muscles and thereby creates a calming effect. Now more popular than ever, massage can be performed by chiropractors, physiotherapists, reflexologists, acupuncturists, and other professionals. Non-professionals can also learn massage. Some types of therapies include:

- *Deep tissue massage,* which focuses on deeper layers of muscle tissue in an attempt to release chronic patterns of tension in the body through slow strokes and deep pressure.
- *Swedish massage,* which is a superficial gentle message that is designed to relax muscles and increase circulation.
- *Lymphatic massage,* which is a light touch technique used to promote health and aid recovery from illness by removing toxic metabolic waste.
- *Cranial massage,* which is a delicate manual technique used to release the muscles around the neck, jaw, and skull. This method is used to help temporal-mandibular joint dysfunction.
- *Reflexology massage,* which helps bring about balance, ease, and soundness of mind, body, and spirit by massaging the feet and hands.
- *Aromatherapy,* which is the use of essential oils combined with massage to provide a powerful calming and energizing effect.
- *Acupuncture,* which is the technique of placing needles at key points on the body to unblock and redirect energy flow to relieve tension and relief from pain.

Hydrotherapy

Hydrotherapy—soaking in a hot tub, warm bath, or hot shower—is a great way to relax at the end of the day. Warm water (about 38 °C) appears to quiet and soothe the body while slowing down the activity of internal organs. Water seems to have the ability to get rid of stress and rejuvenate the body. Whirlpool baths appear to have higher stress-relief benefits, including reducing anxiety. Herbal baths with lavender, linden, passionflower, and chamomile also appear to be effective.

Ultimately, it is up to you to discover what helps you relax and brings your stress level down. You may need to try a particular method a few times before you become comfortable with it.

Also realize that if you do not allow time for yourself, mentally and physically, you will begin to experience symptoms of stress. I wish you luck in developing coping strategies for stress.

KEY TERMS

- stress
- general adaptation syndrome (GAS)
- psychosomatic symptoms
- stressor
- critical incident
- post-traumatic stress disorder (PTSD)
- five Cs

EXERCISES

Review

1. Define stress.

2. What are the differences among neustress, eustress, and distress?

3. What are some of the general symptoms of stress?

4. List five stressors associated with law enforcement work.

5. What is a critical incident?

6. Describe post-traumatic stress disorder (PTSD).

7. What are some of the signs and symptoms of PTSD?

8. What can you do for a colleague who is suffering from critical incident stress or PTSD?

9. Explain how type A, B, and C personalities cope with stress.

10. Briefly explain five relaxation techniques for coping with stress.

Multiple Choice

1. Which of the statements about stress is *incorrect*?
   a. Stress can be self-induced.
   b. Stress can be pleasurable.
   c. Stress can cause psychological disorders.
   d. Individuals differ in what they find stressful.
   e. Your ability to handle stress is hereditary and fixed.

2. A technique of relaxation that uses a machine to monitor body processes is called
   a. yoga
   b. autogenic feedback
   c. biofeedback
   d. transcendental meditation
   e. progressive relaxation

3. Which of the following is *least* likely to be helpful in relieving tension?
   a. taking a brisk walk after sitting for a long time
   b. doing slow stretching exercises
   c. doing rhythmical exercises
   d. drinking alcohol
   e. getting a massage

4. How did Selye label the negative level of stress?
   a. hyperstress
   b. distress
   c. eustress
   d. burnout
   e. neustress

5. What is the first step in managing stress?
   a. Use a relaxation technique.
   b. Recognize symptoms and causes.
   c. Be as fit and healthy as possible.
   d. Get eight hours of sleep a night.
   e. Control lifestyle and avoid stressors.

6. Which is a good way to manage stress?
   a. Allow more time for work.
   b. Avoid talking about your problems.
   c. Think positively.
   d. Insist that things should go your way.
   e. Pretend that the problem will just go away.

7. Why might those in law enforcement be more likely to suffer from critical incident stress?
   a. Their personalities predispose them to PTSD.
   b. Jumping in front of traffic causes problems.
   c. Their job involves facing dangerous situations.
   d. They are more sensitive than the general population.
   e. They enjoy the "buzz" of constant stress.

8. Which behaviour type is characterized by an angry, hostile, and impatient personality?
   a. type A
   b. type B
   c. type C
   d. type E
   e. type AB

9. Jacobson's method of relaxation emphasizes
   a. imagery
   b. visualization
   c. autogenic training
   d. meditation
   e. progressive relaxation

10. Post-traumatic stress disorder refers to
   a. a positive ability to handle stress
   b. the result of completing all your credits in first year
   c. an overwhelming response to stress
   d. the response to completing an assignment on time
   e. none of the above

11. Any physical, social, or psychological event or condition that causes our body to have to adjust to a specific situation is known as a(n):
    a. obstacle
    b. PTSD
    c. stressor
    d. strain
    e. obstacle

12. During which phase of general adaptation syndrome does the brain prepare the body for the "fight or flight" response?
    a. resistance
    b. adaptation
    c. exhaustion
    d. alarm
    e. homeostasis

13. Working out when stressed can help by:
    a. increasing energy
    b. improving mental alertness
    c. allowing you to step back from the situation to view it in a different way
    d. reducing hostility
    e. all of the above

14. General adaptation syndrome explains
    a. the pattern followed by our physiological responses to stress
    b. the path of our autonomic nervous system when we are aroused by a stressful situation
    c. a means of dealing with post-traumatic stress disorder
    d. how to achieve homeostasis
    e. how well we adapt to new situations

15. With a full load of college courses and a part-time job, Steve suffers from excessive time pressure, excessive responsibility, and excessive expectations to succeed. Steve is suffering from
    a. neustress
    b. burnout
    c. eustress
    d. overload
    e. inconsistent goals and behaviours

16. The physiological arousal response in which the body prepares to combat a real or perceived threat is called
    a. the response phase
    b. the resistance phase
    c. homeostasis
    d. the fight or flight response
    e. distress response

17. The characteristics that have been associated with an increased risk for heart disease in a type A personality are
    a. compulsiveness and impatience
    b. competitiveness and fastidiousness
    c. hostility, anger, and cynicsim
    d. perfectionism, impatience, and hostility
    e. competitiveness and introversion

REFERENCES

American Psychiatric Association (APA). (2000). *Diagnostic and statistical manual of mental disorders* (4th ed.). Washington, DC: APA.

Benson, H. (1975). *The relaxation response.* New York: Morrow.

Boyd, N. (1995). Violence in the workplace in British Columbia: A preliminary investigation. *Canadian Journal of Criminology, 37*(4), 491-519.

Brown, H. (2003). The effects of post traumatic stress disorder (PTSD) on the officer and the family. Police Stresline. Available at http://www.geocities.com/stressline_com/ptsd-family.html.

Choe, H.M., Townsend, K.A., Blount, G., Lo, C.H., Sadowski, L., & Standiford, C.J. (2007). Treatment and control of blood pressure in patients with diabetes mellitus. *American Journal of Health System Pharmacy, 64*(1), 97-103.

Connor, K.M., & Butterfield, M.I. (2003). Posttraumatic stress disorder. *Focus, 1*(30), 247-263.

Ellis, D., Choi, A., & Blaus, C. (1993). Injuries to police officers attending domestic disturbances: An empirical study. *Canadian Journal of Criminology, 35*(2), 149-168.

Everly, G.S., & Mitchell, J.T. (2000). The debriefing "controversy" and crisis intervention: A review of lexical and substantive issues. *International Journal of Emergency Mental Health, 2*(4), 211-225.

Figley, C. (Ed). (1995). *Compassion fatigue: Coping with secondary traumatic stress disorders in those who treat the traumatized.* New York: Brunner-Routledge.

Finn, P. (1997). Reducing stress: An organization-centered approach. *Law Enforcement Bulletin* [Department of Justice, Federal Bureau of Investigations] (August). Available at http://www.fbi.gov/publications/leb/1997/aug975.htm.

Friedman, M., & Rosenman, R.H. (1994). *Type A behavior and your heart.* New York: Knopf.

Fullerton, C., Ursano, R.J., Vance, K., & Wang, L. (2006). Debriefing following trauma. *American Psychiatric Association Disaster Psychiatry.* Available at http://www.psych.org/psych_pract/debriefing_following_trauma3501.cfm.

Ghahramanlou, M., & Boradbeck, C. (2000). Predictors of secondary trauma in sexual assault counselors. *International Journal of Emergency Mental Health, 4,* 229-240.

Goldfarb, D.A. (1999). The effects of stress on police officers. Available at http://www.heavybadge.com/efstress.htm.

Gyi, D.E., & Porter, J.M. (1998). Musculoskeletal problems and driving in police officers. *Occupational Medicine (London), 48*(3), 152-160.

Jacobson, E. (1938). *Progressive relaxation.* Chicago: Chicago University Press.

Kabat-Zinn, J. (1991). *Full catastrophe living.* New York: Delacorte.

Kiecolt-Glaser, J.K. (1999). Stress, personal relationships and immune function: Health implications. *Brain Behavior Immunology, 13,* 61-72.

Kobasa, S.C. (1982). The hardy personality: Toward a social psychology of stress and health. In R.S. Sanders and J. Suls (Eds.), *Social psychology of health and illness* (pp. 3-32). Hillsdale, NJ: Erlbaum.

Kohan, A., & O'Connor, B.P. (2002). Police officer job satisfaction in relation to mood, well-being and alcohol consumption. *The Journal of Psychology, 136,* 307-318.

Loo, R. (2003). A meta-analysis of police suicide rates: Findings and issues. *Suicide and Life Threatening Behaviour, 33*(3), 313-325.

Morse, D.R., & Furst, M.L. (1979). *Stress for success: A holistic approach to stress and its management.* New York: Van Nostrand Reinhold.

Myrtek, M. (2001). Meta-analyses of prospective studies on coronary heart disease, type A personality and hostility. *International Journal of Cardiology, 79*, 245–251.

Paul-Labrador, M., Polk, D., Dwyer, J.H., Velasquez, I., Nidich, S., Rainforth, M., Schneider, R., & Merz, C.N. (2006). Effects of a randomized controlled trial of transcendental meditation on components of the metabolic syndrome in subjects with coronary heart disease. *Archives of Internal Medicine, 166*(11), 1218-1224.

Parsons, J. (2004). *Occupational health and safety issues of police officers in Canada, the United States and Europe: A review essay.* International Council of Police Representative Association. Available at http://www.ilecnet.org/resources.htm.

Samuels, M., & Samuels, N. (1975). *Seeing with the mind's eye: The history, techniques and uses of visualization.* New York: Random House.

Seaward, B.L. (2005). *Managing stress* (5th ed.). Sudbury, MA: Jones and Bartlett Publishers.

Selye, H. (1956). *The stress of life.* New York: McGraw-Hill.

Selye, H. (1974). *Stress without distress.* Philadelphia: Lippincott.

Shafer, W. (1996). *Stress management for wellness* (3rd ed.). Fort Worth, TX: Holt, Rinehart and Winston.

Van Netten, C., Brands, R.H., Hoption Cann, S.A., Spinelli, J.J., & Sheps, S.B. (2003). Cancer cluster among police detachment personnel. *Environment International, 28*, 567-572.

World Health Organization. (2003). *The solid facts: The social determinants of health.* Available at http://www.who.dk/document/E59555.pdf.

CHAPTER 14

Shift Work

CHAPTER OBJECTIVES

After completing this chapter, you should be able to:

- Identify the physiological, psychological, and social effects of shift work.
- Identify the physiological stages of sleep.
- Explain the importance of proper sleep for shift workers.
- Develop shift work coping strategies.

It is estimated that 25 to 43 percent of all workers work non-traditional hours. Emergency service and crisis intervention workers, especially, have chosen careers tied to round-the-clock availability. This non-standard schedule includes evening or night shifts, rotating shifts, and extended hours on the job. Your task is to determine whether you are able to withstand the effects of shift work and rotating shifts. The mental, physical, and social implications are very challenging. You must learn to cope with shift work in order to assure a safe work environment for you and your co-workers.

In this chapter we look at shift work and its effects. We will also look at the importance of sleep and ways to get better-quality sleep. This chapter also discusses ways to alleviate the stress caused by shift work. First, let's look at some facts and statistics:

- Approximately 20 percent of shift workers quit their job because they cannot adapt to the demands of shift work. Those who persevere even though they cannot adjust suffer the effects of ill health long after they stop working shifts (Brusgard, 1975).
- Shift work limits socialization with people outside the job due to the demands and risks of the job, so that the shift worker's job becomes the shift worker's life (Wienecke, 1999).
- Law enforcement personnel who work the night shift have more accidents (O'Neil, 1986).
- A higher incidence of serious illness and disability is found among police officers and correctional workers who work rotating shifts (Tasto & Colligan, 1978).

- As officers age, their ability to cope with shift changes diminishes. They find it more difficult to fall asleep and are unable to sleep without interruption.
- Shift work may cause fatigue and somatic anxiety, which are independent predictors of strain, either in the form of cardiovascular or digestive symptoms (Smith et al., 1998).

Turn to **assignment 14.1** (in the appendix) to assess your sleep patterns.

SHIFT SCHEDULE

Police work typically involves two types of shift schedules (although there are many variations):

- Three eight-hour shifts, usually beginning at 7 a.m. (the day shift), 3 p.m. (the afternoon shift), and 11 p.m. (the night or "graveyard" shift).
- Two 12-hour shifts, usually beginning at 7 a.m. and 7 p.m.

Most shift work schedules involve four to seven days on and two to four days off. Each police service has its own arrangement. Some arrangements are tailored to times of peak demand for police services (such as rush hour).

A great deal of research into shift work has resulted in these recommendations for devising shift work routines (Wedderburn & King, 1996):

- Minimize permanent nights.
- Minimize the sequence of nights: only two to four night shifts in succession should be worked. Weekly rotating shifts provide insufficient time for the circadian rhythm to adjust and enough time for a sizable "sleep debt" to accumulate. Working four to seven night shifts in a row is now being condemned by experts.
- Consider shorter night shifts (seven or eight hours will minimize errors and accidents).
- Plan rotations with some free weekends.
- Avoid overlong work sequences.
- Avoid early starts (reduced sleep leads to fatigue and increased risk of errors and accidents on the morning shifts).
- Rotate forward (clockwise rotation from mornings to afternoons to nights).

Which shifts are best?

- Fixed shifts offer the least amount of disruption to the circadian rhythm (discussed later in this chapter); however, shift workers have difficulty reverting to normal hours to participate in family or social activities.
- Working rapid rotating shifts (two days/two nights) keeps the circadian rhythm day-oriented since there is insufficient time to adjust and there is less sleep debt; however, individuals may be out of sync and their alertness may be affected.

Ultimately, it is up to the agency, in consultation with the associations, to address what works most effectively for employees.

UNDERSTANDING THE IMPORTANCE OF SLEEP

We need sufficient sleep to work effectively, sustain emotional health, and resist stress. We spend a third of our lives sleeping. Sleep experts say the average amount of sleep we need is 8 hours a night, although some individuals require 10 hours while others seem to get by on 6 hours.

Think of sleep as a slow elevator ride down to the bottom floor. At the bottom is where you sleep deeply, and halfway up is where you take side trips to have dreams. Usually, we ride the elevator about five times each night—every 70 to 90 minutes—as we cycle through the four ever-deeper stages of non-dreaming sleep, then shift into rapid-eye movement (REM) sleep.

There are several stages of sleep, each providing different resources for recovery from the day's demands. Each night you basically go through the same sequence of sleep stages. Your body begins to slow down and muscle tension decreases. As you enter stage 1 of non-REM sleep, mundane thoughts go through your head. If you are awakened at this stage, you may not admit that you were asleep. Your brain waves at this stage are smaller and irregular. As you enter stage 2, your brain waves become larger. There is an occasional burst of electrical energy. At this stage your eyes become unresponsive. In stage 3, your brain waves are about five times larger and much slower, and in stage 4, your brain waves form jagged patterns and you are in such a profound state of unconsciousness that it is very difficult to wake you. Then you shift to REM sleep, where your pulse and breathing quicken, your face and limbs go slack, and your brain temperature and blood flow increase. Your eyes dart back and forth.

Stages 3 and 4, the two deeper stages of sleep, are necessary for recovery from physical fatigue. It is believed that non-REM sleep helps repair cells, rests the body and mind, and boosts the immune system. **REM sleep** allows your body to recover from mental fatigue, and it also helps to store memories and consolidate learning.

REM sleep
a stage of sleep that allows your body to recover from mental fatigue and helps to store memories and consolidate learning

Because the hours they have for sleep do not coincide with natural and social rhythms, shift workers must make a special effort to ensure that they get enough uninterrupted sleep. If their sleep is interrupted, they may not pass through all five stages of sleep and may suffer health problems as a result.

If a new afternoon or night shift worker adheres strictly to a set sleep pattern, his or her body can usually adjust to shift work in about a month. Unfortunately, most of the world adheres to a different schedule. Socially, night shift routines affect dating opportunities, marriage, child care, and dining routines.

Moreover, most courts are open only during the day. This means that a night shift officer must come to court during his or her days off or has to work a night shift and then stay awake to go to court, getting as little as four hours' sleep before being required to go in for the next night shift. Inevitably, night shift officers reduce their sleep time to take advantage of daytime activities on the days they are off duty. This throws the body's sleep adjustment processes into disorder, and the readjustment period must start all over again.

THE EFFECTS OF SHIFT WORK

Let's look more closely at some effects of shift work and lack of sleep.

Physiological and Psychological Effects

circadian rhythm
the 24-hour cycle on which the human biological clock is based

Like most organisms, humans have a biological clock that regulates their periods of activity and inactivity. The human biological clock is based on a 24-hour cycle known as the **circadian rhythm**.

Exposure to light and dark helps establish physiological cycles. The organ that appears to be responsible for this is the suprachiasmatic nuclei (SCN), a small cluster of nerve tissue connected to the point where the optic nerves meet the brain. Stimulated by nerve impulses triggered by exposure to light and dark, this photosensitive nerve centre sets and resets the biological clock. At regular intervals each day, the body becomes hungry and tired, active or lethargic. Body temperature, blood pressure, heart beat, glandular activity, digestion, brain waves, and so on, rise and fall in a rhythmic pattern. Interference with this cycle reduces mental alertness, elevates the heart rate, upsets the stomach, and causes impatience.

Melatonin is a natural hormone made by the pineal gland (located in the midbrain). Darkness stimulates the pineal gland to secrete melatonin, which promotes sleep by making you feel less alert. This usually happens around 9 p.m., when natural light is gone. Unless an individual is subjected to bright artificial indoor lighting, melatonin is generally released for approximately 12 hours. As you age, the amount secreted decreases. People with weak biorhythms are more adaptable to shift work when young, but are more likely to develop intolerance to shift work later in life (Smolensky & Reinberg, 1990).

Shift work interferes with the circadian rhythm, which is why people who start working new shifts, especially night shifts, need a period of adjustment. If they do not get the necessary uninterrupted sleep between shifts, they will always experience problems. One of the serious results of rotating shift work is that 30–50 percent of these shift workers report falling asleep on the job at least once a week.

Jet lag has many of the same effects as shift work. Jet lag can occur when you cross three or more time zones, with the result that your circadian rhythm is no longer synchronized with periods of light and dark. The consequences of jet lag, which can last for days or even weeks, include sleep problems, irritability, loss of appetite, fatigue, and poor memory. Some people are very severely affected.

Officers who work 3 p.m. to 11 p.m. and 7 p.m. to 3 a.m. shifts generally find it very difficult to fall asleep right away (Bahrke, 1995). Many are still alert after hours of trying to fall asleep.

When dayworkers move to the night shift, they sleep an average of 5.5 hours a day, not the 7.0 or 8.0 hours required. As the sleep deficit builds, we see indications of decreased efficiency in reasoning and reaction time. The sleep deficit can lead to brief periods of dozing or "micro-sleeping" where you fall in and out of sleep for only seconds at a time. The symptoms experienced by the sleep-deprived are similar to those of jet lag. Police officers in this situation report decreased appetite, poor attitude, and general fatigue (Bahrke, 1995).

Some police officers affected by shift work sleep disruptions have experienced temporary partial paralysis and temporary memory loss. Some experience peripheral hallucinations and see phantom runners out of the corners of their eyes. Others find it hard to keep their thoughts straight and difficult to speak in complete sentences. It is almost as if they are sleep-drunk. These symptoms usually occur during the early morning hours. Individuals may be too sleep-impaired to drive, putting themselves and others at risk. Some may actually drive faster to try to compensate for their sleepiness by doing riskier, more stimulating things. This is when more accidents happen.

For those driving or carrying firearms, fatigue and reduced alertness can become a life-threatening problem (Vila, 2000). The constant disruption of hormonal balances from shift work may cause elevated reproductive risks (Nurmine, 1998), including spontaneous premature births and lower birth weights, as well as infertility issues. There is also a link between the disruption of the circadian rhythm and poorer survival rates among patients with breast cancer (Filipski, 2002).

Seasonal affective disorder (SAD) is a syndrome associated with decreased light due to climate, latitude, and changes in neurotransmitter function associated with different seasons in the northern hemisphere. More prevalent in women, it is characterized by winter depression, lethargy, and a craving for carbohydrates associated with weight gain (Gysin et al., 1997). During winter, women increase their nightly production of melatonin, while during the summer they produce less. Men's production of melatonin is relatively unchanging (Leutwyler, 1995).

Sleep Disorders

There are a number of sleep disorders that can be triggered by a lack of sleep. These conditions must be assessed and looked after. For more information, visit the National Sleep Foundation website at www.sleepfoundation.org.

Narcolepsy is a disorder that affects one in 2,000 people. It is a malfunction in the part of the brain that decides whether you're awake or asleep. People with narcolepsy suddenly fall asleep without warning while carrying on their usual daytime activities. They may experience sudden loss of muscle control and this may be triggered by strong emotions and vivid dreams. Some of the symptoms include the following (Hayduk, 2005):

narcolepsy
a disorder that causes the malfunctioning of the brain, leading to one's falling asleep without warning

- *Excessive sleepiness.*
- *Cataplexy,* which is a sudden loss in muscle tone and deep tendon reflexes leading to muscle weakness, temporary paralysis, or a complete postural collapse. Cataplexy is usually brought on by an outburst of emotion—notably laughter, anger, or being startled.
- *Sleep paralysis,* which is the temporary inability to move or talk during the episode.
- *Hypnagogic hallucinations,* which are sensory dream-like experiences during the transition from wakefulness to sleep. These can be vivid, bizarre, and frightening to the individual.
- *Disrupted major sleep episodes,* which involve frequent awakening and increased body movement.
- *Automatic behaviour,* which is unaware behaviour when fluctuating between sleep and wakefulness, such as irrelevant words, lapses in speech, and being unable to explain how you got somewhere.

Restless legs syndrome (RLS) is a common and distressing condition that is characterized by an overwhelming urge to move the legs when they are at rest. Symptoms are more profound at night and during sleep (Allen & Mitler, 2005), and include:

restless legs syndrome (RLS)
a condition characterized by an overwhelming urge to move the legs when they are at rest

- uncomfortable feeling in the legs (such as tingling, creeping, itching, or aching)
- involuntary jerking of limbs that is relieved by movement
- difficulty falling or staying asleep due to the symptoms

sleep apnea
a breathing-related sleep disorder in which inappropriate brain signals do not tell the breathing muscles to initiate respiration

Sleep apnea is a breathing-related sleep disorder that is potentially life-threatening. Central sleep apnea occurs when the brain fails to send the appropriate signals to the breathing muscles to initiate respiration. Obstructive sleep apnea, which is far more common, occurs when the air cannot flow into or out of the person's nose or mouth, although efforts to breathe continue. Sleep apnea is connected to cardiovascular problems. Risk factors include snoring, obesity, smoking, and a small upper airway (Phillips, 2005). Symptoms include:

- breathing pauses, which can happen as much as 20 to 60 times per hour
- breathing pauses accompanied by snoring between the episodes
- gasping or choking sensations
- being awakened just enough to inhale and resume breathing
- excessive daytime sleepiness
- early morning headaches

Social Effects

As mentioned earlier, most of the world operates during daytime hours. Society disregards shift workers in planning its schedules. This, of course, poses special problems for shift workers, especially those who work only at night. Most shift workers restrict their workweek non-work activities to sleeping and eating, and do everything else on their days off. This affects leisure activities, volunteer work, and time with family and friends. Thirty percent of police divorces are related to shift work stress. Reduced family time, mismatched energy levels for intimacy, and decreased alertness can result from shift work (Goldfarb & Ausmiller, 1999).

Scheduling is a must if spouses are to cope with shift work. Planning your days and keeping each other informed of family activities are very important. The parent who works shifts misses school functions, birthday parties, sporting events, and family outings. It becomes difficult to explain to a child why you are constantly missing his or her soccer games but are able to attend your other child's games. Young children find it difficult to understand why a parent has to sleep during the day and why they must play quietly in the house; similarly, they cannot understand why a parent must work weekends. The parent who is not a shift worker has to compensate for the other, and at times feels overloaded.

PERSONAL PERSPECTIVE

Shift work not only robs the officer of precious family moments, it also impacts his or her family. While my husband was called away for a homicide, instead of enjoying our 20th anniversary trip, I spent it picking out a ring for myself, by myself. Feeling robbed of special moments and memories can be hard for all concerned. It is really important to maintain open dialogue and to set time aside for both your significant other and family in order to ensure that all feel included.

Single officers find the social aspect difficult. They have a hard time meeting people during their off hours. Due to the time spent at work, shift workers as a whole fall into the trap of socializing only with their own. They tend to lose touch with dayworkers, who in turn have a difficult time understanding shift workers.

There can be a positive side to shift work, however. Law enforcement officers who get four consecutive days off have time for chores and activities around the house that a dayworker may not have. Having days off during the week allows you to go shopping without having to stand in line, to play a round of golf in short order, and to bring school-aged children home for lunch. Some weekends can be extended to four days, and during the week you can go to a fitness facility during off-peak hours. Those officers with hectic family schedules get some quiet time for themselves while their children are at school.

COPING STRATEGIES

The following suggestions will help you cope with the stress of shift work in your professional and personal life.

Eating Nutritious Food

Following *Canada's Food Guide to Healthy Eating* (Health Canada, 2007) is very important (see chapter 8). Fruits and vegetables should replace chocolate bars, chips, and candy, which are high in fat and sugar. Consuming light to moderate amounts of protein is recommended for the beginning of the shift, and complex carbohydrates can help get you through the shift.

Try to have your main meal of the day in the middle of your awake period and a couple of hours before starting night duty. Having a regular eating schedule for the shift you are on will reduce the risk of developing gastrointestinal disorders and diabetes.

Don't go to bed hungry or overly full. Have a light snack about one hour before you hit the pillow. Snacks such as cheese, milk, a banana, slices of turkey, and tuna contain the amino acid tryptophan, which helps you fall asleep. Avoid sugary snacks, which may cause your blood sugar to plummet later, causing you to wake up. Excessive drinking of liquids may increase the need to go to the bathroom during your sleep time.

Avoid caffeinated soft drinks, tea, coffee, chocolate, and aspirin for five hours before going to sleep. Caffeine affects some people for up to 12 hours. Tobacco should also be avoided because nicotine acts as a stimulant. Alcohol and so-called sleep aids interfere with the depth and quality of sleep. Stimulants to counter listlessness and sleepiness create an unhealthy stimulant–depressant cycle. Recreational drugs can cause restlessness and interfere with sleep. Most sleeping pills contain antihistamines, which have a sedative side effect, inducing light sleep but robbing you of deep sleep.

The Role of Light

When you do paperwork, make sure your workspace is well lit. On patrol, take frequent breaks outside the car to stimulate your biological clock. If you are experiencing moodiness or depression during winter, exposing yourself to sunlight (by going south for a holiday) or artificial light will help get you back on track.

When you have to sleep during the day, reduce as much of the light coming into your room as possible. Use dark blinds for your windows, or sleep in a room without windows.

To help you wake up, use a bright lamp with a timer. Set the timer to go off about half an hour before you need to wake up. The light from the lamp will help you wake up by stimulating your body, and is more effective than waking up to the blare of a radio. This should help trick your body into resetting its awake–sleep cycle so you can better cope with changing shifts.

Relaxation Techniques

Meditation and other relaxation techniques (see chapter 13) help combat high blood pressure, asthma, high cholesterol, sleep disturbances, irritability, and muscle jumpiness (Penn & Bootzin, 1990).

It is also important for shift workers to leave work at work. All too often, an officer takes unresolved issues home.

Add a relaxing bath to your routine. Going from a warm (not hot) bath to a cool room will cause you to release heat, lowering your internal body temperature, which is a key step in inducing sleep.

Have a cup of hot milk. Milk contains tryptophan, a protein that helps promote sleep. Milk's carbohydrate mix also helps settle your stomach. It is important not to have your stomach overfull or empty so you can get to sleep.

Using Your Circadian Rhythm to Your Advantage

Shift workers need to monitor their body temperature. When body temperature is rising, the time is ripe for complicated thinking; routine tasks and paperwork are best done when body temperature is falling.

Body temperature passes through two cycles a day. From about 3 a.m. to 6 a.m. there is a trough, or low point. Body temperature rises from 8 a.m. to 10 a.m., when it reaches a peak. After that it falls until reaching a trough around 2 p.m. to 4 p.m., followed by a steady rise until reaching another peak between 7 p.m. and 9 p.m. If you can determine your peaks and troughs, you may be able to cope better with shift work. Do highly skilled tasks when your body temperature reaches its peak and menial tasks when it is in its trough.

Ways to help you stay alert include exercise, walking outside in the cold air, putting on a bright light, splashing your face with cold water, having an interesting conversation, and singing.

Physical Activity

Increase your physical activity to increase energy, alertness, balance, appetite, and stamina, and to facilitate sleeping. Beware of prolonged or high-exertion exercise, which can actually increase fatigue. You should engage in physical activity at least three times a week.

For those working afternoon shifts, it may be effective to work out at the end of the shift, when you are still keyed up. Make sure that you have a warm (not hot) shower and a light meal to help relax you when you are done working out.

Most graveyard shift workers find it extremely difficult to work out in the morning. A more appropriate time for them is the evening, before beginning a shift, or if the employer allows it, during a lunch period. The only difficulty with an early evening workout is that it can interfere with family time, including meals and children's activities.

Power Napping

Learn to nap effectively. The goal is a nap of 10 to 20 minutes at least 8 hours before going to bed (any longer can make you more tired and interfere with REM sleep).

Coping with Noise During Sleep Time

Moderate levels of noise sustain arousal and partially counter the effects of sleep loss. Too much noise, however, can be counterproductive. Ways to reduce noise during the day include adding sound barriers to your bedroom and building a sleeping area in the basement that keeps you secluded from the rest of the family. An alternative is to create white noise. A fan can mask noises inside and outside the house and should help you fall asleep.

Sleeping Effectively

It is important to keep to a rigid sleep schedule. Keep noises to a minimum, make sure the bedroom is dark enough, ask others to respect your sleep time, and use your bedroom only for sleep and intimacy so that other things, such as television, do not distract you. If you have problems falling asleep after 20 minutes, get up and do something mundane so that you have a better chance of falling asleep when you try again. If you can't fall asleep in the morning, wait until early afternoon, when there's a natural energy dip.

Developing New Friendships

Cultivate friendships with other shift worker families for social enjoyment as well as for a support system to help you cope with the unique stresses of shift work.

Remember that shift work will become a part of your life. You will have to make an effort not to let its physical impact interfere with your quality of life. Be aware of what your body is telling you, and take care of your body.

Turn to **assignment 14.2** (in the appendix) to assess how you will cope with shift work.

MORE INFORMATION

For more information on sleep issues, including sleep disorders and treatments, try the following websites:

- National Sleep Foundation: http://www.sleepfoundation.org
- National Center on Sleep Disorders Research—National Heart, Lung and Blood Institute: http://www.nhlbi.nih.gov/about/ncsdr

KEY TERMS

REM sleep

circadian rhythm

narcolepsy

restless legs syndrome (RLS)

sleep apnea

EXERCISES

Review

1. List five negative physiological effects of shift work.

2. List some positive aspects of shift work.

3. How can shift work affect your social life?

4. List six ways to cope with shift work.

Multiple Choice

1. What amount of sleep do shift workers get compared with non-shift workers?
   a. the same
   b. more
   c. less
   d. none of the above

2. How does the most effective shift work rotate?
   a. from days to nights to afternoons
   b. from days to afternoons to nights
   c. from afternoons to days to nights
   d. from nights to afternoons to days
   e. from nights to days to afternoons

3. Which of the following happens during REM sleep?
   a. Your body repairs cells and boosts your immune system.
   b. You don't get a restful sleep.
   c. You recover from mental fatigue.
   d. You can easily wake up.
   e. Your brain waves become larger.

4. The long-term effects of shift work can include
   a. problems with sleep
   b. eating disorders
   c. cardiovascular disorders
   d. reproductive disorders
   e. all of the above

5. Circadian rhythm refers to
   a. your heartbeat
   b. your biological clock
   c. your reproductive clock
   d. a method of birth control
   e. the amount of blood flowing through your heart

6. The possible symptoms experienced by shift workers do *not* include
   a. temporary partial paralysis
   b. poor appetite
   c. peripheral hallucination
   d. difficulty speaking
   e. staying awake easily around sunrise

7. Coping strategies for shift work include
   a. eating healthy foods
   b. exercising before you go to sleep
   c. avoiding caffeine
   d. not drinking alcohol to fall asleep
   e. all of the above

8. To try to sleep during the day with other people around, avoid
   a. putting sound barriers around your bedroom to keep noise out
   b. using white noise to reduce sounds
   c. sleeping in the basement where kids are playing
   d. using relaxation techniques to fall asleep
   e. consuming coffee and chocolate before going to sleep

9. The hormone that helps you feel tired is
   a. serotonin
   b. melatonin
   c. tyroxine
   d. adenosine
   e. cryprochrome

10. Many people have a clear reduction in task performance around which time of day?
    a. midday
    b. early morning
    c. post-lunch
    d. late afternoon
    e. early evening

11. Which type of work is most disruptive in terms of causing harmful effects through major changes to the circadian rhythm?
    a. permanent night work
    b. slowly rotating shift work
    c. rapidly rotating shift work
    d. non-rotating shift work
    e. permanent day work

12. In which stage of sleep does REM sleep occur?
    a. stage 3
    b. stage 2
    c. stage 5
    d. stage 1
    e. stage 4

13. Under which condition is melatonin released, and what is the effect of the release of this hormone?
    a. Melatonin is released when light levels are high, making a person feel sleepy.
    b. Melatonin is released when light levels are high, making a person feel awake.
    c. Melatonin is released when light levels are low, making a person feel sleepy.
    d. Melatonin is released when light levels are low, making a person feel awake.
    e. Melatonin is released when a person wakes up, making a person feel sleepy.

REFERENCES

Allen, R.P., & Mitler, M.M. (2005). *Restless legs syndrome (RLS) symptoms.* National Sleep Foundation. Available at http://www.sleepfoundation.org/site/c.huIXKjM0IxF/b.2464461/apps/nl/content3.asp?content_id={D9527149-5CDA-4D77-882C-5FE9F30C3949}&notoc=1.

Bahrke, M. (1995). Police officers: Shift work solutions. *Muscle and Fitness Magazine.*

Brusgard, A. (1975). Shift work as an occupational health problem. *Studia Laoris et Salutis, 4,* 9-14.

Filipski, E. (2002). Host circadian clock as a control point in tumor progression. *Journal of the National Cancer Institute, 94*(9), 690-697.

Goldfarb, D., & Ausmiller, G. (1999). *Ten reasons cops are different.* Available at http://www.heavybadge.com/10reasons.htm.

Gysin, F., Gysin, F., & Gross, F. (1997). Winter depression and phototherapy: The state of the art. *Acta Médica Portugesa, 10*(12), 887-903.

Hayduk, R. (2005). *Overview of the diagnosis and treatment of narcolepsy.* National Sleep Foundation. Available at http://www.sleepfoundation.org/site/c.huIXKjM0IxF/b.2453615/apps/nl/content3.asp?content_id={772EA7E1-96F0-461A-9FFE-ADDBB148C544}&notoc=1.

Health Canada. (2007). *Eating well with Canada's Food Guide.* Ottawa: Supply and Services Canada. Available at http://www.hc-sc.gc.ca/fn-an/food-guide-aliment/index_e.html.

Leutwyler, K. (1995). Depression's double standard. Reprinted in Mysteries of the Mind, *Scientific American* (special publication), 53-54.

Nurmine, T. (1998). Shiftwork and reproductive health. *Scandinavian Journal of Work Environment, 24*(suppl. 3), 28-34.

O'Neil, P.S. (1986). Shiftwork. In J.T. Reese & H.A. Godstein (Eds.), *Psychological services for law enforcement* (pp. 471-475). Washington, DC: US Government Printing Office.

Penn, P.E., & Bootzin, R.R. (1990). Behavioural techniques for enhancing alertness and performance in shift work. *Work and Stress, 4,* 213-226.

Phillips, B. (2005). *Sleep apnea basics.* National Sleep Foundation. Available at http://www.sleepfoundation.org/site/c.huIXKjM0IxF/b.2418929/k.89A5/Sleep_Apnea.htm.

Smith, C.S., Robie, C., Folkard, S., Barton, J., Spelten, E., Totterdell, P., Smith, L., & Costa, G. (1998). *The effects of shiftwork on health in the older worker.* APA-NIOSH Work Stress and Health 99 Organization Work in a Global Economy. Available at http://www.apa.org/pi/wpo/niosh/abstract12.html.

Smolensky, M.H., & Reinberg, A. (1990). Clinical chronobiology: Relevance and applications to the practice of occupational medicine. *Occupational Medicine, 5*(2), 273-299.

Tasto, D., & Colligan, M. (1978). *Health consequences of shift work.* Department of Health, Education, and Welfare (NIOSH) Publication 78–154. Washington, DC: US Government Printing Office.

Vila, B. (2000). *Tired cops: The importance of managing police fatigue.* Washington, DC: Police Executive Research Forum.

Wedderburn, A.A.I., & King, C. (1996). Shiftworker's health: Evaluation of a self-help guidebook. *The shiftworker's guide.* Edinburgh: Heriot-Watt University.

Wienecke, A. (1999). *The role of the police subculture in the police suicide epidemic.* Available at http://www.work-warrior.net/policesuicide.html.

CHAPTER 15

Common Injuries

CHAPTER OBJECTIVES

After completing this chapter, you should be able to:

- Describe delayed-onset muscle soreness (DOMS) and common sport-related injuries.
- Explain the causes and the signs and symptoms of injuries.
- Describe the treatments that are available for injuries.
- Understand the risks associated with heat- and cold-related injuries.
- Explain the signs and symptoms of heat- and cold-related injuries.
- Describe treatments for heat- and cold-related injuries.

Exercise-related injuries can be painful and frustrating. They always seem to happen when we're the most motivated to participate in an exercise program. It's no secret why this happens—people who have not exercised for a long time try to push their body past a safe level in an attempt to get back what they had. Many people try to achieve their training goals in too short a period of time. Some people have left training for the PARE test to just weeks prior to the scheduled test. Overtraining has resulted in many injuries. This chapter will look at various injuries, their causes, and treatments for them.

GENERAL TREATMENTS FOR INJURIES

Many sport injuries are the result of too much too soon. By overdoing it, you increase your risk for sprained joints, strained muscles, and other minor injuries. One important but simple way to decrease your risk of injury is to make sure that you properly warm up before exercising or doing sports and cool down after. A good warm-up consists of performing your regular activity at a lesser intensity. Refer to chapter 7, "Flexibility and Stretching," for more information. Remember that there is a difference between feeling uncomfortable because you are out of shape and being in pain. Don't believe that "no pain, no gain" is true. Trying to exercise through pain will likely just create an injury or make an existing injury worse.

General treatment for an injury involves backing off. Proper care during the first day or two after the injury may reduce the time it takes to heal. Remember that even though something may hurt only slightly while you are exercising, it may get worse when you stop. Endorphins, a chemical released by the brain during exercise, tend to dull the sensation of pain. After an injury occurs, the damaged area may bleed (internally or externally) and become inflamed. Healing starts as collagen, the primary component of scar tissue, replaces the damaged tissue. In order for an individual to return to the activity, ideally, the scar tissue should be completely repaired. In the case of acute injuries, follow the RICE principle when you are injured.

The RICE Principle

The RICE principle (rest, ice, compression, and elevation) is immediate, simple treatment for an injury. You can ease pain and assist the healing process if you act quickly. If you are unsure of the extent of your injury, keep the affected part of your body immobilized, follow the RICE principle, and seek medical help as soon as possible.

REST

Reduce regular exercise or daily activities as needed. Rest is important to protect the injured muscle, tendon, ligament, or other tissue from further damage. Rest is also important in order to conserve the energy needed to heal the injury most effectively. Depending on the severity of the injury, do not put any weight on an injured area for 48 hours. If you cannot put weight on an ankle or knee, crutches may help.

ICE

To reduce swelling, apply an ice pack (a plastic bag of ice or a bag of frozen peas wrapped in a towel) to the injured area for 20 minutes at a time, four to eight times a day. Never put ice directly on the tissue, as it may damage your skin.

COMPRESSION

Compression of an injured ankle, knee, or wrist may help reduce swelling. You might use elastic wraps, compression bandages, special boots, air casts, and splints. Ask your doctor for advice on which one to use.

ELEVATION

If possible, keep the injured part elevated on a pillow, above the level of your heart, to help decrease swelling.

SORTING OUT MUSCLE SORENESS

delayed-onset muscle soreness (DOMS) soreness of muscles 12 hours or more after exercise

Aside from the pain of muscle injuries such as strains, there are two common kinds of exercise-related muscle soreness: acute soreness, which occurs during or immediately after exercise, and **delayed-onset muscle soreness (DOMS)**, which develops 12 hours or more after exercise.

Acute muscle soreness during and immediately after exercise usually reflects simple fatigue caused by a buildup of chemical waste products (lactic acid and hydrogen ions). The discomfort will often subside after a minute or two of rest when the muscles can replace energy substrates and oxygen. Once the soreness goes away, you can usually continue exercising with no residual effects. If discomfort persists despite a rest period, stop your activity and rest the part of the body that is hurting. Don't proceed with your workout until you're able to exercise that area without pain.

DOMS after a workout is common, particularly if you aren't used to the activity. If, for example, you haven't exercised for six months, and then you suddenly jump on the treadmill for 5 km and do some push-ups and sit-ups, you may feel soreness throughout much of your body the next morning. You may also notice muscle stiffness and weakness. Such symptoms are a normal response to unusual exertion and are part of an adaptation process that leads to greater strength once the muscles recover. The soreness is generally at its worst in the first two days following the activity and subsides over the next few days.

DOMS is thought to be a result of microscopic tearing of the muscle fibres. The amount of tearing depends on how hard and long you exercise and what type of exercise you do. For example, exercises in which muscles forcefully contract while they are lengthening tend to cause the most soreness. These eccentric contractions (explained in chapter 6) provide a braking action. Examples include running down stairs, running downhill, lowering weights, and performing the downward movements of squats, chin-ups, and push-ups.

In addition to microscopic tearing, swelling may take place in and around a muscle, which can contribute to delayed soreness. Such swelling increases pressure on the neighbouring structures, resulting in greater muscle pain and stiffness.

Preventing and Treating DOMS

Try these tips to prevent and treat DOMS:

- Warm up and stretch the muscles that you will be using and do a few minutes of a light, low-impact aerobic activity such as walking or biking. This should help to increase blood flow to the affected muscles and help to reduce soreness.
- Build up slowly in terms of intensity, duration, and frequency of the exercise. In weight lifting, for example, start with lighter weights, fewer sets, and fewer repetitions.
- Avoid the weekend warrior approach, where you only play a pickup game of football or basketball without some type of aerobic activity during the week.
- Applying ice, gently stretching, and massaging the affected muscles can help.
- Non-steroidal anti-inflammatory medications may reduce the soreness temporarily, but they won't speed healing.
- Try yoga. There is some evidence that yoga may reduce DOMS (Boyle et al., 2004).
- Rest. Let your muscles heal before you attempt to go back to the activity.

COMMON SPORT-RELATED INJURIES

Sprain

sprain
an injury to a ligament—a stretching or tearing

A **sprain** is an injury to a ligament—a stretching or tearing. The severity of the injury depends on the extent of injury to a single ligament (whether the tear is partial or complete) and the number of ligaments involved. A sprain can result from a fall, a sudden twist, or a blow to the body that forces a joint out of its normal position. This results in overstretching or tearing of the ligament supporting that joint. Typically, sprains occur when people fall and land on an outstretched arm, slide into base, land on the side of their foot, or twist a knee with the foot planted firmly on the ground when involved in an altercation with a suspect. The three most common sites of sprains are ankles, knees, and wrists.

There are three levels of sprains:

- *Mild sprains* happen when ligaments are stretched excessively or torn slightly. They are somewhat painful, especially with movement. There is not a lot of swelling and you can put weight on the joint.
- *Moderate sprains* occur when there is partial rupture of the fibres. The area is painful and tender. There is swelling and discolouration, and it is hard to move and bear weight on the joint.
- *Severe sprains* take place when one or more ligaments are torn. You can't put weight on the joint or move it easily. There is swelling, discolouration, and pain. It is hard to distinguish a severe sprain from a fracture or dislocation. You may need a brace to stabilize the joint, and surgery may be required to repair the ligaments.

SIGNS AND SYMPTOMS OF A SPRAIN

The usual signs and symptoms of a sprain include the following:

- varying degrees of pain
- swelling
- bruising
- inability to move and use the joint

Sometimes people feel a pop or tear when the sprain happens. An X-ray may be needed to determine whether a fracture is causing the pain and swelling.

Strain

strain
an injury to a muscle or tendon—a twisting or pulling

Twisting or pulling a muscle or tendon causes a **strain**. Strains can be acute or chronic. An acute strain is caused by trauma or an injury such as a blow to the body; improperly lifting heavy objects or overstressing the muscles can also cause it. Chronic strains are usually the result of overuse—prolonged, repetitive movement of the muscles and tendons.

The two most common sites for a strain are the back and the hamstring muscle (located in the back of the thigh). Law enforcement officers risk injury when they go from prolonged sitting in a cruiser and then are faced with a physical confrontation or other demand on their body. Contact sports such as soccer, football, hockey, boxing, and wrestling put people at risk for strains. Gymnastics, tennis, rowing, golf, and other sports that require extensive gripping can increase the risk of hand and forearm strains. Elbow strains sometimes occur in people who participate in racquet sports, throwing, and contact sports.

SIGNS AND SYMPTOMS OF A STRAIN

Signs and symptoms of a strain include the following:

- pain, muscle spasm, and muscle weakness
- localized swelling, cramping, or inflammation and, with a minor or moderate strain, usually some loss of muscle function
- pain in the injured area and general weakness of the muscle when you try to move it
- in the case of severe strains that partially or completely tear the muscle or tendon, extreme pain due to significant bleeding, swelling, and bruising around the muscle
- a complete lack of muscle function, if the muscle has been torn away completely from the bone

Treatment for Sprains and Strains

You should see a doctor about a sprain or strain if you have severe pain, you cannot move the joint, it is tender to touch, there are lumps and bumps (other than swelling), you are experiencing numbness, and you cannot put any weight on the injured joint. You may see redness or red streaks spreading out from the injury.

Treatment for sprains and strains is similar and can be thought of as having two stages. The goal during the first stage is to reduce swelling and pain. At this stage, doctors usually advise patients to follow the RICE formula (rest, ice, compression, and elevation) for the first 24–48 hours after the injury. A doctor may prescribe a non-steroidal anti-inflammatory drug, such as acetylsalicylic acid (Aspirin) or ibuprofen, to help decrease pain and inflammation.

For people with a moderate or severe sprain, particularly of the ankle, a hard cast may be applied. Severe sprains and strains may require surgery to repair the torn ligaments, muscle, or tendons.

The second stage of treating a sprain or strain is rehabilitation, whose overall goal is to improve the condition of the injured part and restore its function. An exercise program designed to prevent stiffness, improve range of motion, and restore the joint's normal flexibility and strength is key. Some people may need physical therapy during this stage.

Tendinitis, Impingement Syndrome, and Bursitis of the Shoulder

These conditions are closely related and may occur alone or in combination. Repeated motion involving the arms, or the aging process, may irritate and wear down the tendons, muscles, and surrounding structures.

tendinitis
inflammation of a tendon

impingement syndrome
squeezing of the rotator cuff (the group of muscles that surrounds the shoulder)

bursitis
inflammation of a bursa (a sac of fluid near a joint)

Tendinitis is inflammation (redness, soreness, and swelling) of a tendon. In tendinitis of the shoulder, the rotator cuff (the group of muscles that surround the shoulder) and/or biceps tendon become inflamed, usually as a result of being pinched by surrounding structures. The injury may vary from mild to severe inflammation. When the rotator cuff tendon becomes inflamed and thickened, it may get trapped under the outer edge of the shoulder blade, where the collarbone is attached. Squeezing of the rotator cuff is called **impingement syndrome.**

Tendinitis and impingement syndrome are often accompanied by inflammation of the bursa sacs (sacs of fluid near joints) that protect the shoulder. An inflamed bursa is called **bursitis**. Inflammation caused by a disease such as rheumatoid arthritis may cause rotator cuff tendinitis and bursitis. Sports that involve overuse of the shoulder and occupations that require frequent overhead reaching are other potential causes of irritation to the rotator cuff or bursa and may lead to inflammation and impingement.

SIGNS AND SYMPTOMS

Signs and symptoms of tendinitis, impingement syndrome, and bursitis of the shoulder include the following:

- the slow onset of discomfort and pain in the upper shoulder or upper third of the arm
- difficulty sleeping on the shoulder
- pain when the arm is lifted away from the body or overhead
- if tendinitis involves the biceps tendon (the tendon located in front of the shoulder that helps bend the elbow and turn the forearm), pain in the front or side of the shoulder that may travel down to the elbow and forearm (pain may also occur when the arm is forcefully pushed upward)

TREATMENT

These injuries are treated with rest, ice, and anti-inflammatory medicines. In some cases, the doctor or therapist will use ultrasound (gentle sound wave vibrations) to warm deep tissues and improve blood flow. Gentle stretching and strengthening exercises are added gradually, preceded or followed by use of an ice pack. If there is no improvement, the doctor may inject a corticosteroid medicine into the space under the acromion (these injections must be used with caution because they may lead to tendon rupture). Severe cases may need surgery to repair damage and relieve pressure on the tendons and bursae.

Dislocated Shoulder

As shown in figure 15.1, the shoulder comprises a large number of muscles, tendons, and bones that work together to provide movement, structure, and strength. Fifteen muscles move and stabilize the scapula. Nine muscles stabilize the gleno-humeral joint, and six muscles support the scapula on the thorax. The rotator cuff is made up of a group of four muscles (supraspinatus, infraspinatus, teres minor, and subscapularis) that support the shoulder joint. The muscles attach to the skeletal elements by tendons. The rotator cuff stabilizes the gleno-humeral joint to provide rotation, elevation, depression, protraction, and retraction.

A dislocation of the shoulder joint happens when the ball of the joint (the end of the arm bone, or humerus) and the socket (part of your shoulder blade, or scapula) making up the shoulder move apart. When the ball part of the joint is dislocated in front of the socket, it is called an anterior dislocation, the most common type. When it is dislocated behind the socket, it is called a posterior dislocation. In severe cases, ligaments, tendons, and nerves also can be stretched and injured.

An anterior dislocation can be caused by a fall onto your outstretched hand or onto the shoulder itself. A posterior dislocation may occur as a result of a powerful direct blow to the front of your shoulder. A violent twisting of your upper arm, such as that caused by an electric shock or seizure, may also cause it. Dislocated shoulders are common in contact sports such as football, rugby, hockey, and lacrosse. Other sports that may cause the injury include downhill skiing, volleyball, and soccer. In law enforcement, officers sometimes deal with altercations where someone is pulling at their arms or aggressively pushing or punching.

FIGURE 15.1 Shoulder Joint

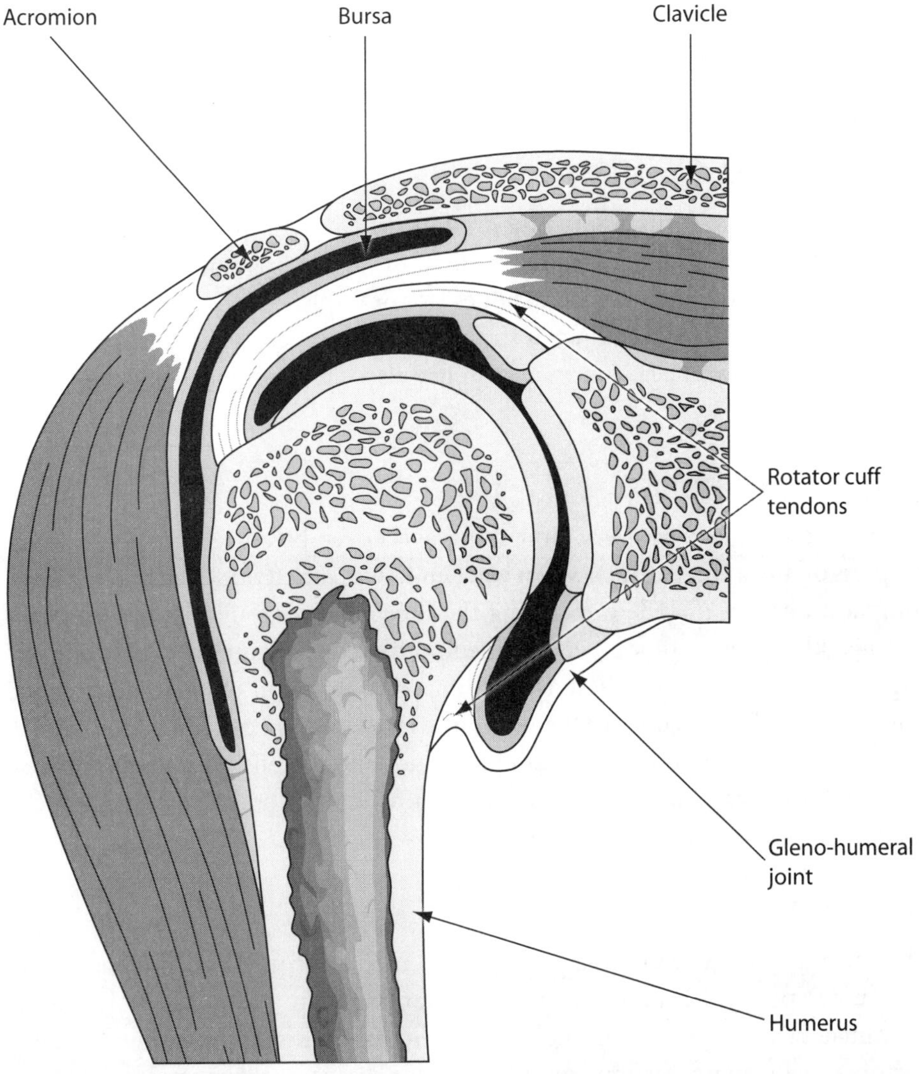

The shoulder joint is the most frequently dislocated joint of the body. It occurs when an impact or force moves the shoulder outward (abduction) or forces extreme rotation of the head of the humerus, causing it to pop out of the socket.

SIGNS AND SYMPTOMS

Signs and symptoms of a dislocated shoulder include the following:

- pain in your shoulder and upper arm that is made worse by movement
- shoulder instability and deformation
- shoulder tenderness and weakness
- possible numbness in the shoulder area, arm, or hand

TREATMENT

Put ice on the shoulder immediately to reduce swelling caused by internal bleeding and the buildup of fluids in and around the injured area, and put the arm in a sling. See a doctor to reposition the head or ball of the joint back in the joint socket. The doctor may give you a prescription for pain, a muscle-relaxant, and anti-inflammatory medication. If your shoulder joint becomes weak because of repeated dislocations, your doctor may recommend an operation to tighten the ligaments that hold the joint together. The healing process may take 4–12 weeks, depending on the extent of your injury. With proper healing and rehabilitation exercise, you should regain full movement of your shoulder.

Broken Ribs

A broken or fractured rib is a common injury when there is trauma to the chest, such as from a fall, a motor vehicle accident, or an impact during an altercation with an individual. Those with weak bones (for example, osteoporosis) have greater risk of ribs breaking when there is strain on the rib cage, such as during a strong coughing spell. As you age, your risk of injury also increases due to lessening elasticity of the ribs.

SIGNS AND SYMPTOMS

When ribs are broken, it is very difficult to take a deep breath. Pain is worse when you press on the injured area or when you bend, twist, or attempt physical exertion. Complications can include puncturing the lungs and surrounding tissue, which can cause blood (hemothorax) or air (pneumothorax) to accumulate between your lungs and the walls of your chest. Depending on the amount of blood or air in the pleural cavity (the closed space that surrounds the lungs), a collapsed lung can result, leading to respiratory and hemodynamic failure (tension pneumothorax). Treatment involves stopping the bleeding, removing the blood and air in the pleural space, and re-expanding the lung.

TREATMENT

It is very important to rest broken ribs, and to use ice for pain and swelling. Over-the-counter pain medication, including acetaminophen and non-steroidal anti-inflammatory drugs such as ibuprofen, can help relieve discomfort while ribs heal. Doctors usually do not recommend compression wraps, as they increase the likelihood of respiratory complications (such as pneumonia). It can take upwards of two months for ribs to heal.

Patello-Femoral Syndrome (Chondromalacia)

Patello-femoral syndrome, or chondromalacia (KON-dro-mah-LAY-she-ah, the old term), refers to softening of the kneecap cartilage. This disorder occurs most often in young adults, especially females, and can be caused by injury, overuse, parts out of alignment, or muscle weakness in the inner thigh. Instead of gliding smoothly across the lower end of the thigh bone, the kneecap rubs against it, roughening the cartilage underneath the kneecap. The damage may range from a slightly abnormal surface of the cartilage to a surface that has been worn away to the bone. It is the result of muscle tightness in the calf, hamstring, or other muscles. The disorder is common in runners and is also seen in skiers, cyclists, and soccer players.

SIGNS AND SYMPTOMS

Signs and symptoms of patello-femoral syndrome include the following:

- dull pain around or under the kneecap that worsens when walking down stairs or hills
- pain when climbing stairs or when the knee bears weight as it straightens
- grinding and clicking in the knee

TREATMENT

Apply the RICE formula (rest, ice, compression, and elevation). Perform low-impact exercises that strengthen muscles, particularly the muscles in the inner part of the quadriceps, without injuring joints and as long as the knee doesn't bend more than 90°. Tape the knee to keep the kneecap in line. Electrical stimulation may also be used to strengthen the muscles. Arthroscopic surgery may be used to smooth the surface of the cartilage and "wash out" the cartilage fragments that cause the joint to catch during bending and straightening. In more severe cases, more invasive surgery may be necessary to correct the angle of the kneecap and relieve friction with the cartilage or to reposition parts that are out of alignment.

Shin Splints

Shin splints are pain along the shin (tibia) and are commonly seen as an overuse injury in runners. They usually develop gradually over a period of weeks to months, but may occur after a single excessive bout of exercise.

Shin splints can be caused by running on the insides of your feet. Shin splints often occur in both legs. This usually happens when someone is beginning a running program, doing excessive downhill running, and engaging in sports that require rapid starts and stops, which cause damage to the muscle, resulting in pain.

SIGNS AND SYMPTOMS

Signs and symptoms of shin splints include the following:

- pain on the side of the shin and the back of the calf (often experienced by runners)
- noticeable pain when exercise starts, which then decreases or goes away as exercise continues; worse after exercise stops or the following morning

TREATMENT

Rest. This means dramatically decreasing both the frequency and the duration of exercise and increasing (doubling or tripling) the time between workouts. Put ice directly on the sore area. Massage the muscles that are affected. A doctor may prescribe anti-inflammatory medications. If the shin splints are caused by the way your feet turn in when you walk or run, you may need a good arch support in the form of an orthotic (a shoe insert that corrects the alignment of the foot). Changing your running shoes every 800 km is another good idea.

Plantar Fasciitis

Plantar fasciitis is the most common cause of pain on the bottom of the heel. The fascia, a thin strip of tissue at the bottom of the foot, stretches to the point of developing small tears. Pain occurs with the onset of activity such as walking and running or even the first few morning steps. The pain subsides as the activity progresses, and usually returns after resting and then resuming activity.

Plantar fasciitis is considered a chronic inflammatory response. It is common in runners, who repetitively flex their feet and toes. It is also common in people who experience sudden weight gain. Shoes with poor cushioning can also contribute to the tearing of the fascia. People who work in occupations that require prolonged standing or weight-bearing activities may also strain the fascia. The leather boots that officers used to wear had no cushion or arch support, which led to this injury.

SIGNS AND SYMPTOMS

Signs and symptoms of plantar fasciitis include the following:

- heel pain that is at its worst during the first steps of the morning
- pain at the start of exercise and when exercise is resumed after resting
- tight Achilles tendon
- sometimes a heel spur, but it is typically not a cause

TREATMENT

Take non-steroidal anti-inflammatory drugs (ask a doctor). Avoid activities that cause pain and avoid walking barefoot on hard surfaces. Lose weight if your weight is a cause of the injury. Stretch the heel cord (Achilles tendon) and plantar fascia. Taping the heel and arch may also help to reduce pain. You may need to wear arch supports if you have flat feet. Massaging the fascia by rolling your foot over a 7–10-cm diameter tube, such as a rolling pin or soup can, has been an effective treatment. Strengthening exercises include scrunching up a hand towel with the toes or pulling a towel weighted with a soup can across the floor. After any physical activity, put ice on the fascia. Buy proper footwear with arch support.

Osgood-Schlatter Disease

Osgood-Schlatter disease is caused by repetitive stress or tension on part of the growth area of the upper tibia (the leg bone between the knee and the ankle). As a result there is inflammation of the tendon in the kneecap and surrounding soft tissues at the point where the tendon is attached to the tibia. The disease may also be associated with an injury in which the tendon is stretched so much that it tears away from the tibia and takes a fragment of bone with it. The body then repairs the bone by depositing calcium, which results in a buildup of bone.

SIGNS AND SYMPTOMS

Signs and symptoms of Osgood-Schlatter disease include the following:

- Pain is experienced just below the knee joint; the pain usually worsens with activity and is relieved by rest.
- A bony bump that is particularly painful when pressed may appear on the upper edge of the tibia, below the kneecap. Although knee motion is usually not affected, it can be very difficult to kneel or sit on your knees.
- Pain may last a few months and may recur until the individual's growth is completed. Teens are especially prone to the pain, which can carry on into their 20s.
- X-rays show that the growth area is in fragments.

TREATMENT

When pain begins, apply ice to the knee to help relieve inflammation. Do stretching and strengthening exercises, and limit your participation in vigorous sports. Wear knee pads for protection when you are taking part in sports, and apply ice to the knee afterward.

Iliotibial Band Syndrome

Iliotibial band syndrome is an overuse condition in which inflammation results when a band of a tendon rubs over the outer bone of the knee. Although iliotibial band syndrome may be caused by direct injury to the knee, it is most often caused by the stress of long-term overuse, such as sometimes occurs in sports training.

SIGNS AND SYMPTOMS

Signs and symptoms of iliotibial band syndrome include the following:

- ache or burning sensation at the outer side of the knee during activity
- pain at the side of the knee or radiating up the side of the thigh
- a snap felt when the knee is bent and then straightened

Note that there is usually no swelling and knee motion is normal.

TREATMENT

Reduce activity and do stretching exercises followed by muscle-strengthening exercises. In rare cases, when the syndrome doesn't disappear, surgery may be necessary to split the tendon so that it isn't stretched too tightly over the bone.

Ligament Injuries of the Knee

Four ligaments connect the leg bones and give the knee joint strength and stability:

1. the medial collateral ligament (MCL), which provides stability to the inner (medial) part of the knee
2. the lateral collateral ligament (LCL), which provides stability to the outer (lateral) part of the knee
3. the anterior cruciate ligament (ACL), in the centre of the knee, which limits rotation and the forward movement of the tibia (the shin bone)
4. the posterior cruciate ligament (PCL), also in the centre of the knee, which limits backward movement of the tibia

The ACL is most often stretched or torn or both (that is, sprained) by a sudden twisting motion (for example, when the feet are planted one way and the knees are turned another). This can happen when you stretch your upper torso while keeping your legs planted, such as when a law enforcement officer must drag someone out of a car. The PCL is most often injured by a direct impact, such as in an automobile accident (trying to brake) or a football tackle. The MCL is more easily injured than the LCL. The cause is most often a blow to the outer side of the knee that stretches and tears the ligament on the inner side of the knee. Such blows frequently occur in contact sports like football or hockey. In law enforcement, they can occur during altercations or when performing self-defence manoeuvres.

SIGNS AND SYMPTOMS

Signs and symptoms of ligament injuries of the knee include the following:

- a popping sound
- swelling
- leg buckling when you try to stand
- top part of leg moves while lower leg remains stationary

Note that there may or may not be pain, depending on which ligament is injured.

TREATMENT

Immediate treatment includes the RICE approach. If there is an incomplete tear, an exercise program can strengthen the surrounding muscles. You may need to wear a brace to protect the knee during activity. You may also need surgery to reattach or reconstruct a ligament that is completely torn.

Injuries to the Meniscus

Separating the bones of the knee are pads of connective tissue called the menisci (muh-NISS-sky), or meniscus (muh-NISS-kus) in the singular. The menisci are divided into two crescent-shaped discs positioned between the leg bones on the outer and inner sides of each knee. They act like shock absorbers, cushioning the lower part of the leg from the weight of the rest of the body, as well as enhancing stability.

(The removal of all four of former hockey player Bobby Orr's menisci, one at a time, left his knees unstable, which eventually led to his retirement from hockey.)

Through degeneration over time or too much concentrated force, the meniscus can be torn, as shown in figure 15.2. The entire rim of the medial meniscus can be torn. Symptoms include pain along the joint line and locking of the leg as it is extended and pulled back. In essence, the knee locks so that it cannot be straightened or fully bent. Swelling occurs as synovial fluid (fluid the body sends as part of a immune response) rushes to the area in response to the deterioration on the surface.

FIGURE15.2 Injuries to the Meniscus

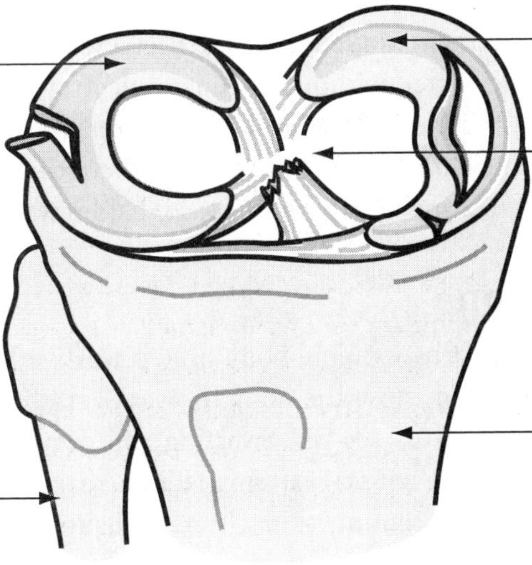

SIGNS AND SYMPTOMS

Signs and symptoms of injuries to the meniscus include the following:

- There may be some pain, particularly when the knee is straightened. If the pain is mild, the person may continue moving. Severe pain may occur if a fragment of the meniscus catches between the leg bones.
- Swelling may occur soon after injury if blood vessels are disrupted, or swelling may occur several hours later if the joint fills with fluid produced by the joint lining as a result of inflammation.
- The knee may click, lock, or feel weak, and pain is persistent.
- On examination, when the leg is rotated outward and inward while extended, there is pain and audible clicking, suggesting a tear. An MRI scan can confirm this.

TREATMENT

Immediate treatment includes the RICE approach for sprains. Muscle-strengthening programs for the knee (quadriceps and hamstrings) can help. Surgery may be needed to repair the tear if there is good blood supply to the area. If the blood supply is poor, parts of or the entire meniscus may need to be removed. Artificial meniscus replacement has met with limited success to date.

HEAT-RELATED INJURIES AND ILLNESSES

Heat-related injuries have become a huge issue in athletics. In the past few summers, a number of athletes have died due to heat-related injuries. You need to be aware of the symptoms. If you do volunteer work with children's sports teams, be especially vigilant, because children's body temperatures easily fluctuate and they can quickly suffer from heat-related injuries.

Heat Cramps

heat cramps
illness caused by a water and sodium deficiency; heat cramps feel like severe muscle pulls

Heat cramps are caused by a deficiency of water and sodium and feel like severe muscle pulls. They occur in worked muscles after exertion, often after profuse sweating and drinking water without adequate electrolyte replacement. Heat cramps cause painful muscle contractions (for example, in the hamstring area). They are usually not life-threatening, but ignoring them can lead to more serious heat-related illnesses. Treatment for heat cramps includes water, cool air, and rest.

Heat Exhaustion

heat exhaustion
illness caused by extreme body heat; excessive heat and dehydration can raise body temperature to 38–40 °C (100–104 °F)

Heat exhaustion is caused by extreme body heat. Excessive heat (a hot environment) and dehydration can cause the body to overreact, thus raising your body temperature to 38–40 °C (102–104 °F). Sweating still occurs. Symptoms of heat exhaustion include paleness, nausea, extreme fatigue, dizziness, light-headedness, vomiting, fainting, and cool, clammy skin. Heat exhaustion is a serious illness and should be carefully monitored.

Treatment includes cool, shady environments; liquids; cool rags or ice packs placed on various areas of the body; and replacement of electrolytes (such as those found in sports drinks). Make sure there is good ventilation. If body temperature remains elevated after treatment or the person is continually vomiting, seek medical treatment.

When body weight drops 1–2 percent (0.7–1.4 kg in a 70-kg person), exercise performance can be impaired and heat exhaustion becomes a possibility.

Heat Stroke

heat stroke
illness caused by failure of the body's heat-regulating mechanism; may lead to permanent disability or death

Heat stroke, the most severe form of heat-related illness, occurs when the body's heat-regulating mechanism fails. Body temperature may be above 40 °C (104 °F) with warm dry skin. The very high body temperature damages tissues, including muscle and brain tissue. Heat stroke may lead to permanent disability or death, and is therefore a medical emergency. Unlike other forms of heat illness, heat stroke does not have to be caused by exercise or exertion. High temperatures, lack of body fluids, and overexposure to the elements can all bring about heat stroke. Very young and very old people are particularly susceptible to the hazards of this illness, especially those playing sports. Symptoms include a red, flushed face; a body temperature of 40 °C (104 °F) or higher; headache; rapid pulse; and unconsciousness.

Anyone exhibiting the signs and symptoms of heat stroke should be rushed to the nearest hospital or clinic. Treat the person with water, cool down his or her body by ventilating the area (fan or windows down in car), and take tight clothing and any hat off the person en route to medical treatment. The person may need fluids pumped into his or her body for rehydration.

Recognizing Dehydration in Individuals

There are signs and symptoms of dehydration that you can watch for. If you identify the condition early enough, you can limit the degree of heat-related illness. Early signs and symptoms include thirst, general discomfort, and irritability, followed by flushed skin, weariness, cramps, and apathy. Greater water deficits result in dizziness, headaches, vomiting, nausea, heat sensations on the head or neck, and decreased performance; dyspnea (difficult or laboured breathing) may also be present (American College of Sports Medicine, 1996; Armstrong & Maresh, 1993).

Preventing Heat-Related Injuries

Sweating is your body's main system for getting rid of extra heat. When you sweat, water evaporates from your skin. The heat that evaporates the sweat comes mainly from your skin. As long as blood is flowing properly to your skin, extra heat from the core of your body is "pumped" to the surface and removed by sweat evaporation. If you do not have good blood flow or do not sweat enough, you cannot get rid of extra heat well. If you are dehydrated, you won't sweat as much, and your body will try to keep blood away from the skin to keep your blood pressure at the right level in the core of your body (your other organs get the needed fluid first). Since you lose water when you sweat, you must make up that water to keep from becoming dehydrated. If the air is humid, it's harder for your sweat to evaporate. This means that your body cannot get rid of extra heat as well when it's muggy out as it can when the air is relatively dry. This is an issue in southern Ontario, with our very humid summers. Here are some ways to prevent heat injuries and illnesses:

- Drink. Staying hydrated is key. Sport drinks are a good choice, but water works fine. As you become heat-acclimatized, you will sweat more, so you'll need more fluids. Two to three hours before exercising, you should drink 500–600 mL of fluid, with another 200–300 mL 10–20 minutes before the event. You should be drinking 200–300 mL every 10–15 minutes during the event. Post-exercise hydration, or rehydration, should aim to correct any fluid loss accumulated during the practice or event. Ideally completed within two hours, rehydration should contain water to restore hydration status, carbohydrates to replenish glycogen stores, and electrolytes to speed rehydration. The primary goal is the immediate return of physiologic function. When rehydration must be quick, you need to replace sweat and urine losses incurred by drinking 25–50 percent more than what was lost to sweat. That means upwards of 500 mL for every half kilogram of weight loss within two hours of finishing training or competition to be at optimal hydration four to six hours after the event (Casa et al., 2000).

- Keep ventilation going (fan, air conditioner, etc.).
- Wear light-coloured, loose-fitting clothing (an issue with sports like football).
- Wear a hat outdoors.
- Limit your activity in hot, humid conditions.

COLD-RELATED INJURIES AND ILLNESSES

hypothermia
condition occurring when the body's control mechanism can no longer maintain a normal body temperature, and the body's temperature drops to an abormally low level

Under most conditions, your body is able to maintain a healthy temperature. But when you are exposed to a cold environment, if you are not dressed appropriately, more heat can escape from your body than you can produce. When the body's control mechanism can no longer maintain normal body temperature, **hypothermia** can set in. Prolonged exposure in cases such as directing traffic in January, overseeing an accident on the highway, or tracking a lost skier may lead to deadly results. Hypothermia can also happen on cool days when it is wet and windy outside and evaporation from your skin helps to drop your core temperature.

Who Is at Risk?

Hypothermia usually comes on gradually. At first, your body shivers (muscles contract) in an attempt to generate heat. Then, as your nervous system is affected, you begin to mumble, fumble, grumble, and stumble. You may lose consciousness and experience loss of fine motor coordination. Additional signs and symptoms include slurred speech, slowed breathing, cold, pale skin, and fatigue that is accompanied by lethargy or apathy. If not dealt with, severe hypothermia can lead to cardiac and respiratory failure and, ultimately, death.

In addition, people who have spent prolonged periods of time in cold environments or cool, wet, and windy environments, those who are of an advanced or very young age, those who are substance abusers, those with impaired mental status, and those who have been immersed in cold water are at increased risk for hypothermia.

One-sixth of Ontario's terrain is covered with lakes, rivers, and streams (Encyclopedia of Canadian Provinces, 2007). Many officers are called upon to assist and rescue individuals who have fallen into the water. Immersion in cold water numbs the extremities quickly to the point that the individual cannot grasp rescue lines, fasten lifejacket straps, or hang on to an object such as a boat. Shivering and the sensation of cold begin when the body temperature decreases from the normal temperature of 37 °C (98.6 °F) to approximately 35.8 °C (96.5 °F). Amnesia can start at approximately 35 °C (95 °F), unconsciousness at 30 °C (86 °F), and death at approximately 26.1 °C (79 °F) (United States Search and Rescue Task Force, n.d.). Cold water robs the body of its heat 32 times faster than cold air. Although it is imperative to get out of the water as soon as possible, physical exertion causes the body to lose heat at a faster rate, as blood is being sent to the extremities and quickly cooled. Survival time can be shortened by more than 50 percent (United States Search and Rescue Task Force, n.d.). See table 15.1 for expected survival times for prolonged exposure to cold water.

TABLE 15.1 Expected Survival Time in Cold Water

Water temperature	Exhaustion or unconsciousness	Expected survival time
21–27 °C (70–80 °F)	3–12 hours	3 hours to indefinitely
16–21 °C (60–70 °F)	2–7 hours	2–40 hours
10–6 °C (50–60 °F)	1–2 hours	1–6 hours
4–10 °C (40–50 °F)	30–60 minutes	1–3 hours
0–4 °C (32.5–40 °F)	15–30 minutes	30–90 minutes
< 0 °C (<32 °F)	under 15 minutes	under 15–45 minutes

Source: United States Search and Rescue Task Force (n.d.).

Signs and Symptoms of a Cold-Water Drowning Victim

Typical symptoms include the following:

- cyanotic (blue) skin coloration
- pupils fully dilated (opened)
- no detectable breathing
- no apparent pulse or heartbeat; remember that heart rates can go down to as little as six to eight beats per minute (diving reflux), so it is important to try resuscitative efforts in accordance with your CPR training.

First Aid Considerations for Cold-Water Victims

It is important to treat hypothermia as quickly as possible. Some treatments include:

- Removing wet clothes and replacing with dry clothes or blankets.
- Using the rescuer's body heat if nothing else is available.
- Avoiding massaging the extremities.
- Laying the semi-conscious person face up with his or her head slightly down to get oxygen back into the brain.
- Rewarming the body in a bath of 40.5–43.3 °C (105–110 °F), but keeping the arms and legs out to prevent cold blood from limbs cooling off the core temperature any further. If a tub is not available, use hot, wet towels or blankets on the victim's head, neck, chest, groin, and abdomen, avoiding warming the arms or legs.
- Beginning CPR if there is no discernible pulse or breathing.

EXERCISING IN COLD TEMPERATURES

As long as we maintain core temperature, it is rarely too cold to exercise. In cold conditions, although we can wear scarves to warm inhaled air, most times the air will naturally warm up to a safe temperature by the time it reaches the lungs. Aerobic exercise helps to maintain core temperature by producing three-quarters of the energy in the form of heat. Aerobic capacity is not adversely affected as long as core temperature is maintained. If we stand around for long periods of time, or stop exercising but stay outside, the cold air begins to affect our body.

As core temperature drops, muscles set off a greater anaerobic metabolism, producing more lactic acid and associated muscle burn in an attempt to maintain core temperature. This results in an overall reduction in the strength and power that can be produced by the muscle tissue in severely cold weather. Combined with cold water in the form of rain, hail, or snow, along with fatigue, these factors allow police officers to become easy targets for hypothermia.

frostnip
a mild form of frostbite, where only the top layer of skin freezes

frostbite
severe condition where both the skin and the underlying tissue (fat, muscle, and bone) are frozen

wind chill index (WCI)
measure representing how the temperature would feel on your skin if the wind were reduced to a walking pace of 4.8 km/h

Frostnip is a mild form of frostbite, where only the top layer of skin freezes. There may be a painful tingling or burning sensation; skin appears yellowish or white, but feels soft to the touch. **Frostbite** is a more severe condition, where both the skin and the underlying tissue (fat, muscle, bone) are frozen. The area is numb. Skin appears white and waxy, and is hard to the touch. At this point, medical attention is necessary.

When headed outdoors, you need to be aware of the **wind chill index (WCI)** instead of just consulting outside air temperatures. The wind chill represents how the temperature would feel on your skin if the wind were reduced to a walking pace of 4.8 km/h.Wind increases the rate at which insulating air surrounding the body is whisked away; the warmer air is then replaced by the colder outside air. When the wind chill index is –27 °C (–18 °F) or warmer, the risk of frostbite is low. At a wind chill factor between –28 °C (–20 °F) and –39 °C (–39 °F), the risk of frostbite rapidly increases. When the wind chill reaches a factor of –40 °C (–40 °F), frostbite will occur in less than 10 minutes on exposed skin for most people. At a wind chill factor of –55 °C (–68 °F), frostbite will occur in two minutes or less on exposed skin for most people. As a general rule, if the WCI is less than –28 °C (–20 °F), caution must be taken to participate in activities outside. See table 15.2 for wind chill and frostbite risk levels, health concerns, and their remedies.

Proper apparel and common sense are key to preventing hypothermia. You can wear up to four layers of clothing, with a ventilation layer next to the skin. It is important to wear gloves and a hat, as large amounts of heat are lost through your head. Keep your neck and throat area covered. Change your socks if your feet get wet.

BIOLOGICAL AND CHEMICAL HAZARDS IN POLICING

Emergency response teams are being faced with hazardous products on a daily basis. Sources of biological hazards include bacteria, viruses, insects, plants, birds, animals, and humans. Methamphetamine laboratories in homes, hepatitis, tuberculosis, anthrax, Lyme disease (bacterial infection acquired from the bite of an infected tick), and AIDS are just a few hazards that officers may face when they respond to a call. Their health can be affected in ways ranging from skin irritation, allergies, and respiratory infections to contraction of diseases, including AIDS and various cancers.

TABLE 15.2 Wind Chill Hazards and Risk of Frostbite

Wind chill	Risk of frostbite	Health concern	What to do
0 to –9 °C (32 to 16 °F)	Low risk	Slight increase in discomfort	Dress warmly with the outside temperature in mind
–10 to –27 °C (14 to 18 °F)	Low risk	Uncomfortable Risk of hypothermia if outside for long periods without adequate protection	Dress in layers of warm clothing, with an outer layer that is wind-resistant Wear hat and mittens
–28 to –39 °C (–20 to –40 °F)	Increasing risk: exposed skin can freeze in 10–30 minutes	Check face and extremities (fingers, toes, ears, and nose) for numbness or whiteness Risk of hypothermia if outside for long periods without adequate protection	Dress in layers of warm clothing, with an outer layer that is wind-resistant Cover exposed skin—wear a hat, mittens, and a scarf, neck tube, or face mask Keep active
–40 to –47 °C (–40 to –54 °F)	High risk: exposed skin can freeze in 5–10 minutes*	Check face and extremities (fingers, toes, ears, and nose) for numbness or whiteness (frostbite) Risk of hypothermia if outside for long periods of time	Dress in layers of warm clothing, with an outer layer that is wind-resistant Cover all exposed skin—wear a hat, mittens, and a scarf, neck tube, or face mask Keep active
WARNING LEVEL** –48 to –54 °C (–56 to –66 °F)	High risk: exposed skin can freeze in 2–5 minutes*	Check face and extremities frequently for numbness or whiteness (frostbite) Serious risk of hypothermia if outside for long periods	Be careful: dress very warmly in layers of clothing, with an outer layer that is wind resistant Cover all exposed skin—wear a hat, mittens, and a scarf, neck tube, or face mask Be ready to cut short or cancel outdoor activities Keep active
–55 °C and colder (–68 °F and colder)	High risk: exposed skin can freeze in less than 2 minutes	DANGER! Outdoor conditions are hazardous	Stay indoors

* In sustained winds over 50 km/h, frostbite can occur faster than indicated.

** In parts of the country with a milder climate (such as southern Ontario and the Atlantic provinces, except Labrador), a wind chill warning is issued at about –35 °C (–32 °F). Further north, people have grown more accustomed to the cold, and have adapted to the more severe conditions. Because of this, Environment Canada issues warnings at progressively colder wind chill values as you move north. Most of Canada hears a warning at about –45 °C (–50 °F). Residents of the Arctic, northern Manitoba, and northern Quebec are warned at about –50 °C (–58 °F), and those of the high Arctic, at about –55 °C (–68 °F).

Source: Meteorological Service of Canada (2003).

Workplace Hazardous Materials Information System (WHMIS)
a system that familiarizes workers with safety information about potentially hazardous products in their workplace

Chemical hazards include individual chemicals, mixtures like petroleum solvents, and synthetic polymers (plastics). In 1988, the national **Workplace Hazardous Materials Information System (WHMIS)** was developed to familiarize workers with safety information about the potential hazardous products in their workplace (Canadian Centre for Occupational Health and Safety [CCOHS], 2007). Workers are required to learn the WHMIS symbols and their meanings, the labels on products, and material safety data sheets. These sheets provide information about the physical, chemical, and environmental characteristics of a material, along with information regarding toxicity and potential hazards (such as whether it is reactive, flammable, combustible, or toxic). Data sheets will also include preparation and production information about the substance, as well as the appropriate first aid measures that should be taken upon exposure.

The aim of the program is to provide basic health and safety measures to protect individuals, and to prevent workplace injuries and illness. It provides information on supplier and workplace labels, material safety data sheets, fundamentals of chemical safety and emergency first aid, and other helpful resources. The New Jersey State Department of Health and Senior Services (www.state.nj.us/health/) provides a database of approximately 1,700 fact sheets on important hazardous substances found in the workplace and the environment.

The CCOHS provides information on biological and chemical hazards. Each police service and community is required to develop an emergency response plan based on risk assessment (what is in a community that could expose its members to hazardous materials). Each community must develop a comprehensive emergency preparedness policy and response program to deal with each emergency in the safest and most efficient manner possible. For more information, go to the CCOHS website at www.ccohs.ca.

KEY TERMS

delayed-onset muscle soreness (DOMS)

sprain

strain

tendinitis

impingement syndrome

bursitis

heat cramps

heat exhaustion

heat stroke

hypothermia

frostnip

frostbite

wind chill index (WCI)

Workplace Hazardous Materials Information System (WHMIS)

EXERCISES

Review

1. What is the RICE principle?

2. Why do people suffer from delayed-onset muscle soreness?

3. Differentiate between a sprain and a strain.

4. How do you treat a sprain or a strain?

5. What are shin splints? How do you prevent shin splints?

6. Name and briefly explain the three heat-related illnesses.

7. How do you treat heat-related illnesses?

8. What is hypothermia? What are some of its signs and symptoms?

9. How do you treat someone who has developed hypothermia?

10. What are some of the biological or chemical hazards that an officer may face while working?

Multiple Choice and True or False

1. The most common preventable cause of exercise injury is
   a. overuse
   b. poor nutrition
   c. sudden trauma
   d. dehydration
   e. muscular endurance

2. To help prevent overuse of muscles, you should
   a. work through the soreness
   b. increase the length of your workout each day to toughen your muscles
   c. exercise seven days a week to toughen your muscles
   d. alternate days spent on aerobic and strength conditioning
   e. do two-a-day workouts to toughen your muscles

3. According to the RICE principle, for a mild ankle sprain you should
   a. rest the injured area for 12 hours
   b. apply ice for 20 minutes after 24 hours
   c. apply tape and leave it wrapped for 12 hours
   d. keep exercising unless there is extreme pain
   e. raise the ankle up and apply ice

4. Injury to a ligament caused by a sudden force is called a
   a. cramp
   b. bursitis
   c. sprain
   d. strain
   e. plantar fasciitis

5. Injury to a tendon caused by a sudden force is called a(n)
   a. pull
   b. sprain
   c. strain
   d. inversion
   e. eversion

6. Heat cramps may be treated by
   a. increased salt intake
   b. increased fluid intake and gentle stretching
   c. alternating heat with ice on the affected area
   d. wrapping the affected muscle
   e. applying more clothes to keep the muscle warm

7. Overuse problems are more common when someone is beginning a fitness program and account for the majority of injuries.
   a. True
   b. False

8. Alternating a high-impact activity with a low-impact activity may prevent overuse of specific muscle groups.
   a. True
   b. False

9. Being fatigued during a workout will not make you more susceptible to developing an injury.
   a. True
   b. False

10. Mild muscle soreness that develops at the beginning of a new exercise program will usually disappear in one to three days.
    a. True
    b. False

REFERENCES

American College of Sports Medicine. (1996). Position stand: Heat and cold illnesses during distance running. *Medicine & Science in Sports & Exercise, 28*(12), i-x.

Armstrong, L.E., & Maresh, C.M. (1993). The exertional heat illness: A risk of athletic participation. *Medicine, Exercise, Nutrition and Health, 2,* 125-134.

Boyle, C.A., Sayers, S.P., Jensen, B.E., Headley, S.A., & Manos, T.M. (2004). The effects of yoga training and a single bout of yoga on delayed onset muscle soreness in the lower extremity. *Journal of Strength and Conditioning Research, 18*(4), 723-729.

Canadian Centre for Occupational Health and Safety (CCOHS). (2007). *What is WHMIS?* Available at http://www.ccohs.ca/headlines/text51.html.

Casa, D.J., Armstrong, L.E., & Hillman, S.K. (2000). National Athletic Trainer's Association position statement: Fluid replacement for athletes. *Journal of Athletic Training, 35*(2), 212-224.

Encyclopedia of Canadian Provinces. (2007). *Ontario.* Available at http://www.nationsencyclopedia.com/canada/Nunavut-to-Yukon/Ontario.html.

United States Search and Rescue Task Force. (n.d.). *Cold water survival.* Available at http://www.ussartf.org/cold_water_survival.htm.

PART V

Preparing to Meet Law Enforcement Fitness Standards

CHAPTER 16

Preparing to Meet Law Enforcement Fitness Standards

CHAPTER OBJECTIVES

After completing this chapter, you should be able to:

- Briefly describe the purposes of the Physical Readiness Evaluation for Police (PREP) test, the Physical Abilities Requirement Evaluation (PARE) test, the Ontario Police Fitness Award (OPFA) Standards, and the Peel Regional Police Service Fitness Standards.
- Briefly describe the main features of the PREP test, the PARE test, and the OPFA Standards.
- Identify exercises that can help you prepare for the PREP test, the PARE test, and the OPFA Standards.

The Ontario Police College first developed physical fitness standards in the 1970s based on the fitness levels of the general Canadian population. Until the late 1970s, minimal height requirements and weight standards were used as part of police service selection criteria. The tests typically had the effect of excluding many women and some minority groups.

In the late 1980s, the RCMP, and in 1992, the Ontario Ministry of the Solicitor General and Correctional Services, began developing Bona Fide Occupational Requirements (BFOR) for assessing recruits' job readiness in Ontario. They looked at the specific demands of policing and corrections, respectively, to determine what physical components were essential to perform the job. These BFOR standards were implemented to address human rights issues so that one standard is applied to all applicants, regardless of age, sex, or race. It was critical to eliminate the adverse impact of entry-level physical assessment, so it included all successful candidates without excluding qualified visible minorities.

The RCMP and Ontario Ministry of the Attorney General and Correctional Services documented the physical activities that are essential for policing (content validity) and predict successful job performance (criterion-related validity). After looking at other BFOR protocols in Canada and around the world, the ministry's policing and fitness experts spent two years developing the Physical Readiness Evaluation for Police (PREP) test. In January 1999, the PREP test became the required standard in Ontario for police applicant physical fitness testing.

In the 1980s the Justice Institute of British Columbia developed the Police Officer's Physical Abilities Test (POPAT) for use in British Columbia. The RCMP's Physical Abilities Requirement Evaluation (PARE) test is a modified version of the POPAT. The PARE is used for applicant and recruit testing, and as a motivational tool for RCMP staff. Currently, incumbents with the RCMP are required to run through the protocol, with specialized units being required to meet certain standards.

The Ontario Police Fitness Award (OPFA) is a provincial incentive program developed to motivate Ontario police officers and police service employees to remain physically fit throughout their entire careers. The OPFA program is sanctioned by the policing services division of the Ministry of the Solicitor General and the Ontario Association of Chiefs of Police. It incorporates several tests: curl-ups, push-ups, sit and reach, and the 1.5-mile run or the shuttle run. Those individuals who achieve a 75 percent grade are awarded the OPFA pin.

Over a three-year period (March 1996 to March 1999), Mr. Peter Shipley, Physiological Health Science Coordinator at the Provincial Police Academy, conducted a cost–benefit analysis within the Ontario Provincial Police (Shipley, 2000). His research indicated that OPP officers who had earned their five-year OPFA pin used, on average, 4.24 less sick days per year than the average OPP officer. With all these benefits in mind, it is felt that police services should be concerned about their officers' physical fitness levels, not just during the initial hiring phase but throughout their careers. The Ontario Police Fitness Award program was designed to assist police services in monitoring and motivating their officers' physical health.

The following pages reproduce testing protocols from the PREP and PARE tests. Also reproduced are police fitness standards developed by the Ontario Police College and the Peel Regional Police Service. While these fitness standards are only being used by Peel Region as hiring requirements since the introduction of PREP, PARE, and OPFA Standards, they may provide some useful performance benchmarks for your own training program. Many forces still use them as benchmarks in hiring of cadets, special constables, recruit training, and promotions.

PHYSICAL READINESS EVALUATION FOR POLICE (PREP) TEST

Fit to Serve: Preparing for the PREP (Ministry of Public Safety and Security, 2002) is available through Ontario colleges and police services or from the Ontario Association of Chiefs of Police. This is the standard that must be achieved to graduate from the Ontario Police College. It outlines the components of the PREP:

1. pre-exercise clearance (PAR-Q, PARmed-X, blood pressure, informed consent), demonstration, and a period of time to get acquainted with the various equipment used in the test
2. pursuit/restraint circuit
3. aerobic fitness test

Pursuit/Restraint Circuit

The pursuit/restraint circuit (see figure 16.1) simulates a police foot chase that includes obstacles, the control of a person who resists arrest, and the dragging of an incapacitated person. This test assesses your physical and occupational readiness to perform the duties of a police officer in the province of Ontario.

Throughout the pursuit/restraint circuit, you must wear a 9-lb. (4.1 kg) soft belt around the waist to simulate the weight of a police belt plus standard equipment. In the pursuit phase of the test, you run four laps around a 25-m (83-ft.) circuit as quickly as possible for a total distance of 100 m (332 ft.).

The following is the sequence of the pursuit/restraint circuit:

FIGURE 16.1 PREP Test: Pursuit/Restraint Circuit

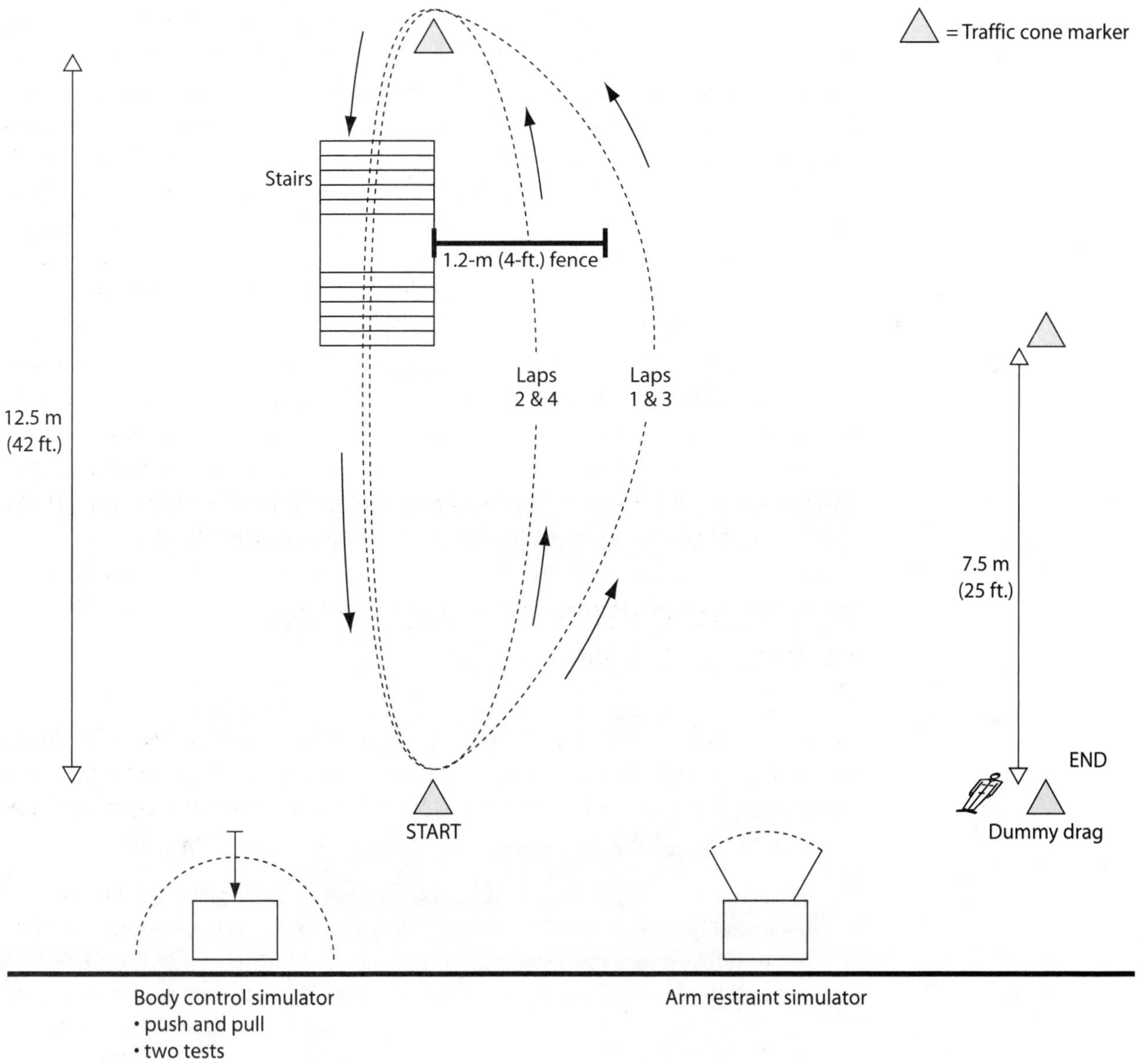

1. You begin from the start point on the command "ready, go."
2. On the first and third of the four rotations of the 25-m circuit, you run around the right end of the fence and over the stairs back to the start point. On the second and fourth rotations, you scale a 1.2-m (4-ft.) solid fence and then return over the stairs to the start point.
3. After completing the pursuit portion, you move quickly to the body-control simulator and push a pair of handles away from you to raise a 32-kg (70-lb.) weight off the floor. Keeping the weight elevated, you side-step through 180°, first to the left and then to the right, completing a total of six half-circles. You then move to the arm-restraint simulator, where you depress the handles on the grips of both arms of the simulator. Keeping the grips depressed, you force the arms together and then return them to their starting position. You then return to the body-control simulator and this time pull the pair of handles to raise the 32-kg (70-lb.) weight off the floor. Again, keeping the weight elevated, you rotate left and then right through 180°, completing six half-circles. You then return to the arm-restraint simulator and repeat the exercise, depressing the grips, forcing the arms together, and returning them to their starting position.
4. Finally, you grasp a 68-kg (150-lb.) dummy and drag it for 15 m (50 ft.). You may grasp the dummy either by the wrists or around the chest and under the arms.

A time of 162 seconds or less is required for successful completion of the pursuit/restraint circuit.

Note: Participants are allowed a 10-minute rest following the pursuit/restraint circuit before beginning the aerobic fitness test.

Aerobic Fitness Test

The aerobic fitness test consists of a 20-m shuttle run to evaluate your aerobic fitness and work capability during physically demanding policing tasks as well as everyday policing activities (Léger & Lambert, 1982). In this test, you run back and forth between two marked lines over a 20-m (67-ft.) course in time with a recorded audio signal. The time permitted to cover the 20 m decreases progressively until you are unable to maintain the pace. The time permitted to cover the 20 m initially requires a slow jog. In each leg of the run, warning lines, placed 2 m (7 ft.) from each of the 20-m lines, must be reached before the permitted time elapses. You will be cautioned when you miss a warning line. The test is terminated when two consecutive warning lines are missed. To successfully complete the minimum requirement of the aerobic fitness test for the PREP, you must achieve stage 6.5 in the 20-m shuttle run.

Instructions for the shuttle run are given prior to the test and are as follows:

> This test is an evaluation of aerobic fitness. A warm-up is included as part of the test and only the last portion of the test may require maximal effort. The objective is to follow the progressively faster pace over a 20-metre course. Successful completion of stage 6.5 must be reached to complete the minimum requirement.
>
> At every signal you must have reached one of the 20-metre lines at each end marked by the pylons. One foot must be on or over the line, then upon hearing the

signal, reverse your direction and arrive at the other line in time for the next signal. To turn, *pivot* on the ball of your foot. DO NOT MAKE WIDE TURNS. At the start it will be very slow, so you may reach the line with time to spare. However, YOU MUST WAIT FOR THE SIGNAL BEFORE YOU LEAVE. *Two metres* in front of the end lines are *warning lines*. IF TWICE IN A ROW YOU HAVE NOT CROSSED THE WARNING LINE WHEN THE SIGNAL SOUNDS, THE LAST STAGE ANNOUNCED ON THE TAPE IS THE LAST COMPLETED STAGE AND YOU ARE FINISHED. You will be cautioned clearly when you miss the first warning line. However, you must still reach the end line before starting the next leg. If you miss the warning line at one end but you make it at the other end, the warnings start over. The *two misses must be consecutive.* When you finish, remain in your lane and exit out the end. DO NOT CROSS INTO ANOTHER PERSON'S LANE.

Remember to successfully complete the minimum requirement of the aerobic fitness test you must achieve Stage 6.5 in the 20-metre Shuttle Run.

PHYSICAL ABILITIES REQUIREMENT EVALUATION (PARE) TEST

PARE measures the essential physical occupational capacities to perform satisfactory police work. On the basis of task analysis, the RCMP developed PARE for its Bona Fide Occupational Requirement (BFOR).

The RCMP Physical Abilities Requirement Evaluation (PARE) is an occupational test used to assess a person's ability to perform the physical demands of police work. There are nine essential physical activities required of police officers in the pursuit of their duties: walking, carrying, jumping, pushing, lifting, climbing (stairs, hills), pulling, vaulting, and running. These nine essential tasks are included in the PARE, which simulates a scenario where a police officer must get to the scene of a problem or occurrence (the obstacle course), physically solve the problem (the push/pull activity), and remove objects or persons from the scene (the torso bag carry) (RCMP, 2005).

The PARE is a BFOR that assesses whether you can perform the basic physical skills necessary to do the job, based on your level of fitness. It is a job-specific physical ability evaluation, designed to assess a person's capacity to meet the physical demands of police work (RCMP, 2005). The PARE test sections are described in detail below and are illustrated in figure 16.2.

PARE is divided into three sections:

1. Obstacle Course
2. Push/Pull Station
3. Torso Bag Carry

The first two stations (Obstacle Course and Push/Pull) are timed and must be completed in less than/equal to 4 minutes 45 seconds for applicants, and less than/equal to 4 minutes for members applying for specialized duties and cadets before graduating from Depot. [For example, as of spring 2002, air marshals in the Canadian Air Career Protective Service must be fit for duty at the PARE standard of four minutes; as of 2007, VIP bodyguards must also pass the standard (Séguin, 2007).] The last section, the torso bag carry, is a pass or fail activity and is not timed. [Note: Penalties are handed out to those who commit an error in performance (such as knocking down a stick, throwing a bag over the shoulders, or walking with the bag resting on the knees). Participants may be required to re-perform a manoeuvre or given a time penalty.]

Screening

Prior to attempting PARE all participants must pass a health screening using PAR-Q. Regular members must provide current medical clearance. Applicants must provide medical clearance and signed informed consent.

Participants with any of the following may not participate in PARE:

a. Heart Rate > 99 bpm
b. Systolic Blood Pressure > 144 mm Hg
c. Diastolic Blood Pressure > 94 mm Hg

FIGURE 16.2 PARE Test Stations

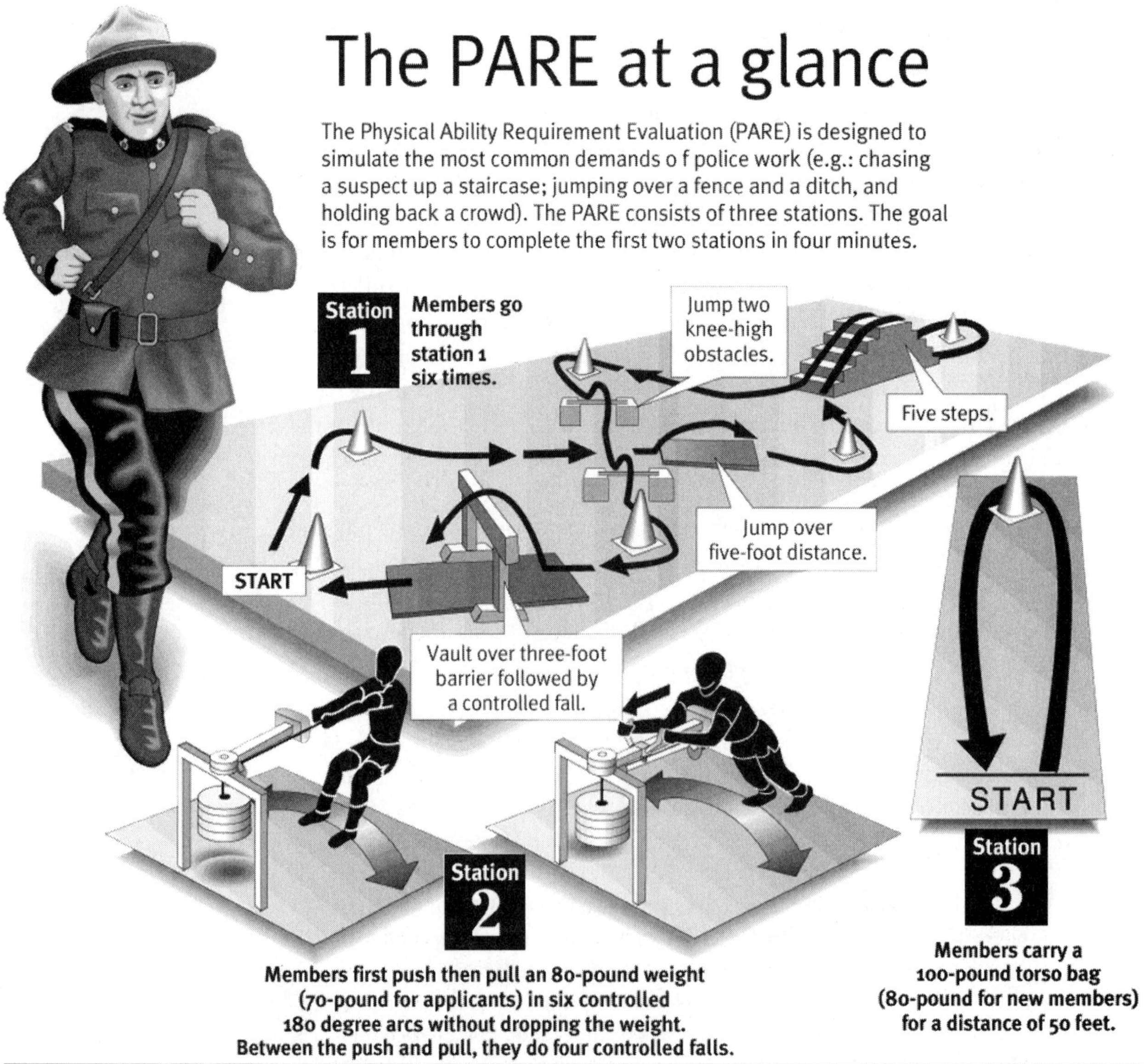
The PARE at a glance
The Physical Ability Requirement Evaluation (PARE) is designed to simulate the most common demands o f police work (e.g.: chasing a suspect up a staircase; jumping over a fence and a ditch, and holding back a crowd). The PARE consists of three stations. The goal is for members to complete the first two stations in four minutes.
Station 1
Members go through station 1 six times.
Jump two knee-high obstacles.
Five steps.
Jump over five-foot distance.
START
Vault over three-foot barrier followed by a controlled fall.
START
Station 3
Station 2
Members first push then pull an 80-pound weight (70-pound for applicants) in six controlled 180 degree arcs without dropping the weight. Between the push and pull, they do four controlled falls.
Members carry a 100-pound torso bag (80-pound for new members) for a distance of 50 feet.

Source: Reprinted with the permission of the RCMP.

In many cases, anxiety may be influencing the above. If attempts to relax the participant bring the values under the limits they may participate. Applicants are required to have a medical prior to being tested by a force-appointed physician.

Pursuit Course: Agility Run

The first part of PARE consists of a 1148 ft (350 metre) obstacle run where the participant must demonstrate gross motor ability such as mobility, agility, flexibility, power and general endurance. [The course is typically performed in about two minutes and 30 seconds (25 seconds/lap).]

The course is laid out in the following manner [see figure 16.3]:

1. From the start marker (#1), the participant runs diagonally to the left, towards #2 marker placed 20 ft (6.1 metres) out from #1, and 10 ft (3.05 metres) to the left of the centre line.
2. Going around the left side of this marker (#2), the participant runs inside diagonally towards the #3 marker. Before reaching marker #3, the participant must jump over and clear a 5 ft (1.52 metre) mat. Upon landing, the participant turns left around marker #3 and proceeds towards the stairs. The last edge of the mat is placed 5 ft (1.52 metres) from marker #3.
3. The stairs are placed in the centre of the course in such a manner that the centre of the top platform is exactly 60 ft (18.29 metres) from the start marker (#1), 20 ft (6.1 metres) from marker #4 and directly in line with the centre. The participant must run up and down the stairs, stepping on at least one step on the way up, the top platform, and one step on the way down. This is for the participant's safety.
4. Marker #4 is set on the centre line exactly 80 ft (24.38 metres) from the start marker (#1). The participant runs around this marker, from either the right or left side and runs back towards the stairs going up and down again with the same safety precautions as previously mentioned. He/she then proceeds towards marker #5.
5. Marker #5 is placed 40 ft (12.19 metres) from the start marker (#1) and 10 ft (3.05 metres) to the left of the centre line. The participant runs around the right side of marker #5, turns left diagonally heading towards marker #6. The first hurdle is 5 ft (1.52 metres) from marker #5. The second hurdle is located 10 ft (3.05 metres) from the first hurdle. The participant must leap over the 2 hurdles raised 18 in (45 cm) from the floor, which are lined up straight with each other and between marker #5 and #6.
6. Reaching marker #6, the participant runs around the left side of the marker and turns right heading towards the start marker (#1). Before reaching marker #1, the participant traverses a 3 ft (0.91 metre) high railing vault **halfway between markers #6 and #1**. The participants must land in control on their feet on the opposite side of the obstacle, then perform a controlled fall on either their chest (chest, stomach, hips must be flat on the ground) or back (both shoulder blades must touch the ground simultaneously), alternating after each lap as per tester instructions. After each controlled fall, the participant must get up without assistance (may not touch the vault rail) and proceed around marker #1 to complete the lap. Six laps must be completed before proceeding to the Push/Pull station which should be located within 20 ft (6.1 metres) from marker #1 before starting Section 2.

FIGURE 16.3 PARE Test Obstacle Course

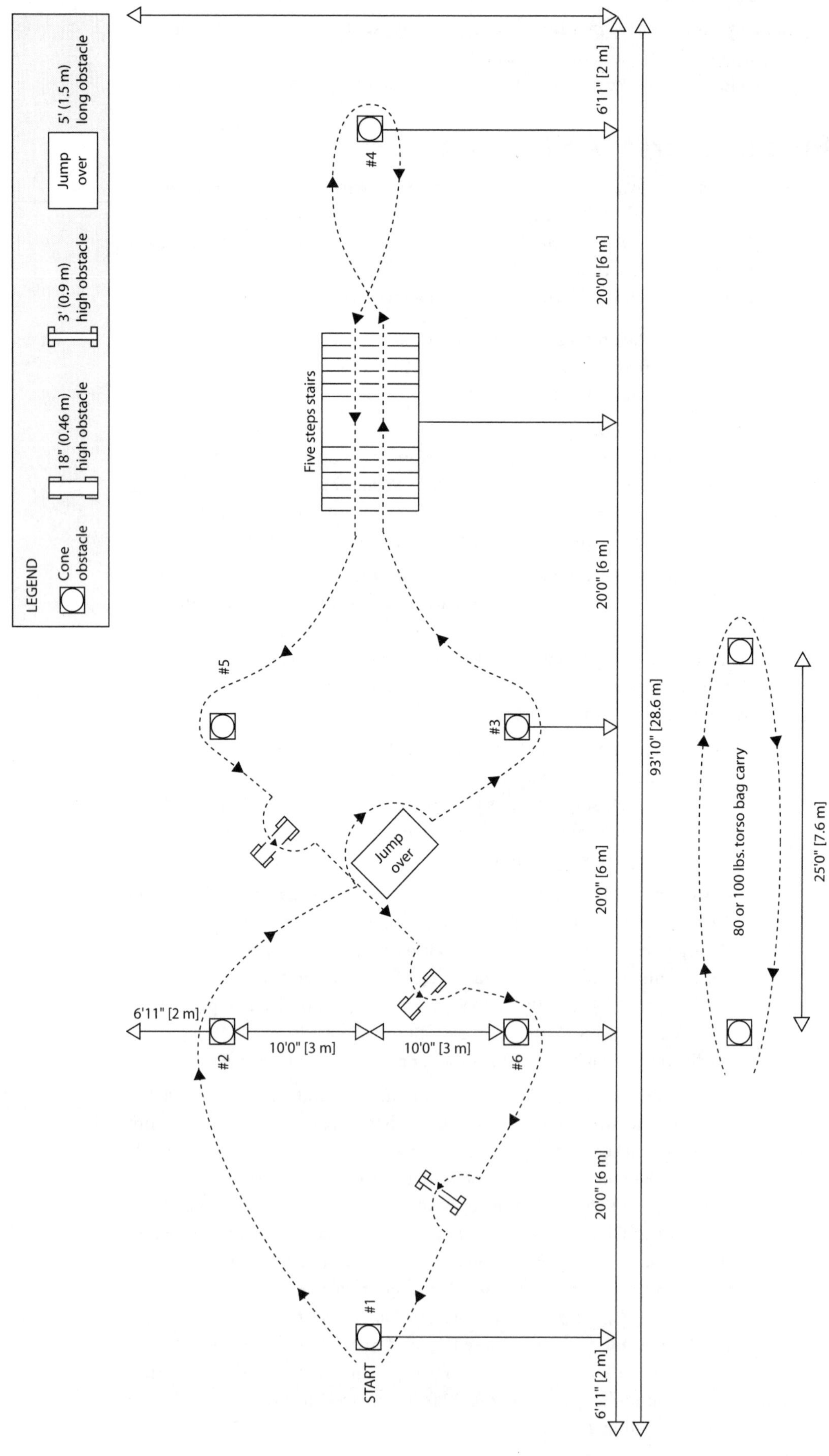

Remarks Related to the Performance of the Obstacle Course

To perform the PARE in 4:45 minutes (for applicant testing), and 4 mnutes (for members applying for specialized duties and cadets before graduating from Depot), the Obstacle Course portion should typically be performed in no more than two minutes and thirty seconds (approximately 25 seconds/lap). Test administrators should provide the participant with lap times and encouragement throughout the test. Faults can occur during the Obstacle Course and will result in penalties:

FAULTS AND PENALTIES

i. **Markers (going around):** A participant failing to go around the outside of a marker must come back and go around the outside of the marker.

ii. **Mat:** A participant not clearing the 5 foot mat will be penalized 5 seconds.

iii. **Stairs:** Participants are instructed to follow proper protocol for safety reasons.

iv. **Hurdles (knocking down):** If one of the hurdles is knocked down, the penalty is 2 seconds. The tester replaces the stick.

v. **Hurdles (going outside):** A participant jumping over the hurdle with his/her trail leg outside the cone will be assessed a 2 second penalty.

vi. **Vault (traversing):** If a participant is unable to traverse the vault, the test is terminated. The way a participant traverses the vault is not specifically directed; however, it must be in a controlled manner. The participant may touch the vault with any parts of his/her body but must remain in control at all times.

vii. **Vault (landing):** A participant not landing in a controlled manner after traversing the vault is required to go back and traverse the vault again, landing in control on both feet.

viii. **Controlled falls (getting up):** Using the vault or mat to pull oneself to a standing position will require the participant to repeat the controlled fall.

ix. **Controlled falls (proper form):** A participant not touching his/her chest, stomach, hips or both shoulder blades during the front and back falls, must repeat the controlled fall.

Once the sixth lap is completed [the pursuit section is typically performed in about 2 minutes and 30 seconds], the participant proceeds to the push/pull machine, to begin Section 2. Please note that the push/pull machine should be mounted to a wall within 20 ft (6.1 metres) from the start marker.

Apprehension Section

Upon finishing the obstacle run, the participant moves immediately to the push/pull station, which consists of a push/pull unit and a mat 6.6 × 23 ft (2 × 7 metres). The maximum allowed distance between the end of the obstacle course (marker #1) and the push/pull apparatus is 20 ft (6 metres). In the case where it is physically impossible to locate the station within 20 ft (6 metres) of the end of the run, then the amount of time it reasonably takes to reach the push/pull must be deducted from the participant's total time.

The participant may perform this activity in the order he/she chooses (i.e., push first, then pull, or vice versa). Since the push is more difficult to perform, it is recommended to do this activity first. [This second part of the test is typically performed in 65 to 70 seconds.]

PUSH ACTIVITY

Upon reaching the push/pull unit, the participant grasps the handles and pushes the weight, 70 lb (32 kg) for applicants or 80 lb (36 kg) for members, *off the base of the machine*, then proceeds to complete six controlled 180° arcs. In order to complete an arc, the participant's body and the arm of the machine must be directly in line with the frame of the push/pull machine.

The participant's chest may or may not touch the pad on the lever arm. This is a question of choice and comfort for the participant. The arms must remain bent at the elbow throughout the performance of the activity. The elbows or hands must not be touching the chest or shoulders. The pad cannot be held under the arm pit nor the chin locked onto the pad. The "handle" of the unit must be maintained in a neutral position and not locked left or right in order to "steer" the unit.

This activity should typically last no longer than 30 seconds. It is important to watch that the abdominal muscles are contracted and the back is maintained in a neutral position. If after one reminder the participants fail to correct their technique and form, the specific arc must be repeated.

CONTROLLED FALLS

After six arcs are completed, the weight is lowered with control. The participant then moves away from the unit about 3 feet (1 metre) and faces the pad or wall (marked at pad height). The participant must perform a controlled fall on their front with chest, stomach and hips on the ground and get up executing a push-up like movement. The participant must then come to a standing ready position, touch the pad or wall with two hands and execute a second fall, this time on their back, both shoulder blades on the ground. A sit-up like manoeuvre is required to come back up to the standing ready position. This sequence—front and back falls returning to a ready position between each—is repeated until the participant has completed two front falls and two back falls. This procedure should be demonstrated by the tester and practised by the participant before the test. The participant **must not use the pad or wall for assistance to get up** from the falls. This activity should typically last no longer than 30 seconds.

The participant must always face the wall or the machine. Turning the back to the machine or wall is considered a fault and the participant is asked to repeat the fall. This activity typically lasts 20 seconds.

PULL ACTIVITY

Once the sequence of falls is completed, the participant grasps the rope (on any portions of the rope) using both hands and pulls so the weight plates lift off the base of the machine. The participant then proceeds to completing six 180° arcs.

In order to complete an arc, the participant's body (head and trunk) must face the push/pull machine at all times during this activity (i.e., shoulders not turning away from the machine). The participant must remain in control throughout the arcs while keeping his/her elbows, hips and knees bent and his/her shoulders facing the machine. The participant may not lean back during the pull activity as it would demonstrate a lack of control. The pull activity should typically last no longer than 30 seconds.

The administrator should advise the participant to "sit down," keeping the back straight and knees bent. If proper technique is not maintained, the participant is provided a warning. Failing to comply will result in repeating the arc.

The tester stops the clock once the sixth arc is completed when the participant puts the weight down in a control fashion and touches the pad.

The timed section of PARE is finished when the participant completes the [Apprehension] Section.

Remarks Related to Performance of the Push/Pull Section

To perform the PARE in 4 minutes or less, the Push/Pull section should typically be performed in no more than one minute and thirty seconds. Test administrators should provide direction and encouragement to the participant throughout this section. Faults can occur during the Push/Pull section and will result in penalties.

Faults and Penalties

ARCS

i. **Dropping weights:** A participant failing to maintain the weight off the base of the machine during a controlled arc will be asked to perform an additional correct arc.

ii. **Straight elbows:** A participant failing to maintain elbows bent in the push or pull activity (participant is allowed one warning) will be asked to perform an additional arc.

iii. **Steering or locking the handles:** A participant "steering" or locking the handles during the push activity (participant is allowed one warning) will be asked to perform an additional arc.

iv. **Leaning back:** A participant leaning back during the pull activity (participant is allowed one warning) or failing to keep the elbows, hips and knees bent at 90° (participant is allowed one warning) will be asked to perform an additional arc.

v. **Incomplete arc:** A participant failing to complete an entire 180° arc will be asked to perform an additional arc.

vi. **Holding the pad:** Participant holding the pad under the arm pit or locking the chin onto the pad during the push (participant is allowed one warning) will be asked to perform an additional arc.

FALLS

When a fault of the following nature occurs, the participant must repeat the controlled fall.

vii. **Proper position:** Participant failing to come to a controlled, ready position between falls will be required to redo the controlled fall.

viii. **Touching the pad/wall:** Participant not touching the pad or wall with both hands between the falls will be required to redo the controlled fall.

ix. **Not facing the pad:** Participant falling and turning away from the pad or wall will be required to redo the controlled fall.

x. **Getting up:** Participant using the push/pull apparatus to assist with getting up will be required to redo the controlled fall.

xi. **Proper technique:** Participant not touching their chest, stomach, hips or both shoulder blades during the front and back falls, will be required to redo the controlled fall.

Torso Bag Carry Section

The Torso Bag Carry section of PARE is a pass/fail untimed activity. The participant must be able to pick up a weight, 80 lb (36 kg) for applicants or 100 lb (45 kg) for members, and carry it using arms only, over a distance of 50 ft (15 metres). This activity should begin 60 to 120 seconds after completion of the timed part of the test.

The resistance is placed within a bag made of waterproof material. On either side of the bag, enough material is provided to allow the participant a secure grip. Being able to lift the bag demonstrates good muscular strength in the forearms, wrists and fingers. Participants are allowed to wrap their arms around the bag and lift. The lift must be with the legs, and not the back, to avoid injury. The bag must be carried in front of the participant, NOT over the shoulders (fireman carry) *and not resting on the knees while walking.*

Once the torso bag is lifted, the participant must carry it to a cone placed 25 ft (7.6 metres) from the start cone, go around it and come back to the start cone where the bag is lowered to the floor, **in a controlled manner**.

Remarks Related to the Performance of the Torso Bag Carry

The participant must demonstrate sufficient strength and endurance to manipulate, lift and carry heavy objects. The participant will have a maximum of three trials to complete the torso bag carry in the proper manner over a distance of 50 feet (15 metres). Faults can occur during the weight carry activity and will trigger penalties.

FAULTS AND PENALTIES

i. **Unable to lift the bag:** Participant failing to pick up the bag will be given a maximum of three trials to complete the weight carry.

ii. **Dropping the bag:** Participant picking up the bag but dropping it before completing the task must redo the entire weight carry section.

iii. **Improper carry:** Participant throwing the bag over the shoulder or walking with the bag resting on the thighs will be asked to redo the entire weight carry section.

iv. **Lowering the bag:** Participant failing to lower the bag in a controlled manner at the end of the activity will be asked to redo the entire weight carry section.

An unsuccessful carry *after three failed attempts* will constitute a PARE failure.

ONTARIO POLICE FITNESS AWARD (OPFA) STANDARDS

The OPFA Standards, developed in the early 1980s, are used to assess the fitness level of police officers. The standard of comparison is the general population of

Canada. Whereas BFOR standards are for assessing your physical readiness for the job, the OPFA Standards are for assessing your general fitness level.

The charts on the following pages are adapted from the OPFA Standards. They cover four fitness assessments—push-ups, curl-ups, trunk forward flexion, and the 1.5-mile run—that can help you prepare for the PREP and similar tests. Each chart provides benchmarks that allow you to score your performance and gauge your improvement as you work toward your goal of meeting law enforcement fitness standards. Descriptions of push-ups, curl-ups, trunk forward flexion, and the 1.5-mile run precede each set of charts. Officers who meet 75 percent of the OPFA Standards receive a fitness pin that they wear on their uniform, sponsored by the Police Fitness Personnel of Ontario (PFPO) and the Ontario Association of Chiefs of Police. Some services require recruits to meet this fitness level in order to attend recruit training at OPC. Some services require cadets to meet the 75 percent standard in order to be hired. However, the PREP is the graduation standard for the Ontario Police College.

Push-ups

Push-ups are a test of muscular endurance, which is defined as the ability of a muscle to perform repeated contractions over a period of time.

Push-ups

Number of push-ups (males)/modified push-ups (females), by age

	Age 20–29		Age 30–39		Age 40–49		Age 50–59		Age 60+	
Score	Males	Females	Males	Females	Males	Females	Males	Females	Males	Females
20	49+	38+	37+	37+	31+	33+	29+	31+	28+	31+
19	48	37	36	36	30	32	28	30	25–27	30
18	36–47	30–36	30–35	27–35	22–29	24–31	21–27	21–29	18–24	17–29
17	32–35	24–29	25–29	22–26	20–21	20–23	15–20	15–20	13–17	13–16
16	29–31	21–23	22–24	20–21	17–19	15–19	13–14	11–14	11–12	12
15	27–28	20	21	17–19	16	14	11–12	10	10	10–11
14	25–26	18–19	20	16	15	13	11	10	10	9
12	24	16–17	19	14–15	13–14	12	10	9	9	6–8
10	21–23	14–15	16–18	12–13	12	10–11	9	5–8	7–8	4–5
8	18–20	11–13	14–15	10–11	10–11	7–9	7–8	3–4	6	2–3
6	16–17	9–10	11–13	7–9	8–9	4–6	5–6	1–2	4–5	1
4	11–15	5–8	8–10	4–6	5–7	2–3	4	—	2–3	—
2	10	4	7	3	4	1	3	—	1	—
0	≤9	≤3	≤6	≤2	≤3	0	≤2	0	0	0

Source: Adapted with permission from Reeves, M. (2002). *Peel Regional Police recruit fitness standards*. Brampton, ON: Peel Regional Police Service.

PROCEDURE

It is imperative that the participant is well instructed in the correct performance of the push-up prior to beginning the test. The push-ups are to be performed consecutively and without a time limit. The test is terminated when the participant has completed as many push-ups as possible, the form deviates too much from the procedure, or there is more than a two-second pause between repetitions. If the upper body does not stay in a straight line, or the individual does not go to full extension, or the individual is forcibly straining over two consecutive repetitions, the test is terminated.

MALES

The participant lies on his stomach, legs together. His hands, *pointing forward*, are positioned under the shoulders. To begin, the participant pushes up from the mat by fully straightening the elbows, using the toes as the pivotal point. The upper body must be kept in a straight line. The participant returns to the starting position, chin to the mat. Neither the stomach nor the thighs should touch the mat.

FEMALES

The participant lies on her stomach, legs together. Her hands, *pointing forward*, are positioned under the shoulders. She then pushes up from the mat by fully straightening the elbows, using the knees as the pivot point. The upper body must be kept in a straight line. The participant returns to the starting position, chin to the mat. The stomach should not touch the mat. The participant *must* have the lower leg remain in contact with the mat, ankles plantar-flexed. The participant may not bend her lower legs up at the knees.

It is not acceptable for either males or females to have their feet against a wall or for a mat to be placed under their chin.

Curl-ups

Endurance is the ability to sustain an effort for an extended period of time. The curl-up tests the muscular endurance of the abdominal muscles. The test is terminated if the participant is unable to maintain required cadence, or unable to maintain the proper curl-up technique (for example, heels come off the floor) over two repetitions despite cautions by the appraiser. The appraiser before termination of the test allows a maximum of three corrections.

STARTING POSITION

Participants lie in a supine position with the head resting on the mat, arms straight at sides and parallel to the trunk, palms of hands in contact with the mat, and the middle finger tip of both hands at the 0 mark. Knees are bent at 90 degrees and the heels are kept in contact with the mat. The test is performed with shoes on.

PROCEDURE

Use the cadence provided on a metronome (50 beats per minute). A slow curling up of the upper spine far enough so that the middle finger tips of both hands reach

Curl-ups

Number of curl-ups, by age and distance

	Age 20–29/12 cm		Age 30–39/12 cm		Age 40–49/8 cm		Age 50–59/8 cm		Age 60+/8 cm	
Score	Males	Females	Males	Females	Males	Females	Males	Females	Males	Females
20	65–75	56–70	72–75	49–55	75	46–50	67–74	38–48	42–53	39–50
19	54–64	44–55	66–71	42–48	74	41–45	58–66	30–37	33–41	30–38
18	45–53	40–43	52–65	37–41	70–73	36–40	49–57	25–29	28–32	26–29
17	38–44	36–39	43–51	33–36	62–69	32–35	42–48	21–24	24–27	23–25
16	32–37	33–35	37–42	29–32	52–61	29–31	36–41	17–20	20–23	20–22
15	31	31–32	35–36	27–28	48–51	28	33–35	15–16	19	18–19
14	28–30	28–30	32–34	22–26	40–47	26–27	28–32	10–14	17–18	14–17
12	25–27	22–27	27–31	17–21	32–39	21–25	24–27	6–9	10–16	10–13
10	21–24	18–21	20–26	13–16	27–31	15–20	20–23	5	7–9	5–9
8	14–20	13–17	14–19	4–12	23–26	6–14	14–19	4	4–6	4
6	5–13	6–12	3–13	3	14–21	3–5	3–13	3	3	3
4	4	5	2	2	13	2	2	2	2	2
2	1–3	4	1	1	1–12	1	1	1	1	1
0	0	≤3	0	0	0	0	0	0	0	0

Source: Adapted with permission from Reeves, M. (2002). *Peel Regional Police recruit fitness standards.* Brampton, ON: Peel Regional Police Service.

the 12 cm (or 8 cm if 40 years or older) mark follows this. During the curl-up the palms and heels must remain in contact with the mat. Anchoring of the feet is not permitted. On return, the shoulder blades and head must contact the mat and the finger tips of both hands must touch the 0 mark. The movement is performed in a slow, controlled manner so that the time to perform the lifting and lowering stages of the curl-up is the same at a rate of 25 curl-ups per minute. The curl-ups should be performed at a steady rate, without pausing, to a maximum of 75.

The following are some matters to ensure during the curl-up test.

Do

- Verify metronome accuracy with a stopwatch (50 beats/minute).
- Keep knees at 90 degrees.
- Keep heels in contact with the mat.
- Make sure the shoulders are relaxed, neither depressed nor elevated.
- Return to the starting position with head on the mat.
- Keep arms straight.

Don't

- Slide the seat from the starting position.
- Lift or slide the heels.
- Use your neck to curl up your trunk.
- Bend elbows or lose contact between the palms of the hand and the mat.
- Slide the finger tips past the 12 cm (or 8 cm if 40 years or older) mark on the mat.
- Pause during the movement at top or bottom position.
- Go ahead or fall behind the correct cadence.

The test is terminated if the individual is

- Experiencing undue discomfort.
- Unable to maintain proper curl-up technique (that is, lifting shoulder blades off the ground, only moving arms, heels coming off the ground, head not returning to mat, and palm of hands not maintaining contact with the mat).
- Unable to maintain required cadence.

Trunk Forward Flexion (Sit and Reach)

The trunk forward flexion test measures the flexibility of the hamstring and lower back muscles. Flexibility depends upon the elasticity of the muscles, tendons, and ligaments, and is the ability to bend without injury.

Trunk forward flexion

	Distance in cm									
	Age 20–29		Age 30–39		Age 40–49		Age 50–59		Age 60+	
Score	Males	Females	Males	Females	Males	Females	Males	Females	Males	Females
10	45+	46+	44+	46+	41+	44+	42+	44+	45+	41+
9.5	44	45	43	45	40	43	41	43	44	40
9	40–43	41–44	38–42	41–44	35–39	38–42	35–40	39–42	33–43	35–39
8.5	37–39	39–40	35–37	38–40	32–34	36–37	30–34	36–38	28–32	33–34
8	34–36	37–38	33–34	36–37	29–31	34–35	28–29	33–35	25–27	31–32
7.5	33	36	32	35	28	33	27	32	24	30
7	32	35	31	34	26–27	32	26	31	23	28–29
6	31	34	29–30	33	25	31	25	30	22	28
5	29–30	32–33	27–28	31–32	23–24	29–30	22–24	29	18–21	26–27
4	26–28	29–31	24–26	28–30	20–22	26–28	18–21	26–28	16–17	24–25
3	23–25	26–28	21–23	25–27	16–19	24–25	15–17	23–25	14–15	23
2	18–22	22–25	17–20	21–24	12–15	19–23	12–14	19–22	11–13	18–22
1	17	21	16	20	11	18	11	18	10	17

Source: Adapted with permission from Reeves, M. (2002). *Peel Regional Police recruit fitness standards.* Brampton, ON: Peel Regional Police Service.

PROCEDURE

Participants warm up for this test by performing slow stretching movements before taking the actual measurements. Participants, without shoes, sit with legs fully extended and the soles of the feet placed flat against the flexometer. Keeping the knees fully extended, arms evenly stretched, and palms down, participants bend and reach forward (without jerking). The position of maximum flexion must be held for approximately two seconds. Participants are advised to lower their heads during the motion to maximize the distance reached. Each participant takes a turn and then the procedure is repeated. Both results are recorded with the higher result scored.

The trial does not count if

- The knees are bent.
- The participant is attempting to do a bouncing or jerking motion to reach the board.
- The participant is unable to hold the position for two seconds.

1.5-Mile Run

The 1.5-mile run is a test of aerobic fitness or cardiovascular endurance. It tests the combined efficiency of the lungs, heart, bloodstream, and local muscles in getting oxygen to the muscles and putting it to work.

PROCEDURE

Participants are required to cover an accurately measured 1.5-mile distance in as short a time as possible.

PEEL REGIONAL POLICE SERVICE FITNESS STANDARDS

The Peel Regional Police Service's Fitness Standards for the bench press, chin-ups, and 100-yard sprint can be used to supplement the standards given above. The bench press tests upper-body strength, the chin-ups test muscular endurance, and the 100-yard sprint tests anaerobic capacity (the body's ability to use energy stored in the muscles without having to draw on inhaled oxygen).

Bench Press

The bench press—with standards set for a selectorized plate machine—provides an indication of upper-body strength. Each plate on the bench press machine used by Peel Regional Police is 10 pounds (4.5 kg) with all scoring correspondingly in 10-pound increments. If you do not have access to a bench press machine, you can train using the formula in the next paragraph, by establishing goals based on your body weight.

The bench press chart that follows shows the score that you earn when you lift a certain amount of weight. All scoring is based on your body weight. First, weigh yourself and then round the amount to the closest 10-pound increment (for example,

1.5-Mile run

Time to complete (minutes)

Score	Age 20–29		Age 30–39		Age 40–49		Age 50–59		Age 60+	
	Males	Females	Males	Females	Males	Females	Males	Females	Males	Females
50	≤9:00	<10:35	≤9:20	<11:00	≤10:06	<11:53	≤10:54	<13:04	≤11:59	<14:22
47.5	9:01–9:30	10:36–11:10	9:21–9:50	11:01–11:05	10:07–10:37	11:54–12:31	10:55–11:41	13:05–13:46	12:00–12:51	14:23–15:08
45	9:31–10:00	11:11–11:52	9:51–10:20	11:36–12:10	10:38–11:10	12:32–13:08	11:42–12:18	13:47–14:27	12:52–13:31	15:09–15:53
42.5	10:01–10:30	11:53–12:34	10:21–10:50	12:11–12:45	11:11–11:42	13:09–13:46	12:18–12:52	14:28–15:08	13:32–14:07	15:54–16:38
40	10:31–10:56	12:35–13:00	10:51–11:20	12:46–13:20	11:43–12:14	13:47–14:24	12:53–13:28	15:09–15:50	14:08–14:49	16:39–17:25
37.5	10:57–11:22	13:01–13:26	11:21–11:50	13:21–13:55	12:15–12:47	14:25–15:02	13:29–14:04	15:51–16:32	14:50–15:28	17:26–18:11
35	11:23–11:46	13:27–13:42	11:51–12:20	13:56–14:30	12:48–13:19	15:03–15:40	14:05–14:39	16:33–17:14	15:29–16:07	18:12–18:57
30	11:47–12:10	13:43–13:57	12:21–12:50	14:31–15:05	13:20–13:52	15:41–16:17	14:40–15:15	17:15–17:55	16:08–16:47	18:58–19:42
25	12:11–12:35	13:58–14:12	12:51–13:20	15:06–15:40	13:53–14:24	16:18–16:55	15:16–15:50	17:56–18:21	16:48–17:25	19:43–20:11
20	12:36–12:59	14:13–14:27	13:21–13:50	15:41–16:15	14:25–14:56	16:56–17:33	15:51–16:26	18:22–19:18	17:26–18:05	20:12–21:14
15	13:00–13:30	14:28–14:42	13:51–14:20	16:16–16:50	14:57–15:29	17:34–18:11	16:27–17:02	19:19–20:06	18:06–18:44	21:15–22:00
10	13:31–14:00	14:43–14:57	14:21–14:50	16:51–17:25	15:30–16:01	18:12–18:29	17:03–17:37	20:07–20:41	18:45–19:23	22:01–22:45
5	14:01–14:30	14:58–15:12	14:51–15:20	17:26–18:00	16:02–16:34	18:30–19:50	17:38–18:13	20:42–21:22	19:24–20:02	22:46–23:30
0	Did not attempt.									

Source: Adapted with permission from Reeves, M. (2002). *Peel Regional Police recruit fitness standards*. Brampton, ON: Peel Regional Police Service.

176 pounds is rounded to 180 pounds). Next, subtract 20 pounds—this amount (body weight minus 20 pounds) will give you a score of 10 out of 10. All other scores can be determined based on the number of plates lifted above or below this amount. For example, one plate less (body weight minus 30 pounds) will give a score of 9, two plates less would be a score of 8, and so on.

Bench press — Muscular strength test

Score (out of 10)	Age 20–29		Age 30–39	
	Males	Females	Males	Females
+1	+8 plates	+5 plates	+6 plates	+4 plates
+1	+5 plates	+4 plates	+4 plates	+3 plates
10	100% BW	100% BW	100% BW	100% BW
9	−1 plate	−1 plate	−1 plate	−1 plate
8	−2 plates	−2 plates	−2 plates	−2 plates
7	−3 plates	−3 plates	−3 plates	−3 plates
6	−4 plates	−4 plates	−4 plates	−4 plates
5	−5 plates	−5 plates	−5 plates	−5 plates
4	−6 plates	−6 plates	−6 plates	−6 plates
3	−7 plates	−7 plates	−7 plates	−7 plates
2	−8 plates	−8 plates	−8 plates	−8 plates
1	−9 plates	−9 plates	−9 plates	−9 plates

Source: Adapted with permission Reeves, M. (2002). *Peel Regional Police recruit fitness standards*. Brampton, ON: Peel Regional Police Service.

Plate Weights for Bench Press

These weights are used on the selectorized plate machine used by Peel Regional Police. Select your starting plate by using your body weight as a guide.

330 lb.	182 lb.
315 lb.	165 lb.
296 lb.	149 lb.
279 lb.	132 lb.
265 lb.	115 lb.
248 lb.	100 lb.
231 lb.	83 lb.
215 lb.	66 lb.
198 lb.	50 lb.

This test requires the applicant to lie supine on a flat bench either with knees bent up and feet flat on the bench or with legs bent at the knees such that the feet are in contact with the ground. Assistance is given to the applicant to lift the chosen weight until he or she has arms fully extended. When the participant indicates readiness, he or she will flex the arms, bringing the weight down until an angle of 90 degrees at the elbow is achieved at which time the weight will then be pressed back to the starting position. One maximum repetition only is required at the weight chosen by the applicant. You are permitted at total of three repetitions *if* you are successful on the previous.

Chin-ups

This test requires a functional range of flexibility, good elbow flexor strength, and back shoulder girdle strength. The participant is required to pull him- or herself off the ground by fully flexing the arms. The chin must be brought up above the level of the bar and the body is lowered until the angle at the elbow joint is approximately 90 degrees. The hands grip the bar in an underneath grip position while the movement is repeated continually over a period of 30 seconds.

Chin-ups — Muscular endurance test

Number of chin-ups completed in 30 seconds

Score (out of 10)	Age 20–29		Age 30–39	
	Males	Females	Males	Females
+1	30	20	27	16
+1	24	15	22	13
10	18	10	17	10
9	17	9	16	9
8	16	8	15	8
7	15	7	14	7
6	14	6	13	6
5	13	5	12	5
4	12	4	11	4
3	11	3	10	3
2	10	2	9	2
1	9	1	8	1

Source: Adapted with permission from Reeves, M. (2002). *Peel Regional Police recruit fitness standards.* Brampton, ON: Peel Regional Police Service.

100-Yard Sprint

Applicants are required to demonstrate their ability to have an adequate anaerobic capacity. A 100-yard sprint demonstrates an applicant's ability to pursue an individual.

Make sure that you have adequately warmed up. It is important to stretch your quadriceps and hamstring muscles adequately to ensure that you do not strain your muscles as you run the test.

PHYSICAL FITNESS LOG

As part of your physical fitness training goals, you should chart your progress throughout the two years. At the end of your first semester, you may have to change those goals that you have not been able to meet. Ultimately, it is your responsibility to know where you stand with your grades. Depending on the college, you will have certain standards to meet depending on which semester you are in. By charting your results, you will know where you stand and what areas you will have to address each semester.

Assignment 16.1 (in the appendix), "Physical Fitness Log," allows you to chart your progress.

100-Yard sprint — Anaerobic capacity test

Time to complete (seconds)

	Age 20–29		Age 30–39	
Score	Males	Females	Males	Females
20	10.5	13.0	11.0	13.5
19	11.0	13.5	11.5	14.0
18	11.5	14.0	12.0	14.5
17	12.0	14.5	12.5	15.0
16	12.5	15.0	13.0	15.5
15	13.0*	15.5*	13.5*	16.0*
14	13.5	16.0	14.0	16.5
12	14.0	16.5	14.5	17.0
10	14.5	17.0	15.0	17.5
8	15.0	17.5	15.5	18.0
6	15.5	18.0	16.0	18.5
4	16.0	18.5	16.5	19.0
2	16.5	19.0	17.0	19.5

* denotes standard.

Source: Adapted with permission from Reeves, M. (2002). *Peel Regional Police recruit fitness standards*. Brampton, ON: Peel Regional Police Service.

REFERENCES

Léger, L.A., & Lambert, J. (1982). A maximal multistage 20m shuttle run test to predict VO2max. *European Journal of Applied Physiology, 49*, 1–5.

Ministry of Public Safety and Security. (2002). *Fit to serve: Preparing for the PREP—The physical readiness evaluation for police.* Toronto: Queen's Printer for Ontario.

Ontario Police College. (2001, April). *Ontario Police College fitness standards.* Aylmer, ON: Author.

Police Fitness Personnel of Ontario. (1989). *The Ontario police fitness award program.* Toronto: Queen's Printer for Ontario.

Police Fitness Personnel of Ontario. (1998). *The Ontario police fitness award program.* Toronto: Police Services Division of the Ministry of the Solicitor General and Correctional Services and the Ontario Association of Chiefs of Police.

RCMP. (2005). The Royal Canadian Mounted Police Physical Abilities Requirement Evaluation (PARE) PARE PROTOCOL (updated June 2005).

Reeves, M. (2002). *Peel Regional Police recruit fitness standards.* Brampton, ON: Peel Regional Police Service.

Séguin, R. (2007). Division fitness lifestyle adviser, RCMP, Central Region, London, ON.

Shipley, Peter D. (2000, November). Cost benefit analysis of Ontario Provincial Police, OPFA. Toronto: Queen's Printer for Ontario.

APPENDIX

Assignments

ASSIGNMENT 1.1 WELLNESS

Complete the following questionnaires to determine how ready you are to make healthier choices concerning habits, nutrition, stress management, and physical activity.

F•A•N•T•A•S•T•I•C LIFESTYLE CHECKLIST

INSTRUCTIONS:

Unless otherwise specified, place a ✓ beside the box which best describes your behavior or situation in the past month.

*See back for instructions

F AMILY RIENDS	I have someone to talk to about things that are important to me	almost always	fairly often	some of the time	seldom	almost never
	I give and I receive affection	almost always	fairly often	some of the time	seldom	almost never
A CTIVITY	I am physically active (gardening, climbingstairs,walking,housework)	almost always	fairly often	some of the time	seldom	almost never
	I actively exercise for at least 20 min.eg.running,cycling,fast walk	5 or more times/week	4 times/week	3 times/week	1-2 times /week	less than once/week
N UTRITION	*I eat a balanced diet (See over)	almost always	fairly often	some of the time	seldom	almost never
	I often eat excess sugar or salt or animal fats or junk foods	none of these	one of these	two of these	three of these	four of these
	I am within ____ lbs. of my ideal weight	5 lbs (2 kg)	10 lbs (4 kg)	15 lbs (6 kg)	20 lbs (8 kg)	not within 20 lbs
T OBACCO TOXICS	I smoke tobacco	never smoked	quit over 5 yrs. ago	quit over a year ago	quit in past year	currently smoke
	I usually smoke ____ cigarets per day	none	5 or less	6-20	21-40	more than 40
	I use drugs such as marijuana, cocaine	never	almost never	only occasionally	fairly often	almost daily
	I overuse prescribed or "over the counter" drugs	never	almost never	only occasionally	fairly often	almost daily
	I drink caffeine-containing coffee, tea, or cola	never	1-2/day	3-6/day	7-10/day	more than 10/day
A LCOHOL	*My average alcohol intake per week is (See over)	0 - 7 drinks	8 - 10 drinks	11 - 13 drinks	14 - 20 drinks	more than 20 drinks
	I drink more than four drinks on an occasion	never	almost never	only occasionally	fairly often	almost daily
	I drive after drinking	never	almost never	only occasionally	once a month	often
S LEEP EATBELTS TRESS	I sleep well and feel rested	almost always	fairly often	some of the time	seldom	almost never
	I use seatbelts	always	most of the time	some of the time	seldom	never
	I am able to cope with the stresses in my life	almost always	fairly often	some of the time	seldom	almost never
	I relax and enjoy leisure time	almost always	fairly often	some of the time	seldom	almost never
T YPE OF PERSON ALITY	I seem to be in a hurry	almost never	seldom	some of the time	fairly often	almost always
	I feel angry or hostile	almost never	seldom	some of the time	fairly often	almost always
I NSIGHT	I am a positive or optimistic thinker	almost always	fairly often	some of the time	seldom	almost never
	I feel tense or uptight	almost never	seldom	some of the time	fairly often	almost always
	I feel sad or depressed	almost never	seldom	some of the time	fairly often	almost always
C AREER	I am satisfied with my job or role	almost always	fairly often	some of the time	seldom	never

STEP 1	Total the ✓s in each column	☐	☐	☐	☐	☐
STEP 2	Multiply the totals by the numbers indicated (Write in box below)	X4	X3	X2	X1	0
STEP 3	Add your scores across the bottom for your grand total	☐ +	☐ +	☐ +	☐ =	☐ % GRAND TOTAL

Name____________________________ Age__________ Sex M☐ F☐

FANTASTIC LIFESTYLE

***A balanced diet each day consists of:**

Milk and Milk Products

Children up to 11 years 2-3 servings
Adolescents 3-4 servings
Pregnant and nursing women 3-4 servings
Adults 2 servings

Meat, Fish, Poultry and Alternates 2 servings

Breads and Cereals 3-5 servings whole grain or enriched

Fruits and Vegetables 4-5 servings Include at least two vegetables

---

***1 DRINK =**

		CANADIAN	METRIC	U.S.
1 bottle beer	5% alcohol	12 oz.	340.8 ml	10 oz.
1 glass wine	12% alcohol	5 oz.	142 ml	4.5 oz.
1 shot spirits	40% alcohol	1.5 oz.	42.6 ml	1.25 oz.

What does your score mean?
If you score:

85-100%—Congratulations—You are in control.

70- 84%—Good work—You are on the right track.

60- 69%—Fair

40- 59%—Somewhat low—you could take more control.

0- 19%—You are in the danger zone (but honesty is your real strength).

Note: The total score does not mean that you have failed. There is always the chance to change your lifestyle—starting now. Look at the areas where you scored a **0** or **1** and decide which areas you want to work on first.

Tips:
1. Don't try to change all the areas at once. This will be too overwhelming for you.
2. Writing down your proposed changes and your overall goal will help you to succeed.
3. Make changes in small steps towards the overall goal.
4. Enlist the help of a friend to make similar changes and/or to support you in your attempts.
5. Congratulate yourself for achieving each step. Give yourself appropriate rewards.
6. Ask your family physician, nurse or health department for more information on any of these areas.

Source: © 1985 Dr. Douglas Wilson, Department of Family Medicine, McMaster University, Hamilton, Ontario, Canada, L8N 3Z5.

Physical Activity Readiness Questionnaire - PAR-Q (revised 2002)

PAR-Q & YOU

(A Questionnaire for People Aged 15 to 69)

Regular physical activity is fun and healthy, and increasingly more people are starting to become more active every day. Being more active is very safe for most people. However, some people should check with their doctor before they start becoming much more physically active.

If you are planning to become much more physically active than you are now, start by answering the seven questions in the box below. If you are between the ages of 15 and 69, the PAR-Q will tell you if you should check with your doctor before you start. If you are over 69 years of age, and you are not used to being very active, check with your doctor.

Common sense is your best guide when you answer these questions. Please read the questions carefully and answer each one honestly: check YES or NO.

YES	NO	
☐	☐	**1. Has your doctor ever said that you have a heart condition and that you should only do physical activity recommended by a doctor?**
☐	☐	**2. Do you feel pain in your chest when you do physical activity?**
☐	☐	**3. In the past month, have you had chest pain when you were not doing physical activity?**
☐	☐	**4. Do you lose your balance because of dizziness or do you ever lose consciousness?**
☐	☐	**5. Do you have a bone or joint problem (for example, back, knee or hip) that could be made worse by a change in your physical activity?**
☐	☐	**6. Is your doctor currently prescribing drugs (for example, water pills) for your blood pressure or heart condition?**
☐	☐	**7. Do you know of any other reason why you should not do physical activity?**

If you answered

YES to one or more questions

Talk with your doctor by phone or in person BEFORE you start becoming much more physically active or BEFORE you have a fitness appraisal. Tell your doctor about the PAR-Q and which questions you answered YES.

- You may be able to do any activity you want — as long as you start slowly and build up gradually. Or, you may need to restrict your activities to those which are safe for you. Talk with your doctor about the kinds of activities you wish to participate in and follow his/her advice.
- Find out which community programs are safe and helpful for you.

NO to all questions

If you answered NO honestly to all PAR-Q questions, you can be reasonably sure that you can:

- start becoming much more physically active – begin slowly and build up gradually. This is the safest and easiest way to go.
- take part in a fitness appraisal – this is an excellent way to determine your basic fitness so that you can plan the best way for you to live actively. It is also highly recommended that you have your blood pressure evaluated. If your reading is over 144/94, talk with your doctor before you start becoming much more physically active.

DELAY BECOMING MUCH MORE ACTIVE:

- if you are not feeling well because of a temporary illness such as a cold or a fever – wait until you feel better; or
- if you are or may be pregnant – talk to your doctor before you start becoming more active.

PLEASE NOTE: If your health changes so that you then answer YES to any of the above questions, tell your fitness or health professional. Ask whether you should change your physical activity plan.

Informed Use of the PAR-Q: The Canadian Society for Exercise Physiology, Health Canada, and their agents assume no liability for persons who undertake physical activity, and if in doubt after completing this questionnaire, consult your doctor prior to physical activity.

No changes permitted. You are encouraged to photocopy the PAR-Q but only if you use the entire form.

NOTE: If the PAR-Q is being given to a person before he or she participates in a physical activity program or a fitness appraisal, this section may be used for legal or administrative purposes.

"I have read, understood and completed this questionnaire. Any questions I had were answered to my full satisfaction."

NAME ____

SIGNATURE ____ DATE ________________________

SIGNATURE OF PARENT ________________________________ WITNESS ________________________
or GUARDIAN (for participants under the age of majority)

Note: This physical activity clearance is valid for a maximum of 12 months from the date it is completed and becomes invalid if your condition changes so that you would answer YES to any of the seven questions.

continued on other side...

...continued from other side

PAR-Q & YOU

Physical Activity Readiness Questionnaire - PAR-Q (revised 2002)

Canada's Physical Activity Guide to Healthy Active Living

Physical activity improves health.

Every little bit counts, but more is even better – everyone can do it!

Get active your way – build physical activity into your daily life...

- at home
- at school
- at work
- at play
- on the way

...that's active living!

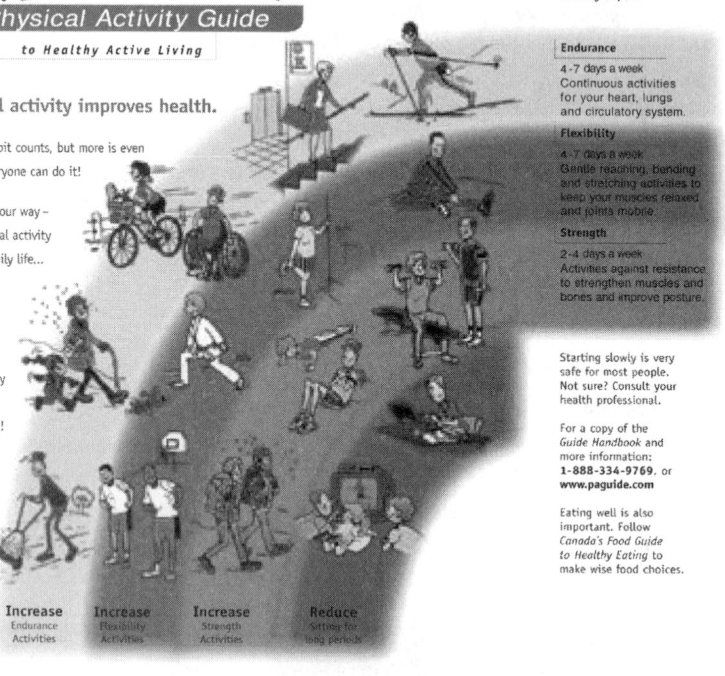

Choose a variety of activities from these three groups:

Endurance
4-7 days a week
Continuous activities for your heart, lungs and circulatory system.

Flexibility
4-7 days a week
Gentle reaching, bending and stretching activities to keep your muscles relaxed and joints mobile.

Strength
2-4 days a week
Activities against resistance to strengthen muscles and bones and improve posture.

Starting slowly is very safe for most people. Not sure? Consult your health professional.

For a copy of the *Guide Handbook* and more information: **1-888-334-9769**, or **www.paguide.com**

Eating well is also important. Follow *Canada's Food Guide to Healthy Eating* to make wise food choices.

Get Active Your Way, Every Day–For Life!

Scientists say accumulate 60 minutes of physical activity every day to stay healthy or improve your health. As you progress to moderate activities you can cut down to 30 minutes, 4 days a week. Add-up your activities in periods of at least 10 minutes each. Start slowly... and build up.

Time needed depends on effort

Very Light Effort	Light Effort *60 minutes*	Moderate Effort *30-60 minutes*	Vigorous Effort *20-30 minutes*	Maximum Effort
• Strolling • Dusting	• Light walking • Volleyball • Easy gardening • Stretching	• Brisk walking • Biking • Raking leaves • Swimming • Dancing • Water aerobics	• Aerobics • Jogging • Hockey • Basketball • Fast swimming • Fast dancing	• Sprinting • Racing

Range needed to stay healthy

You Can Do It – Getting started is easier than you think

Physical activity doesn t have to be very hard. Build physical activities into your daily routine.

- Walk whenever you can – get off the bus early, use the stairs instead of the elevator.
- Reduce inactivity for long periods, like watching TV.
- Get up from the couch and stretch and bend for a few minutes every hour.
- Play actively with your kids.
- Choose to walk, wheel or cycle for short trips.
- Start with a 10 minute walk – gradually increase the time.
- Find out about walking and cycling paths nearby and use them.
- Observe a physical activity class to see if you want to try it.
- Try one class to start – you don t have to make a long-term commitment.
- Do the activities you are doing now, more often.

Benefits of regular activity:

- better health
- improved fitness
- better posture and balance
- better self-esteem
- weight control
- stronger muscles and bones
- feeling more energetic
- relaxation and reduced stress
- continued independent living in later life

Health risks of inactivity:

- premature death
- heart disease
- obesity
- high blood pressure
- adult-onset diabetes
- osteoporosis
- stroke
- depression
- colon cancer

Health Canada Santé Canada — Canadian Society for Exercise Physiology

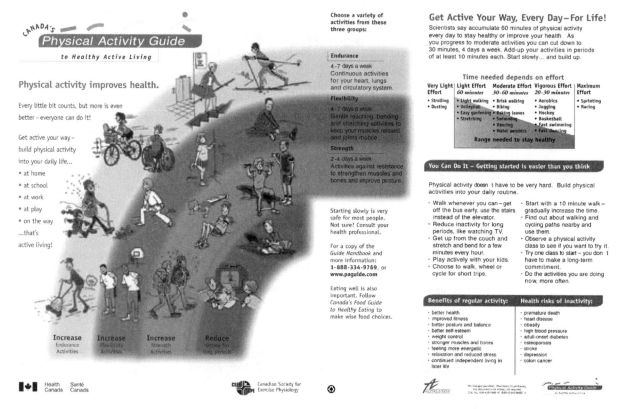

Source: Canada's Physical Activity Guide to Healthy Active Living, Health Canada, 1998 http://www.hc-sc.gc.ca/hppb/paguide/pdf/guideEng.pdf

FITNESS AND HEALTH PROFESSIONALS MAY BE INTERESTED IN THE INFORMATION BELOW:

The following companion forms are available for doctors' use by contacting the Canadian Society for Exercise Physiology (address below):

The **Physical Activity Readiness Medical Examination (PARmed-X)** – to be used by doctors with people who answer YES to one or more questions on the PAR-Q.

The **Physical Activity Readiness Medical Examination for Pregnancy (PARmed-X for Pregnancy)** – to be used by doctors with pregnant patients who wish to become more active.

References:

Arraix, G.A., Wigle, D.T., Mao, Y. (1992). Risk Assessment of Physical Activity and Physical Fitness in the Canada Health Survey Follow-Up Study. **J. Clin. Epidemiol.** 45:4 419-428.

Mottola, M., Wolfe, L.A. (1994). Active Living and Pregnancy, In: A. Quinney, L. Gauvin, T. Wall (eds.), **Toward Active Living: Proceedings of the International Conference on Physical Activity, Fitness and Health**. Champaign, IL: Human Kinetics.

PAR-Q Validation Report, British Columbia Ministry of Health, 1978.

Thomas, S., Reading, J., Shephard, R.J. (1992). Revision of the Physical Activity Readiness Questionnaire (PAR-Q). **Can. J. Spt. Sci.** 17:4 338-345.

For more information, please contact the:

Canadian Society for Exercise Physiology
202-185 Somerset Street West
Ottawa, ON K2P 0J2
Tel. 1-877-651-3755 • FAX (613) 234-3565
Online: www.csep.ca

The original PAR-Q was developed by the British Columbia Ministry of Health. It has been revised by an Expert Advisory Committee of the Canadian Society for Exercise Physiology chaired by Dr. N. Gledhill (2002).

Disponible en français sous le titre «Questionnaire sur l'aptitude à l'activité physique - Q-AAP (revisé 2002)».

Supported by: Health Canada Santé Canada

Source: Physical Activity Readiness Questionnaire (PAR-Q) © 2002. Used with permission from the Canadian Society for Exercise Physiology www.cesp.ca.

Physical Activity Readiness
Medical Examination
(revised 2002)

PARmed-X PHYSICAL ACTIVITY READINESS MEDICAL EXAMINATION

The PARmed-X is a physical activity-specific checklist to be used by a physician with patients who have had positive responses to the Physical Activity Readiness Questionnaire (PAR-Q). In addition, the Conveyance/Referral Form in the PARmed-X can be used to convey clearance for physical activity participation, or to make a referral to a medically-supervised exercise program.

Regular physical activity is fun and healthy, and increasingly more people are starting to become more active every day. Being more active is very safe for most people. The PAR-Q by itself provides adequate screening for the majority of people. However, some individuals may require a medical evaluation and specific advice (exercise prescription) due to one or more positive responses to the PAR-Q.

Following the participant's evaluation by a physician, a physical activity plan should be devised in consultation with a physical activity professional (CSEP-Professional Fitness & Lifestyle Consultant or CSEP-Exercise Therapist™). To assist in this, the following instructions are provided:

PAGE 1: • Sections A, B, C, and D should be completed by the participant BEFORE the examination by the physician. The bottom section is to be completed by the examining physician.

PAGES 2 & 3: • A checklist of medical conditions requiring special consideration and management.

PAGE 4: • Physical Activity & Lifestyle Advice for people who do not require specific instructions or prescribed exercise.

• Physical Activity Readiness Conveyance/Referral Form - an optional tear-off tab for the physician to convey clearance for physical activity participation, or to make a referral to a medically-supervised exercise program.

This section to be completed by the participant

A PERSONAL INFORMATION:

NAME ______

ADDRESS ______

______

TELEPHONE ______

BIRTHDATE ______ GENDER ______

MEDICAL No. ______

B PAR-Q: Please indicate the PAR-Q questions to which you answered YES

- ❑ Q 1 Heart condition
- ❑ Q 2 Chest pain during activity
- ❑ Q 3 Chest pain at rest
- ❑ Q 4 Loss of balance, dizziness
- ❑ Q 5 Bone or joint problem
- ❑ Q 6 Blood pressure or heart drugs
- ❑ Q 7 Other reason: ______

C RISK FACTORS FOR CARDIOVASCULAR DISEASE:

Check all that apply

- ❑ Less than 30 minutes of moderate physical activity most days of the week.
- ❑ Currently smoker (tobacco smoking 1 or more times per week).
- ❑ High blood pressure reported by physician after repeated measurements.
- ❑ High cholesterol level reported by physician.
- ❑ Excessive accumulation of fat around waist.
- ❑ Family history of heart disease.

Please note: *Many of these risk factors are modifiable. Please refer to page 4 and discuss with your physician.*

D PHYSICAL ACTIVITY INTENTIONS:

What physical activity do you intend to do?

______

______

______

This section to be completed by the examining physician

Physical Exam:

Ht	Wt	BP i) /
		BP ii) /

Conditions limiting physical activity:

- ❑ Cardiovascular ❑ Respiratory ❑ Other
- ❑ Musculoskeletal ❑ Abdominal

Tests required:

- ❑ ECG ❑ Exercise Test ❑ X-Ray
- ❑ Blood ❑ Urinalysis ❑ Other

Physical Activity Readiness Conveyance/Referral:

Based upon a current review of health status, I recommend:

Further Information:
- ❑ Attached
- ❑ To be forwarded
- ❑ Available on request

- ❑ No physical activity
- ❑ Only a medically-supervised exercise program until further medical clearance
- ❑ Progressive physical activity:
  - ❑ with avoidance of: ______
  - ❑ with inclusion of: ______
  - ❑ under the supervision of a CSEP-Professional Fitness & Lifestyle Consultant or CSEP-Exercise Therapist™
- ❑ Unrestricted physical activity–start slowly and build up gradually

Physical Activity Readiness
Medical Examination
(revised 2002)

PARmed-X PHYSICAL ACTIVITY READINESS MEDICAL EXAMINATION

Following is a checklist of medical conditions for which a degree of precaution and/or special advice should be considered for those who answered "YES" to one or more questions on the PAR-Q, and people over the age of 69. Conditions are grouped by system. Three categories of precautions are provided. Comments under Advice are general, since details and alternatives require clinical judgement in each individual instance.

	Absolute Contraindications	Relative Contraindications	Special Prescriptive Conditions	ADVICE
	Permanent restriction or temporary restriction until condition is treated, stable, and/or past acute phase.	Highly variable. Value of exercise testing and/or program may exceed risk. Activity may be restricted. Desirable to maximize control of condition. Direct or indirect medical supervision of exercise program may be desirable.	Individualized prescriptive advice generally appropriate: • limitations imposed; and/or • special exercises prescribed. May require medical monitoring and/or initial supervision in exercise program.	
Cardiovascular	❑ aortic aneurysm (dissecting) ❑ aortic stenosis (severe) ❑ congestive heart failure ❑ crescendo angina ❑ myocardial infarction (acute) ❑ myocarditis (active or recent) ❑ pulmonary or systemic embolism—acute ❑ thrombophlebitis ❑ ventricular tachycardia and other dangerous dysrhythmias (e.g., multi-focal ventricular activity)	❑ aortic stenosis (moderate) ❑ subaortic stenosis (severe) ❑ marked cardiac enlargement ❑ supraventricular dysrhythmias (uncontrolled or high rate) ❑ ventricular ectopic activity (repetitive or frequent) ❑ ventricular aneurysm ❑ hypertension—untreated or uncontrolled severe (systemic or pulmonary) ❑ hypertrophic cardiomyopathy ❑ compensated congestive heart failure	❑ aortic (or pulmonary) stenosis—mild angina pectoris and other manifestations of coronary insufficiency (e.g., post-acute infarct) ❑ cyanotic heart disease ❑ shunts (intermittent or fixed) ❑ conduction disturbances • complete AV block • left BBB • Wolff-Parkinson-White syndrome ❑ dysrhythmias—controlled ❑ fixed rate pacemakers	• clinical exercise test may be warranted in selected cases, for specific determination of functional capacity and limitations and precautions (if any). • slow progression of exercise to levels based on test performance and individual tolerance. • consider individual need for initial conditioning program under medical supervision (indirect or direct).
			❑ intermittent claudication	progressive exercise to tolerance
			❑ hypertension: systolic 160-180; diastolic 105+	progressive exercise; care with medications (serum electrolytes; post-exercise syncope; etc.)
Infections	❑ acute infectious disease (regardless of etiology)	❑ subacute/chronic/recurrent infectious diseases (e.g., malaria, others)	❑ chronic infections ❑ HIV	variable as to condition
Metabolic		❑ uncontrolled metabolic disorders (diabetes mellitus, thyrotoxicosis, myxedema)	❑ renal, hepatic & other metabolic insufficiency	variable as to status
			❑ obesity ❑ single kidney	dietary moderation, and initial light exercises with slow progression (walking, swimming, cycling)
Pregnancy		❑ complicated pregnancy (e.g., toxemia, hemorrhage, incompetent cervix, etc.)	❑ advanced pregnancy (late 3rd trimester)	refer to the "PARmed-X for PREGNANCY"

References:

Arraix, G.A., Wigle, D.T., Mao, Y. (1992). Risk Assessment of Physical Activity and Physical Fitness in the Canada Health Survey Follow-Up Study. **J. Clin. Epidemiol.** 45:4 419-428.

Mottola, M., Wolfe, L.A. (1994). Active Living and Pregnancy, In: A. Quinney, L. Gauvin, T. Wall (eds.), **Toward Active Living: Proceedings of the International Conference on Physical Activity, Fitness and Health**. Champaign, IL: Human Kinetics.

PAR-Q Validation Report, British Columbia Ministry of Health, 1978.

Thomas, S., Reading, J., Shephard, R.J. (1992). Revision of the Physical Activity Readiness Questionnaire (PAR-Q). **Can. J. Spt. Sci.** 17: 4 338-345.

The PAR-Q and PARmed-X were developed by the British Columbia Ministry of Health. They have been revised by an Expert Advisory Committee of the Canadian Society for Exercise Physiology chaired by Dr. N. Gledhill (2002).

No changes permitted. You are encouraged to photocopy the PARmed-X, but only if you use the entire form.

Disponible en français sous le titre
«Évaluation médicale de l'aptitude à l'activité physique (X-AAP)»

Continued on page 3...

Physical Activity Readiness
Medical Examination
(revised 2002)

	Special Prescriptive Conditions	ADVICE
Lung	❑ chronic pulmonary disorders	special relaxation and breathing exercises
	❑ obstructive lung disease ❑ asthma	breath control during endurance exercises to tolerance; avoid polluted air
	❑ exercise-induced bronchospasm	avoid hyperventilation during exercise; avoid extremely cold conditions; warm up adequately; utilize appropriate medication.
Musculoskeletal	❑ low back conditions (pathological, functional)	avoid or minimize exercise that precipitates or exasperates e.g., forced extreme flexion, extension, and violent twisting; correct posture, proper back exercises
	❑ arthritis—acute (infective, rheumatoid; gout)	treatment, plus judicious blend of rest, splinting and gentle movement
	❑ arthritis—subacute	progressive increase of active exercise therapy
	❑ arthritis—chronic (osteoarthritis and above conditions)	maintenance of mobility and strength; non-weightbearing exercises to minimize joint trauma (e.g., cycling, aquatic activity, etc.)
	❑ orthopaedic	highly variable and individualized
	❑ hernia	minimize straining and isometrics; stregthen abdominal muscles
	❑ osteoporosis or low bone density	avoid exercise with high risk for fracture such as push-ups, curl-ups, vertical jump and trunk forward flexion; engage in low-impact weight-bearing activities and resistance training
CNS	❑ convulsive disorder not completely controlled by medication	minimize or avoid exercise in hazardous environments and/or exercising alone (e.g., swimming, mountainclimbing, etc.)
	❑ recent concussion	thorough examination if history of two concussions; review for discontinuation of contact sport if three concussions, depending on duration of unconsciousness, retrograde amnesia, persistent headaches, and other objective evidence of cerebral damage
Blood	❑ anemia—severe (< 10 Gm/dl) ❑ electrolyte disturbances	control preferred; exercise as tolerated
Medications	❑ antianginal ❑ antiarrhythmic ❑ antihypertensive ❑ anticonvulsant ❑ beta-blockers ❑ digitalis preparations ❑ diuretics ❑ ganglionic blockers ❑ others	NOTE: consider underlying condition. Potential for: exertional syncope, electrolyte imbalance, bradycardia, dysrhythmias, impaired coordination and reaction time, heat intolerance. May alter resting and exercise ECG's and exercise test performance.
Other	❑ post-exercise syncope	moderate program
	❑ heat intolerance	prolong cool-down with light activities; avoid exercise in extreme heat
	❑ temporary minor illness	postpone until recovered
	❑ cancer	if potential metastases, test by cycle ergometry, consider non-weight bearing exercises; exercise at lower end of prescriptive range (40-65% of heart rate reserve), depending on condition and recent treatment (radiation, chemotherapy); monitor hemoglobin and lymphocyte counts; add dynamic lifting exercise to strengthen muscles, using machines rather than weights.

*Refer to special publications for elaboration as required

The following companion forms are available online: http://www.csep.ca/forms.asp

The **Physical Activity Readiness Questionnaire (PAR-Q)** - a questionnaire for people aged 15-69 to complete before becoming much more physically active.

The **Physical Activity Readiness Medical Examination for Pregnancy (PARmed-X for PREGNANCY)** - to be used by physicians with pregnant patients who wish to become more physically active.

For more information, please contact the:

Canadian Society for Exercise Physiology
202 - 185 Somerset St. West
Ottawa, ON K2P 0J2
Tel. 1-877-651-3755 • FAX (613) 234-3565 • Online: www.csep.ca

Note to physical activity professionals...

It is a prudent practice to retain the completed Physical Activity Readiness Conveyance/Referral Form in the participant's file.

Supported by: Health Canada Santé Canada

Continued on page 4...

Physical Activity Readiness
Medical Examination
(revised 2002)

PARmed-X PHYSICAL ACTIVITY READINESS MEDICAL EXAMINATION

Canada's Physical Activity Guide to Healthy Active Living

Physical activity improves health.

Every little bit counts, but more is even better – everyone can do it!

Get active your way – build physical activity into your daily life...

- at home
- at school
- at work
- at play
- on the way

...that's active living!

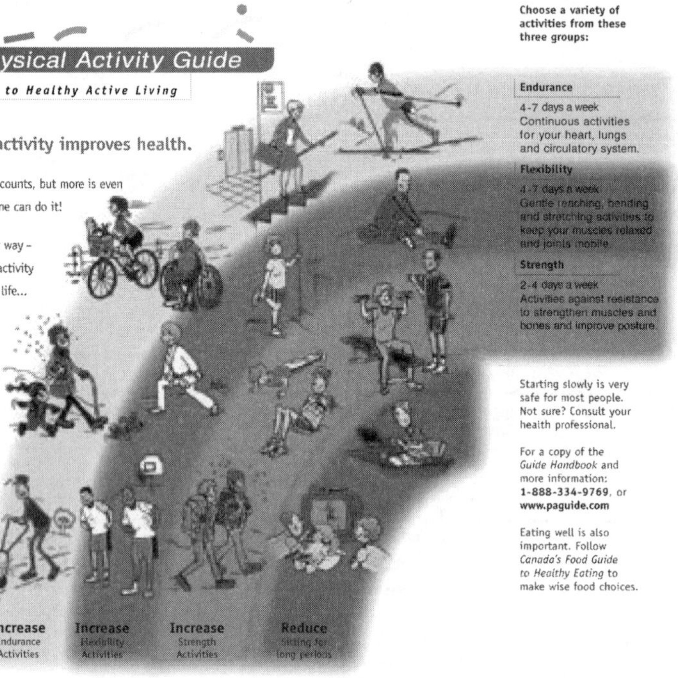

Choose a variety of activities from these three groups:

Endurance
4-7 days a week
Continuous activities for your heart, lungs and circulatory system.

Flexibility
4-7 days a week
Gentle reaching, bending and stretching activities to keep your muscles relaxed and joints mobile.

Strength
2-4 days a week
Activities against resistance to strengthen muscles and bones and improve posture.

Starting slowly is very safe for most people. Not sure? Consult your health professional.

For a copy of the *Guide Handbook* and more information: **1-888-334-9769**, or **www.paguide.com**

Eating well is also important. Follow *Canada's Food Guide to Healthy Eating* to make wise food choices.

Get Active Your Way, Every Day–For Life!

Scientists say accumulate 60 minutes of physical activity every day to stay healthy or improve your health. As you progress to moderate activities you can cut down to 30 minutes, 4 days a week. Add-up your activities in periods of at least 10 minutes each. Start slowly... and build up.

Time needed depends on effort

Very Light Effort	Light Effort *60 minutes*	Moderate Effort *30-60 minutes*	Vigorous Effort *20-30 minutes*	Maximum Effort
• Strolling • Dusting	• Light walking • Volleyball • Easy gardening • Stretching	• Brisk walking • Biking • Raking leaves • Swimming • Dancing • Water aerobics	• Aerobics • Jogging • Hockey • Basketball • Fast swimming • Fast dancing	• Sprinting • Racing

Range needed to stay healthy

You Can Do It – Getting started is easier than you think

Physical activity doesn t have to be very hard. Build physical activities into your daily routine.

- Walk whenever you can – get off the bus early, use the stairs instead of the elevator.
- Reduce inactivity for long periods, like watching TV.
- Get up from the couch and stretch and bend for a few minutes every hour.
- Play actively with your kids.
- Choose to walk, wheel or cycle for short trips.
- Start with a 10 minute walk – gradually increase the time.
- Find out about walking and cycling paths nearby and use them.
- Observe a physical activity class to see if you want to try it.
- Try one class to start – you don t have to make a long-term commitment.
- Do the activities you are doing now, more often.

Benefits of regular activity:	Health risks of inactivity:
· better health · improved fitness · better posture and balance · better self-esteem · weight control · stronger muscles and bones · feeling more energetic · relaxation and reduced stress · continued independent living in later life	· premature death · heart disease · obesity · high blood pressure · adult-onset diabetes · osteoporosis · stroke · depression · colon cancer

Health Canada Santé Canada

Canadian Society for Exercise Physiology

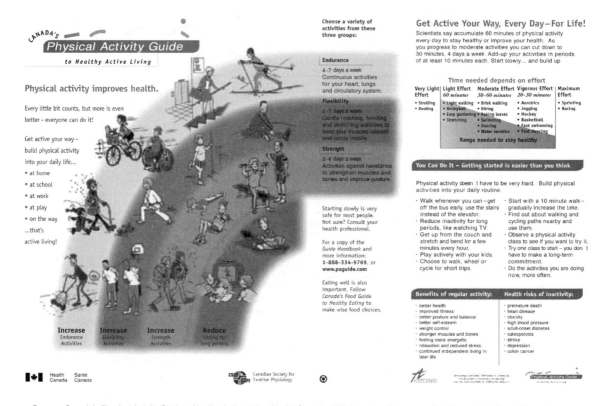

Source. Canada's Physical Activity Guide to Healthy Active Living, Health Canada, 1998 http://www.hc-sc.gc.ca/hppb/paguide/pdf/guideEng.pdf

PARmed-X Physical Activity Readiness Conveyance/Referral Form

Based upon a current review of the health status of ______________________________, I recommend:

- ❑ No physical activity
- ❑ Only a medically-supervised exercise program until further medical clearance
- ❑ Progressive physical activity
  - ❑ with avoidance of: ______________________________
  - ❑ with inclusion of: ______________________________
  - ❑ under the supervision of a CSEP-Professional Fitness & Lifestyle Consultant or CSEP-Exercise Therapist™
- ❑ Unrestricted physical activity — start slowly and build up gradually

Further Information:
- ❑ Attached
- ❑ To be forwarded
- ❑ Available on request

Physician/clinic stamp:

______________________________ M.D.

______________________________ 20______
(date)

NOTE: This physical activity clearance is valid for a maximum of six months from the date it is completed and becomes invalid if your medical condition becomes worse.

4

Source: Physical Activity Readiness Medical Examination (PARmed-X) © 2002. Used with permission from the Canadian Society for Exercise Physiology www.cesp.ca.

ASSIGNMENT 1.2 INFORMED CONSENT FOR TRAINING AND BFOR TESTING

After filling out the PAR-Q and prior to starting your fitness class, read and fill out this informed consent. Make sure to ask your instructor if you have any questions. If you have answered yes to any of the questions in the PAR-Q, please see your instructor.

Informed Consent to Undertake Training to Be Fit for ____________________ Course at ______________ College

I, ____________________________________, understand that ______________ Fitness Class evaluates my physical capacity as it applies to police work. I understand that I will participate in training and testing of policing job simulation tests, metabolic assessments (shuttle run, timed 1.5-mile runs, runs, sprints, stairs), and fitness assessments (e.g., curl-ups, push-ups, chin-ups, bench press). The successful completion of this training and testing shows that I possess the minimal physical abilities deemed essential for the performance of police work.

Physical Demands

I understand that we will work at training and testing that is physically demanding. During training and testing my heart rate may reach its maximal level, and may remain there for several minutes, thus placing me under heavy physical stress. The training and testing of various Bona Fide Occupational Requirement (BFOR) assessments will also challenge my muscular strength, agility, and coordination skills. I will be required to run various distances, run stairs, carry heavy objects (36–45 kg), climb over a 1.2-m (4-ft.) wall, run up and down stairs, drag a 68-kg (150-lb.) victim, grasp a 15-kg (33-lb.) mechanism and move the arms of the machine, and push/pull 32–36 kg (70–80 lb.), jump hurdles, jump over a vault rail, and wear weighted vests.

I state that I have no known medical or physical problems that may place me at risk during or following my performance of the test. I have read and signed the PAR-Q. I have not taken any medication, supplements, or stimulants other than whole food prepared naturally today. (If on medication that is approved, it is indicated on my medical clearance.) My health has not changed since my last medical examination. Prior to each class, I have followed the training/test preparation instructions, which include abstinence from alcohol and vigorous exercise for at least six hours prior to the test, abstinence from caffeinated products (including drinks that profess to provide you with energy and help keep you alert) for at least two hours prior to the test, avoidance of a *heavy* meal within three to four hours of the test, and abstinence from smoking for at least two hours prior to the test.

I understand the training/test as it has been explained and demonstrated to me, and I have had the opportunity to ask questions and practise on equipment. I will follow all safety procedures as outlined. Heart rate and blood pressure screening will be required and I will remain at the testing session until successfully screened after the test. It is my obligation to immediately inform the appraiser of any pain, discomfort, fatigue, or other symptoms that I may suffer during or immediately following the test. My understanding is that there are potential risks associated with training and testing, such as light-headedness, fainting, chest discomfort, and nausea. I willfully assume those risks.

No Compulsion

Any attempt of the BFOR or fitness training will be considered adherence to the college policy and will be recorded as such for my student file. I understand that UNDER NO CIRCUMSTANCES am I compelled to continue to complete the test should I decide to stop. I also will follow the instructions about safety, including slowing down or stopping immediately, IF INSTRUCTED TO DO SO by the test administrator and/or fitness instructor.

Full Effort

If I participate at full effort, I acknowledge that I have participated in physical activities such as sports or exercise requiring maximal exertion in the last two months and have a current medical clearance. If I am not used to maximal effort (last two months) then a maximal effort is NOT RECOMMENDED at this time.

Participant's Acknowledgement: ______________________________

Date: ______________________________

Witness: ______________________________

Date: ______________________________

Test Administrator/Fitness Instructor: ______________________________

______________________________ College

ASSIGNMENT 2.1 ASSESSING YOUR VALUES

Determine what values are important to you at this point in your life. Rank the following values on a scale of 1 (most important) to 5 (least important). Two or more values can share the same ranking. Space is provided at the end for adding values not mentioned in the list, if you wish. Knowing which values are most important to you will help you build short-term and long-term goals.

Value	Rank
Education	____
Lifelong learning	____
Keeping current on everyday legal issues	____
Mental health	____
Physical health	____
Fitness and exercise	____
Learning a new sport/skill	____
Being employed in law enforcement	____
Continuing education	____
Being well-paid	____
Being financially stable	____
Staying organized	____
Volunteering your time	____
Getting involved in student life	____
Joining college sports teams	____
Serving on student council	____
Time for yourself	____
Time for family and friends	____
Spiritual/religious life	____
Creative/artistic endeavours	____
A balanced lifestyle	____
A healthy diet	____
Free time/vacations	____
Reading/studying	____
Self-improvement	____
____________________	____
____________________	____
____________________	____
____________________	____
____________________	____

What are your five most important values?

1. ________________________________
2. ________________________________
3. ________________________________
4. ________________________________
5. ________________________________

Return to "Short- and Long-Term Goals" in chapter 2.

ASSIGNMENT 2.2 DETERMINING WHAT SUCCESS MEANS TO YOU

Most people define "success" as fulfilling their goals in life. To set a path for success, it is important to set goals and work toward achieving them. Try to set goals that you would like to achieve in your life by using the values from assignment 2.1 that you determined were important to you.

Fill in five of your goals in each of the following sections:

Personal Goals

What are your personal goals? What commitment do you have to fitness? Do you have goals relating to your health? What courses do you want to take to improve yourself (e.g., self-confidence, public speaking)? What type of fame—if any—do you want to achieve?

1. ______________________________
2. ______________________________
3. ______________________________
4. ______________________________
5. ______________________________

Family and Relationship Goals

What kinds of relationships do you want with your friends, parents, co-workers, and others? Do you want to be married, have children? How many close friends do you want?

1. ______________________________
2. ______________________________
3. ______________________________
4. ______________________________
5. ______________________________

Professional Goals

What kind of work do you want to do? What skills do you need to prepare for a job interview? Do you have the basic skills that employers are looking for? Name specific career areas or occupations.

1. ______________________________
2. ______________________________
3. ______________________________
4. ______________________________
5. ______________________________

Financial Goals

Are you choosing a career that will support your lifestyle? What type of material items do you want in life? Can you handle loans, credit cards, and other financial obligations? Do you have enough money to make it through the school year? Have you demonstrated a good credit rating (imperative for applying to a police agency)?

1. ______________________________
2. ______________________________
3. ______________________________
4. ______________________________
5. ______________________________

Lifestyle Goals

What types of leisure activities do you want to pursue? What interests do you want to develop? What kinds of vacations do you want to take? What type of community involvement do you want (volunteer work is paramount when applying to a law enforcement agency)?

1. ______________________________
2. ______________________________
3. ______________________________
4. ______________________________
5. ______________________________

Now try to rate your goals.

1. Choose the 10 goals you consider most important. Decide which of the 10 is most important, and write it down beside number 1 in the table below. Write your second most important goal beside number 2, and so on.
2. Rate the difficulty of achieving each of your 10 goals according to the following scale. Write these rating in the table.

   3 – I will have to work very hard to reach this goal.

   2 – I can reach this goal if I work at it.

   1 – I can reach this goal fairly easily.
3. Complete the Effects on Other Goals column as follows:
   - If the goal is likely to conflict with other goals on your list, write *conflicts with* in the column.
   - If the goal will probably have no effect on your other goals, write *none* in the column.
   - If working toward the goal will probably help you achieve another goal on your list, write *helps with* in the column.

Remember: if goals are in conflict, you must either find ways for them to work together or decide which goal to achieve first before moving on to the next one.

	Goal	Difficulty	Effects on Other Goals
1.			
2.			
3.			
4.			
5.			
6.			
7.			
8.			
9.			
10.			

Based on the goals that you have listed, comment on what success means to you.

ASSIGNMENT 2.3 DEVELOPING YOUR SHORT-TERM GOALS TO ACHIEVE LONG-TERM GOALS

Now that you have assessed your values, formulate one or two goals for each of the areas mentioned in assignment 2.2 (personal, family and relationship, professional, financial, and lifestyle). These goals should be tied to the values you ranked the highest. Below are a number of questions you might want to ask yourself before writing down the goals and action plans to accomplish the ones you chose. Remember that you need to reassess at the end of each semester if they are specific goals. Some of the questions that you may want to ask yourself include:

- Have I prioritized the five most important goals for the next two years?
- Do they reflect my most important values?
- Will my goals help me obtain the skills that law enforcement demands?
- Am I physically fit to an acceptable level, and am I committed to maintaining fitness throughout my life?
- Do I meet the academic, medical, and physical requirements for the career I am pursuing?

Now fill out the Smart Goal Setting & Action Planner on the following page. After four weeks, assess your progress using assignment 2.4, Summary of Goal-Setting Results—Successes, Barriers, and Strategies to Overcome Challenges.

SMART GOAL SETTING & ACTION PLANNER — 4-Week Planner

SMART: Specific, Measurable, Attainable, Realistic, Timed

Start Date	Completed Date

NUTRITION GOAL (long term)

Short-Term Goal Statement: *Over the next 4 weeks, I will …*								
Action Steps	**Weekly check box ✓ or ✗ depending on achievement**							
1.								
2.								
3.								
Reward upon Completion								

PHYSICAL ACTIVITY GOAL (long term)

Short-Term Goal Statement: *Over the next 4 weeks, I will …*								
Action Steps	**Weekly check box ✓ or ✗ depending on achievement**							
1.								
2.								
3.								
Reward upon Completion								

TIME-MANAGEMENT GOAL (long term)

Short-Term Goal Statement: *Over the next 4 weeks, I will …*								
Action Steps	**Weekly check box ✓ or ✗ depending on achievement**							
1.								
2.								
3.								
Reward upon Completion								

OTHER GOAL (Long Term)

Short-Term Goal Statement: *Over the next 4 weeks, I will …*								
Action Steps	**Weekly check box ✓ or ✕ depending on achievement**							
1.								
2.								
3.								
Reward upon Completion								

SUCCESS INDICATORS

1.
2.
3.
4.

THINGS TO RE-EVALUATE (for the next four weeks)

1.
2.
3.
4.

Source: Adapted from Canadian Physical Activity, Fitness & Lifestyle Appraisal: CSEP-Health & Fitness Program's Appraisal and Counselling Strategy, Third Edition © 2003.

ASSIGNMENT 2.4 SUMMARY OF GOAL-SETTING RESULTS—SUCCESSES, BARRIERS, AND STRATEGIES TO OVERCOME CHALLENGES

	Goal	Covering Dates of:
What I felt went well and why in the following areas	Nutrition	
	Physical Activity	
	Time Management	
	Other	

	Goal	Covering Dates of:
What I felt did not go well and why in the following areas	Nutrition	
	Physical Activity	
	Time Management	
	Other	

	Goal	Covering Dates of:
Strategies I will try in order to overcome future barriers in the following areas	Nutrition	
	Physical Activity	
	Time Management	
	Other	

What have I learned?	
Where do I need to go from here?	
Who/what can help me accomplish my goals?	

Teacher's Comments

ASSIGNMENT 2.5 MISSION STATEMENT

Prepare a mission statement that incorporates the goals you prioritized earlier.

Five Top Goals (from assignment 2.3)

1. ______________________________

2. ______________________________

3. ______________________________

4. ______________________________

5. ______________________________

Mission Statement

ASSIGNMENT 3.1 WHERE DOES ALL YOUR TIME GO?

Think back over the past seven days and estimate how much time you spent on each of the following activities:

Activity	Hours
Classroom learning	________
Homework	________
Computer use (games, Internet use, word processing, etc.)	________
Time spent in the college cafeteria	________
Library use	________
Fitness training (outside of class)	________
Recreational activities	________
Meal preparation	________
Meal consumption	________
Grocery shopping	________
Other shopping	________
Laundry and other household chores	________
Commuting	________
Waiting in line	________
Speaking on the telephone	________
Text messaging	________
Searching the Web, reading blogs, etc.	________
Chatting online	________
Sleeping	________
Grooming and personal hygiene activities	________
Watching television	________
Reading the newspaper or books unrelated to academic work	________
Time spent with family or significant other	________
Time spent with friends	________
Attending meetings of clubs and other organizations	________
Volunteer work	________
Paid work	________
Other activities:	________
________________________________	________
________________________________	________
________________________________	________
Total time	________

Evaluating Your Time-Management Skills

1. A week has 168 hours. Was your total within 10 percent of this figure? If yes, can you explain why?

____

____

____

____

____

____

2. If your total was well below 168 hours, can you account for the lost time? Does the lost time indicate that there are issues and priorities in your life that are not being addressed? Make specific comments.

____

____

____

____

____

____

3. If your total was well above 168 hours, how do you account for this? Make specific comments.

____

____

____

____

____

____

4. What have you learned about your time-management skills? What skills do you need to work on (avoiding procrastination, prioritizing your time, etc.)?

____

____

____

____

____

____

ASSIGNMENT 3.2 TRACKING YOUR TIME

For the next seven days, use the time-management chart at the end of this assignment to track your activities. Colour-code the chart to analyze where you are spending your time. Confine yourself to the following categories:

- *Black* Time-wasters (wasting time between classes, standing in lines, etc.)
- *Dark blue* Duties, obligations (includes work hours)
- *Light blue* School hours
- *Dark green* Fitness and recreational activities
- *Light green* Physical needs, including grooming and personal hygiene (including the time it takes you to get ready for school, work, dates, etc.) and meal preparation and eating time
- *Pink* Transportation (getting to and from school, work, social activities)
- *Orange* Intellectual needs (reading, studying, doing research)
- *Red* Personal needs (time for yourself)
- *Dark purple* Volunteer work
- *Light purple* Time spent on the phone and Internet for personal reasons
- *Yellow* Fun activities, including social time (at school, and evenings and weekends)
- *Grey* Sleep

You may add additional colours to reflect additional responsibilities. Try to fill the chart out at least three times during the day—we all tend to forget the time we spend doing trivial things like reading junk mail, sitting in the cafeteria talking to classmates, changing for gym class, making meals, doing dishes, tidying up, and talking on the phone. Some people include how they feel periodically during the day, whether they are alert, lethargic, tired, or energetic. This may help you assess whether your circadian rhythm (discussed in chapter 14) affects your productivity or whether you need to look at your eating habits.

Some people who struggle with time management prefer to keep track of 15-minute increments so that they can see more clearly where their time is going. You may want to do this as well. Remember that this assignment takes only a few minutes if you do it over the course of your day. You will not be as accurate if you only try to write it down at the end of each day.

At the end of the seven days, look over your chart and answer the following questions:

1. Do you use your time effectively? Why or why not?

____

____

____

____

____

____

____

____

2. Which time periods do you use most effectively?

____

____

____

____

____

3. Which time periods do you use least effectively?

____

____

____

____

____

4. Were you able to achieve all your goals for the week?

____

____

____

____

____

5. Does the time of day affect your productivity level (i.e., are there times during the day when you are more efficient, more alert, more energetic)?

____

____

____

____

____

6. Does your time management for the week raise any issues that need to be addressed? What could you change to improve your time management?

____

____

____

____

____

____

TIME-MANAGEMENT CHART

Time	Monday	Tuesday	Wednesday	Thursday	Friday	Saturday	Sunday
05:00							
05:30							
06:00							
06:30							
07:00							
07:30							
08:00							
08:30							
09:00							
09:30							
10:00							
10:30							
11:00							
11:30							
12:00							
12:30							
13:00							
13:30							
14:00							
14:30							
15:00							
15:30							
16:00							
16:30							
17:00							
17:30							
18:00							
18:30							
19:00							
19:30							
20:00							
20:30							
21:00							
21:30							
22:00							
22:30							
23:00							
23:30							
24:00							
00:30							
01:00							
01:30							
02:00							
02:30							
03:00							
03:30							
04:00							
04:30							

ASSIGNMENT 3.3 YOUR TO-DO LIST FOR THIS WEEK

Using the acitivity headings below as a guideline, create a to-do list of essential, regular, and optional activities for this week. The list should include all of your formal job duties, special projects you want to complete, your daily/weekly routine responsibilities, and other tasks you would like to see accomplished.

Essential activities

1. ______________________________
2. ______________________________
3. ______________________________
4. ______________________________

Regular activities

1. ______________________________
2. ______________________________
3. ______________________________
4. ______________________________

Optional activities

1. ______________________________
2. ______________________________
3. ______________________________
4. ______________________________

Using the activity chart on the next page, take these tasks and estimate the time for each, their importance, priority, and whether the task could be delegated. Set dates for follow-up and deadlines for each. This can be done on a weekly basis to assist you with developing an action plan for time management.

ACTIVITY CHART FOR WEEK OF :

	Activity Description	Estimated Time	Importance					Potential for Delegation	Person to Whom Task Is to Be Delegated	Follow-up Date	Priority					Deadline	Completed
			1	2	3	4	5				1	2	3	4	5		
1.																	
2.																	
3.																	
4.																	
5.																	
6.																	
7.																	
8.																	
9.																	
10.																	
11.																	
12.																	

ASSIGNMENT 3.4 ASSESSING YOUR LEVEL OF PROCRASTINATION

1. What are your time-wasters? How do you deal with them (e.g., slow start/ procrastination, disorganization, diversion, interruptions)?

Time-waster	Method of dealing with time-waster
•	
•	
•	
•	
•	
•	
•	
•	

2. Everyone procrastinates at some point. How do you get yourself going on a project or completing a task?

3. What techniques do you use to keep yourself going, especially on unpleasant or boring tasks? How do you motivate yourself to complete the task?

4. How do you deal with or minimize interruptions?

5. Do you know how to delegate tasks? Why or why not?

6. Based on the answers above, do you need to work on procrastination skills? If so, what would be a good first step?

ASSIGNMENT 4.1 HEALTH BENEFITS OF PHYSICAL ACTIVITY

Drawing on the information presented in chapter 4 and on your own knowledge, list and explain eight health benefits of physical activity.

1. ______________________________

2. ______________________________

3. ______________________________

4. ______________________________

5. ______________________________

6. ______________________________

7. ______________________________

8. ______________________________

ASSIGNMENT 4.2 PHYSICAL AND PSYCHOLOGICAL BENEFITS OF PHYSICAL ACTIVITY

List five physical benefits of physical activity that are important to you and that you would like to set as fitness training goals. Comment on why they are important to you.

1. ______________________________

2. ______________________________

3. ______________________________

4. ______________________________

5. ______________________________

Now do the same for five psychological benefits of physical activity.

1.

2.

3.

4.

5.

ASSIGNMENT 4.3 REVIEWING YOUR FITNESS TRAINING GOALS

Review the fitness training goals that you set for yourself in assignment 4.2. Do they address some of the principles that we have just examined? If you need to adjust your fitness training goals, go ahead. Be aware that these are short-term goals and therefore a reflection of your long-term goals. Accordingly, they should be continually reassessed and, if necessary, modified. Set a review date three to four months away. Once you pick your goals, use the information that you have learned from chapter 4 to pick training techniques that you can use to accomplish these goals.

Short-Term Goals

1. ______________________________

____

____

____

Physical training techniques needed to accomplish this goal:

____

____

____

2. ______________________________

____

____

____

Physical training techniques needed to accomplish this goal:

____

____

____

3. ______________________________

____

____

____

Physical training techniques needed to accomplish this goal:

____

____

____

Long-Term Goals

1. ______________________________
____
____
____

Physical training techniques needed to accomplish this goal:

____
____
____

2. ______________________________
____
____
____

Physical training techniques needed to accomplish this goal:

____
____
____

3. ______________________________
____
____
____

Physical training techniques needed to accomplish this goal:

____
____
____

______________	______________	______________
Date	Witness	Review date

ASSIGNMENT 5.1 ASSESSING YOUR CARDIORESPIRATORY FITNESS LEVEL

Before you begin training, you should assess your cardiorespiratory fitness level, even if aerobic exercise is already a part of your routine. The following questions are designed to assist you.

1. What, if anything, are you doing to train your cardiorespiratory system?

____

____

____

____

____

____

2. Do your workouts follow the FITT formula? How many times a week do you participate in aerobic activities (*frequency*)? What is the level of your activities (*intensity*)? How long is each session (*time*)? What kinds of activities do you participate in (*type*)?

F (Frequency) times per week ______________________________

I (Intensity) ______________________________

T (Time) minutes per workout ______________________________

T (Type) ______________________________

3. If you are participating in aerobic activities, what do you think are the benefits?

____

____

____

____

____

4. If you do not regularly participate in aerobic activities, what strategies do you think you need to begin participating in a regular program?

____

____

____

____

____

5. What types of aerobic activities do you think will help you train to be successful in the 1.5-mile run, shuttle run, and Bona Fide Occupational Requirements (e.g., PREP, PARE)?

____

____

____

____

____

6. What types of interval aerobic and anaerobic training do you think you have to incorporate to assist you to easily complete jumping the 4-ft. (1.2-m) wall, going over the vault rail, completing the 12 sets of stairs in the PARE test, and completing the running involved in the PARE circuit?

____

____

____

____

____

ASSIGNMENT 5.2
DETERMINING YOUR RESTING HEART RATE AND TARGET HEART RATE

To determine your true resting heart rate, you should test yourself first thing in the morning, before getting out of bed. Test yourself again later in the day.

Resting heart rate = ____________ bpm

Heart rate later in the day = ____________ bpm

Is there a large difference between your resting heart rate and your heart rate later in the day? If so, can you account for it? Be aware that caffeine, smoking, physical activity, stress, and even eating can affect your heart rate. Is your heart rate later in the day at a healthy level (lower than 100 bpm)?

Comment:

____

____

____

____

____

____

Determine Your Target Heart Rate

Your target heart rate should be between 70 and 85% of your maximal heart rate. First, subtract your age from 220 to determine your maximal heart rate (MHR). Then, use your MHR to determine your target heart rate.

MHR = 220 – ____________ = ____________ bpm

70% MHR = 0.70 × ____________ = ____________ bpm

85% MHR = 0.85 × ____________ = ____________ bpm

Your target heart rate is between ____________ bpm and ____________ bpm.

Attempt a few aerobic activities to determine whether you are exercising within your target heart rate. If you are below 70 percent MHR, what can you do to get up to your target range? If you are above 85 percent MHR and not fit, what considerations should you be aware of?

ASSIGNMENT 5.3 SETTING UP YOUR CARDIORESPIRATORY FITNESS PROGRAM

Drawing on the material in chapter 5 and other sources, set up a cardiorespiratory fitness program for the semester. Include the cardiorespiratory exercises you most enjoy and create a program that follows the FITT formula.

Goals (for one semester):

Cardiorespiratory activities you want to engage in (remember to include aerobic and anaerobic activities):

Cardiorespiratory program (based on the FITT formula):

Date to check benchmarks for goals: ______________________

Success markers (based on semester goals):

Strategies for potential barriers (What barriers might you face with your aerobic plan? What can you do to be successful?):

____

____

____

____

____

____

Maintaining a Cardiorespiratory Fitness Log

For each semester you may be required to maintain a fitness profile, including a log of the cardiorespiratory activities you engage in. You are encouraged to record all cardiorespiratory activities, including activities outside class. Use the blank log below (photocopy extra pages as needed). The log includes sections for noting the weather (which can affect outdoor activities) and recording your comments on how the workouts went. Your instructor will advise you on the specific requirements for your fitness profile and log.

CARDIORESPIRATORY FITNESS LOG

Activity	Date	Duration of Activity	Distance (if applicable)	Intensity Check (indicate heart rate monitoring, Borg scale, or talk test)
	 Weather			Comments
	 Weather			Comments
	 Weather			Comments
	 Weather			Comments
	 Weather			Comments
	 Weather			Comments
	 Weather			Comments
	 Weather			Comments
	 Weather			Comments
	 Weather			Comments
	 Weather			Comments
	 Weather			Comments
	 Weather			Comments
	 Weather			Comments

ASSIGNMENT 6.1 DETERMINING YOUR ONE-REPETITION MAXIMUM (1RM) FOR BENCH PRESS

Muscular strength plays a vital role throughout an individual's life. Strength develops quite rapidly during the development years, but as a person get older, strength levels begin to decrease significantly. When assessing an individual's muscular strength, most of the time a hand-held dynamometer is used, which measures grip strength. There is a strong correlation between grip strength and overall body strength. There are established norms for gender and age. You will find standards that are used by Peel Regional Police Service in chapter 16.

There are also one-repetition maximum formulas for various lifts (such as bench press, leg press, or squats) that are used to determine relative strength norms.

The following is the formula for determining a **one-repetition maximum (1RM)** from a submaximal test:

Weight lifted (for 2–20 repetitions) / [1.0 – (# of reps × 0.02)] = 1RM

For example, if an individual bench-presses 225 lb. 10 times, the formula would read:

225 divided by [1.0 – (10 × 0.02)], which is 225 divided by 0.8 = 281.25 lb. 1RM

To determine **relative strength**, take the individual's 1RM and divide it by his or her body weight in pounds.

Example: 281.25/195 = 1.44 (195 lb. being the body weight)

This individual has an upper-body relative strength that is 1.44 times his body weight (or 144 percent of his body weight).

The following are **norms established for relative strength**, with each norm being a percentage of body weight (in pounds).

	Upper Body	**Lower Body**	
	Bench Press	**Squats**	**Leg Press**
Excellent	1.5+	2.0+	3+
Good	1.25	1.75	2.75
Average	1.0	1.5	2.5
Fair	0.85–0.99	1.35	2.25
Poor	Below 0.85	1.25	Below 2.25

Source: Kraemer, W.J., & Fry, A.C. (1995). Strength testing: Development and evaluation of methodology. In P. Maud & C. Foster (Eds.), *Physiological assessment of human fitness* (pp. 115-138). Champaign, IL: Human Kinetics.

Determining Your 1RM for Bench Press

(for 2–20 repetitions)

$$1\text{RM} = \text{weight lifted} / [1.0 - (\text{\# of reps} \times 0.02)]$$

Weight lifted = __________ lb.

# of repetitions = ________

1RM = ___________ lb. / [1.0 – (__________ × 0.02)]

1RM = ___________ lb.

My potential for one maximal repetition for bench press could be _________ lb.

Look up bench press standards to see your potential score for grade (chapter 16).

Determining Your Relative Strength

$$\text{Relative strength} = 1\text{RM} / \text{Body weight}$$

Relative strength = _________ / ________

Relative strength = __________

Now go to the **norms established for relative strength** and determine what level you are at.

____

Comment on your maximal repetition and your relative strength. Are you where you want to be? Are you meeting the standards for bench press? Set a goal as to where you want to be by the end of the year.

____

____

____

____

____

____

____

____

ASSIGNMENT 6.2 DESIGNING YOUR STRENGTH AND ENDURANCE TRAINING PROGRAM

Before designing a strength and endurance training program, determine your training goal. Table 6.1 lists the possible goals.

1. List the goals of your strength and endurance training program, and indicate what sort of workout is necessary for each. Specify the number of exercises associated with each goal. Goals can be general, such as developing greater muscle definition, or specific, such as increasing power to withstand an altercation. If your goal is to develop a specific muscle group, note that as well.

   - ____
   - ____
   - ____
   - ____

2. Based on your goals, choose 6–10 exercises to perform during each weight training session. Pick exercises for each muscle group. Record them on the chart on the next page.
3. Choose starting weights. Follow the guidelines in chapter 6 to determine what you can easily lift for 10–12 repetitions.
4. Choose a starting number of sets and repetitions. The optimal pattern for a weight training workout includes three sets of 10–12 repetitions for each exercise. If your program is focusing on strength alone, your sets can contain fewer repetitions using a heavier load.
5. Choose the number of training sessions per week. Choose a frequency between two and four days per week (three days per week is recommended).
6. Monitor your progress using a workout card. An example that you can photocopy is provided on p. 413.

EXERCISES FOR A WEIGHT TRAINING PROGRAM

Exercise	Muscle(s) developed	Weight (kg or lb.)	Repetitions	Sets	Frequency (check √)						
					S	M	T	W	R	F	S

WORKOUT CARD FOR:

Exercise		Date																							
	Wt																								
	Set																								
	Reps																								
	Wt																								
	Set																								
	Reps																								
	Wt																								
	Set																								
	Reps																								
	Wt																								
	Set																								
	Reps																								
	Wt																								
	Set																								
	Reps																								
	Wt																								
	Set																								
	Reps																								
	Wt																								
	Set																								
	Reps																								
	Wt																								
	Set																								
	Reps																								
	Wt																								
	Set																								
	Reps																								

ASSIGNMENT 7.1 DESIGNING A STRETCHING PROGRAM

1. Determine how flexible you are.

   a. Sit and reach (or trunk forward flexion)

   One of the tests in the Ontario Police Fitness Award (OPFA) Standards is the sit and reach. It is a measure of posterior hip flexibility. Short hip flexors can lead to a higher risk of back problems and injuries.

   Before you attempt the test, warm up your hamstring and back muscles with a light aerobic activity for a few minutes. Add static stretching. When you are ready, take off your shoes and sit in front of the sit-and-reach apparatus with your feet flat against it. With your arms reaching forward, put one hand on top of the other. Reach as far forward as you can along the measurements. Hold the position for at least three seconds. *Do not bounce.* Repeat the test once.

   From your first attempt during class assessment, record how you did and how it compares with the scores in chapter 16. Touching your toes is reaching 26 cm.

   Sit and reach measurement—Attempt 1: ____________________

   Sit and reach measurement—Attempt 2: ____________________

   Score: ____________________

   b. Shoulder flexibility

   Raise your right arm with your elbow bent behind your back. At the same time, bring your left arm over your shoulder and reach down your back as far as you can. Try to cross your left-hand fingers over your right hand. Repeat on the other side.

   Rating: Fail to touch fingers = Below average

   Touch fingers = Average

   Overlap fingers = Above average

   Right shoulder flexibility: ____________________

   Left shoulder flexibility: ____________________

   c. Low-back stretch

   Lie on your back. While bending your knees, grasp the back of your thighs and pull the knees toward your chest. To have good flexibility, your upper legs should touch your chest.

   Pass: ____________________

   Room for improvement: ____________________

   d. Hip flexor stretch

   Lie on your back. With your left leg straight on the floor, try to pull your right knee to your chest by grasping the back of your right thigh. To pass, your right upper thigh must touch your chest while your straight left leg remains in contact with the floor. Repeat on the other side.

Right hip flexor

Pass: ____________________

Room for improvement: ____________________

Left hip flexor

Pass: ____________________

Room for improvement: ____________________

e. Quadriceps stretch

Lie on your stomach with your knees together. Keeping your left leg straight, pull your right heel toward your buttocks by grasping your ankle. To pass, you should be able to touch your heel to your buttocks. Repeat on the other side.

Right quadriceps

Pass: ____________________

Room for improvement: ____________________

Left quadriceps

Pass: ____________________

Room for improvement: ____________________

2. Comment on how you did in these tests and how flexible you are in general. Describe your strengths and weaknesses.

____

____

____

____

____

____

____

____

____

3. Based on your assessment and comments, set some specific goals regarding a stretching program.

Goal 1: ____________________

Goal 2: ____________________

Goal 3: ____________________

4. Based on the information provided in chapter 7 and on the FITT principle, design a stretching program that will fit your needs. Record the exercises on the chart on the next page.

EXERCISES FOR A STRETCHING PROGRAM

Exercise	Muscle(s) stretched	Repetitions	Frequency (check ✓) S	M	T	W	R	F	S

ASSIGNMENT 8.1 PORTION DISTORTION

Restaurants have food portions that have enlarged significantly since the 1950s and 1960s when fast food chains became mainstream. The idea of "super-sizing" portions to attract sales have, in some cases, provided enough food for at least two people. With portion growth have come increasing waistlines and body weight.

Go to the National Heart, Lung and Blood Institute (NHLBI) Portion Distortion Interactive Quizzes at http://hin.nhlbi.nih.gov/portion.

The two Portion Distortion quizzes compare portions now with those that were available 20 years ago. The quizzes address caloric disparity and how much physical activity it would require to burn off the extra calories.

Comment on your results. How well did you do in determining caloric content and the amount of physical activity required to burn off the extra calories provided by today's portions? Do you need to look at what you are consuming more closely?

ASSIGNMENT 8.2 NUTRITIONAL LABELLING

At the Health Canada website, go to the Food and Nutrition page and take the Interactive Nutrition Label and Quiz at www.hc-sc.gc.ca/fn-an/label-etiquet/nutrition/interactive/index_e.html.

First, go to the Interactive Nutrition Label.

List the six components of the new food label that was required for food products in Canada since December 12, 2005.

1. ______________________________
2. ______________________________
3. ______________________________
4. ______________________________
5. ______________________________
6. ______________________________

Now, go the Interactive Nutrition Label Quiz. Comment on the results of your knowledge. Record your score and make two comments regarding what you learned doing the quiz.

____
____
____
____
____
____
____
____
____
____
____
____
____
____
____
____
____
____

ASSIGNMENT 9.1 DETERMINING YOUR BODY MASS INDEX (BMI)

To determine your BMI, follow these steps:

1. Measure your height in metres (m) to the nearest 0.005 m (that is, to the nearest half-centimetre).

   = ______________ m

2. Convert your height to metres squared (that is, multiply the figure by itself—e.g., 1.955 m × 1.955 m).

   = ______________ m^2

3. Measure your weight in kilograms (kg) to the nearest 0.1 kg.

   = ______________ kg

4. Determine your BMI by dividing your weight in kilograms by your height in metres squared.

   BMI = ______________ kg ÷ ______________ m^2

   BMI = ______________ kg/m^2

5. Comment on your BMI. According to the number, do you have to be concerned? Why or why not?

   ____

   ____

   ____

   ____

   ____

   ____

   ____

   ____

   ____

   ____

   ____

   ____

Alternatively, you can use the chart below.

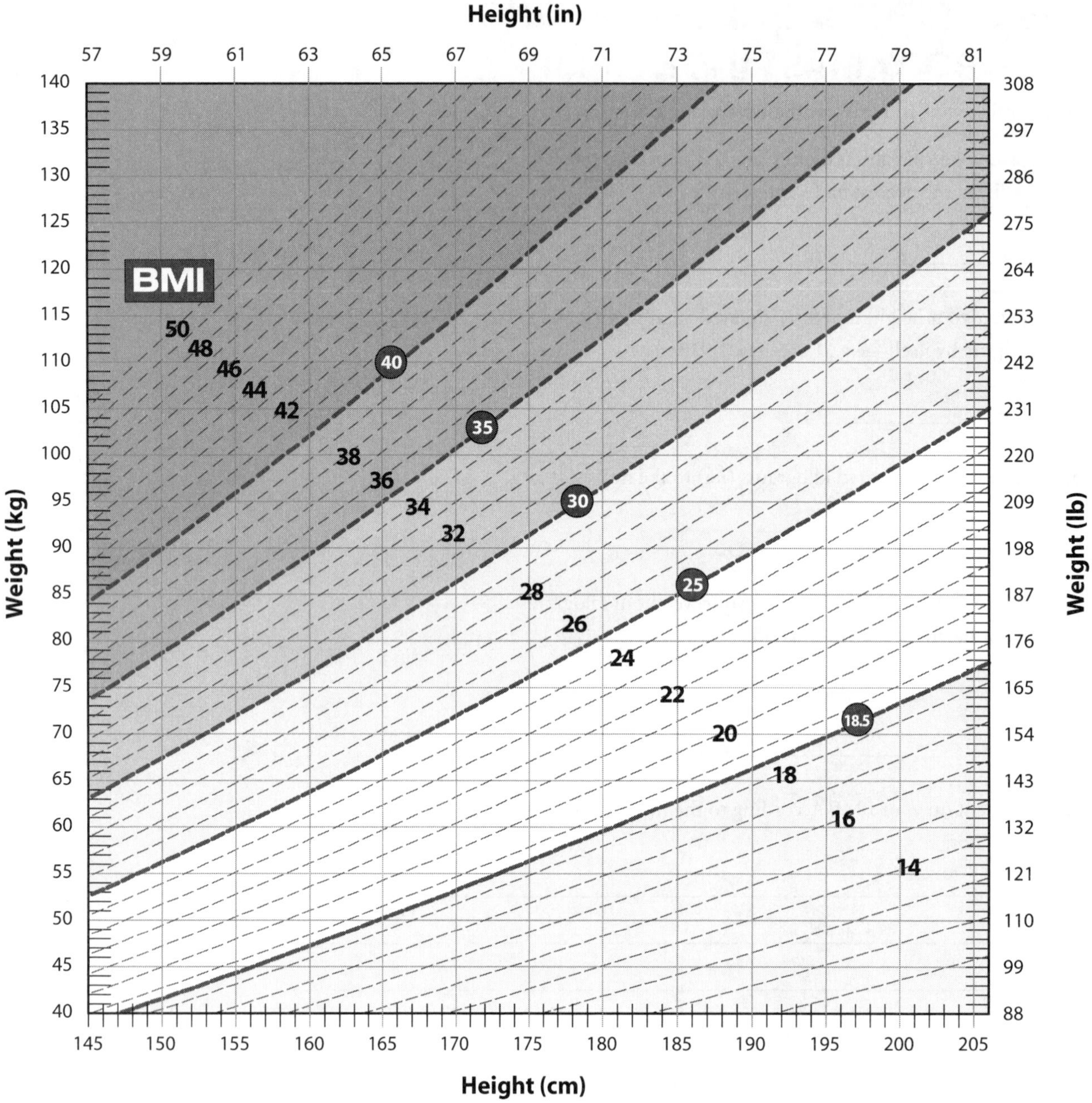

Source: Health Canada. (2003). *Canadian guidelines for body weight classifications in adults.* Catalogue no. H49-179/2003-1E. http://www.hc-sc.gc.ca/fn-an/nutrition/weights-poids/guide-ld-adult/cg_quick_ref-ldc_rapide_ref_e.html. Reproduced with permission of the Minister of Public Works and Government Services Canada, 2007.

ASSIGNMENT 9.2 DETERMINING YOUR WAIST CIRCUMFERENCE (WC)

Excess weight, as measured by BMI, is not the only risk to your health. The location of fat on your body is also a factor. If you carry fat mainly around your waist, you are more likely to develop health problems than if you carry fat mainly on your hips and thighs. This is true even if your BMI falls within the normal range.

To measure your WC, have someone place a tape measure at the part of the torso located midway between the lowest rib and the iliac crest (the top of the pelvic bone). Be sure that the tape is snug, but does not compress your skin and is parallel to the floor. Relax, exhale, and measure your waist. Repeat, to ensure that your WC has been measured accurately. The table below shows measurements that indicate increased risks to your health.

Measurement #1: ______________________________ cm

Measurement #2: ______________________________ cm

Risk for Type 2 Diabetes, Coronary Heart Disease, and Hypertension

WC cut-off points	**Risk of developing health problems**
Males: < 102 cm (40 in) Females: < 88 cm (35 in)	Increased

Source: Adapted from WHO. (2000). *Obesity: Preventing and managing the global epidemic: Report on a WHO consultation on obesity*. Consultation Technical Report Series No. 894. Geneva: Author.

What does your score indicate? Are there any issues you should address? Comment.

____

____

____

____

____

____

____

____

____

____

____

____

____

____

ASSIGNMENT 9.3 DETERMINING YOUR WAIST-TO-HIP RATIO (WHR)

To determine your WHR, follow these steps:

1. Measure the girth of your waist by positioning a metric measuring tape horizontally at the place where the waist is noticeably narrowing, and take the measurement at the end of a normal exhale. Record the measurement to the nearest half-centimetre.

   Girth of waist = _______________ centimetres (cm)

2. Measure the girth of your hips by positioning a metric measuring tape horizontally at the place where the circumference of the hips is the greatest. Record the measurement to the nearest half-centimetre.

   Girth of hips = _______________ cm

3. Determine your WHR by dividing the girth of your waist by the girth of your hips.

   WHR = _______________ cm (waist) ÷ _______________ cm (hips)

   WHR = _______________

4. What does your score indicate? Are there any issues you should address? Comment.

   ____

   ____

   ____

   ____

   ____

   ____

   ____

   ____

   ____

   ____

   ____

   ____

   ____

   ____

   ____

   ____

ASSIGNMENT 10.1 ARE YOU AT RISK FOR DIABETES?

1. Go the Canadian Diabetes Association website at www.diabetes.ca.
2. Click on About Diabetes, and then on Diabetes: Facts.
3. Click on "Are you at risk?"
4. Answer the Risk Assessment questionnaire to determine your level of risk for diabetes.
5. Comment on your results.

____
____
____
____
____
____
____
____

6. Click on Diabetes Facts and read the information provided.
7. Summarize two points that you feel are the most important to someone who lacks any knowledge of diabetes and why.

____
____
____
____
____
____
____
____

ASSIGNMENT 11.1 FIRST AID FOR HEART ATTACK AND STROKE VICTIMS

1. Investigate and describe the first aid procedures for suspected victims of heart attacks and strokes, noting differences and similarities. Why are they important to know?

2. What is CPR? Why is it important to know CPR?

3. Research what an AED is and why law enforcement officers need to know how to use it.

ASSIGNMENT 11.2 ARE YOU AT RISK FOR HEART DISEASE?

1. Go the Canadian Heart and Stroke Foundation of Canada website at http://ww2.heartandstroke.ca.
2. In the Hot Buttons box, click on Risk Assessment.
3. Click on the Take the Heart & Stroke Risk Assessment link to learn what your heart and stroke risks are.
4. After answering the questions in the assessment, make a copy of your Customized Action Plan, which outlines both modifiable and non-modifiable risk factors.
5. Comment on your results. What do you need to be aware of? What changes should you think about? Is there anything you should adjust within your semester fitness/health goals based on your results?

ASSIGNMENT 12.1 HEALTHY BACK ASSESSMENT

Sit and Reach Flexibility Test
(Known as the Trunk Forward Flexion in the Ontario Police Fitness Award [OPFA] Standards)

This test measures the flexibility of the lower back and hamstring muscles. Those with tight hamstrings increase their risk of back problems. The Police Fitness Personnel of Ontario (PFPO) incorporated this test in their OPFA Standards as a result of concerns about the high incidence of low-back pain in police officers.

Procedure

This test involves sitting on the floor with legs out straight ahead. Feet (shoes off) are placed with the soles flat against the box, shoulder-width apart. Both knees are held flat against the floor by the tester. With hands on top of each other and palms facing down, the subject reaches forward along the measuring line as far as possible. After three practice reaches, the fourth reach is held for at least two seconds while the distance is recorded. Make sure there are no jerky movements and that the fingertips remain level and the legs flat.

Refer to the OPFA standards to rate your results in chapter 16 for Trunk Forward Flexion standards.

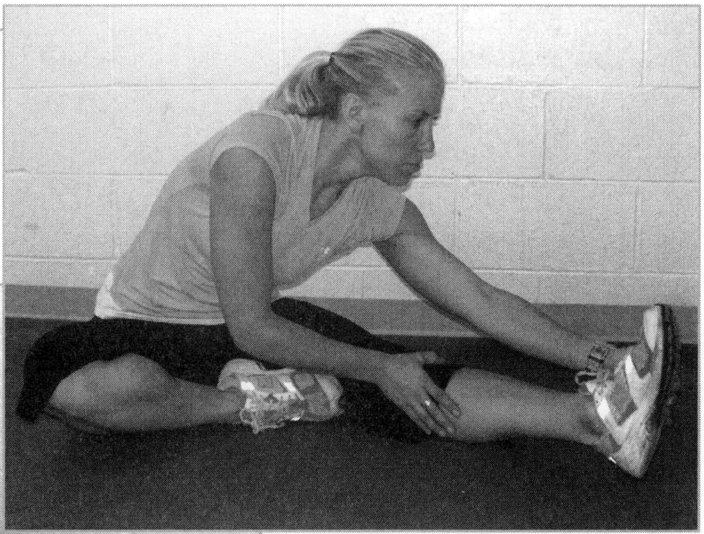

The **modified hurdle stretch** is recommended to be used to help stretch the hip flexors prior to attempting the sit and reach stretch.

Sit and reach stretch

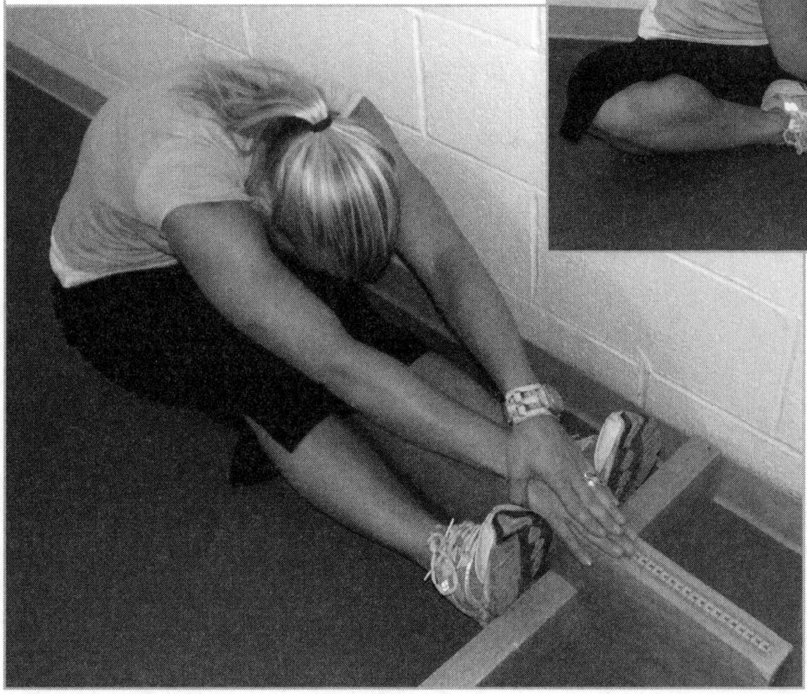

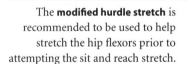

ASSIGNMENT 13.1 THE LIFE EXPERIENCE SURVEY

Listed on the following pages are a number of events that sometimes bring about change in the lives of those who experience them and necessitate social readjustment. Check off those events that you have experienced in the past year and indicate how long ago the event occurred (0–6 months or 7–12 months).

Also, for each item checked off, assign a whole number between –3 and +3 to indicate the extent to which you viewed the event as having either a positive or a negative impact on your life at the time it occurred. A rating of –3 indicates an extremely negative impact, a rating of 0 indicates an impact that is neither positive nor negative, and a rating of +3 indicates an extremely positive impact.

Section I of the test is for everyone. It provides three blanks (items 45, 46, and 47) for you to list any recent experiences that have had an impact on your life but are not covered in items 1–44.

Section II of the test is designed for students only. If there are school-related experiences that have had a noticeable impact on your life but are not listed, you may list them in one or more of the three blanks in section I.

Some items apply only to males and some only to females; these are indicated in the survey.

After you complete the survey, consider the following questions:

1. Was your level of stress close to what you predicted it would be? Why or why not?

____

____

____

____

____

____

____

2. Can you highlight a few stressors that are affecting you, or are you experiencing an overall stress level?

____

____

____

____

____

____

____

3. Recognizing your stressors, are there any that you could work on to relieve your stress level?

4. What can you do to improve your positive stress?

5. Comment on any other observations you have made.

THE LIFE EXPERIENCE SURVEY

Section I	0–6 months	7–12 months	Extremely negative	Moderately negative	Somewhat negative	No impact	Slightly positive	Moderately positive	Extremely positive
1. Marriage	____	____	−3	−2	−1	0	+1	+2	+3
2. Detention in jail or comparable institution	____	____	−3	−2	−1	0	+1	+2	+3
3. Death of spouse	____	____	−3	−2	−1	0	+1	+2	+3
4. Major change in sleeping habits (much more or less sleep)	____	____	−3	−2	−1	0	+1	+2	+3
5. Death of close family member:									
a. mother	____	____	−3	−2	−1	0	+1	+2	+3
b. father	____	____	−3	−2	−1	0	+1	+2	+3
c. brother	____	____	−3	−2	−1	0	+1	+2	+3
d. sister	____	____	−3	−2	−1	0	+1	+2	+3
e. child	____	____	−3	−2	−1	0	+1	+2	+3
f. grandmother	____	____	−3	−2	−1	0	+1	+2	+3
g. grandfather	____	____	−3	−2	−1	0	+1	+2	+3
h. other (specify) ____________	____	____	−3	−2	−1	0	+1	+2	+3
6. Major change in eating habits (much more or much less food intake)	____	____	−3	−2	−1	0	+1	+2	+3
7. Foreclosure on mortgage or loan	____	____	−3	−2	−1	0	+1	+2	+3
8. Death of a close friend	____	____	−3	−2	−1	0	+1	+2	+3
9. Outstanding personal achievement	____	____	−3	−2	−1	0	+1	+2	+3
10. Minor law violations (traffic ticket, disturbing the peace, etc.)	____	____	−3	−2	−1	0	+1	+2	+3
11. *Male:* Wife's/girlfriend's pregnancy *Female:* Pregnancy	____	____	−3	−2	−1	0	+1	+2	+3
12. Changed work situation (different working conditions, working hours, etc.)	____	____	−3	−2	−1	0	+1	+2	+3
13. New job	____	____	−3	−2	−1	0	+1	+2	+3
14. Serious illness or injury of close family member									
a. father	____	____	−3	−2	−1	0	+1	+2	+3
b. mother	____	____	−3	−2	−1	0	+1	+2	+3
c. sister	____	____	−3	−2	−1	0	+1	+2	+3
d. brother	____	____	−3	−2	−1	0	+1	+2	+3
e. grandfather	____	____	−3	−2	−1	0	+1	+2	+3
f. grandmother	____	____	−3	−2	−1	0	+1	+2	+3
g. spouse	____	____	−3	−2	−1	0	+1	+2	+3
h. child	____	____	−3	−2	−1	0	+1	+2	+3
i. other (specify) ____________	____	____	−3	−2	−1	0	+1	+2	+3
15. Sexual difficulties	____	____	−3	−2	−1	0	+1	+2	+3
16. Trouble with employer (in danger of losing job, being suspended, demoted, etc.)	____	____	−3	−2	−1	0	+1	+2	+3
17. Trouble with in-laws	____	____	−3	−2	−1	0	+1	+2	+3
18. Major change in financial status (a lot better off or a lot worse off)	____	____	−3	−2	−1	0	+1	+2	+3
19. Major change in closeness of family members (decreased or increased closeness)	____	____	−3	−2	−1	0	+1	+2	+3

The Life Experience Survey, Section I, continued

Section I (continued)	0–6 months	7–12 months	Extremely negative	Moderately negative	Somewhat negative	No impact	Slightly positive	Moderately positive	Extremely positive
20. Gaining a new family member (through birth, adoption, family member moving in, etc.)	____	____	−3	−2	−1	0	+1	+2	+3
21. Change of residence	____	____	−3	−2	−1	0	+1	+2	+3
22. Marital separation from mate (due to conflict)	____	____	−3	−2	−1	0	+1	+2	+3
23. Major change in church activities (increased or decreased attendance)	____	____	−3	−2	−1	0	+1	+2	+3
24. Marital reconciliation with mate	____	____	−3	−2	−1	0	+1	+2	+3
25. Major change in number of arguments with spouse (a lot more or a lot less arguments)	____	____	−3	−2	−1	0	+1	+2	+3
26. *Married Male:* Change in wife's work outside the home (beginning work, ceasing work, changing to a new job) *Married Female:* Change in husband's work (loss of job, beginning new job, retirement, etc.)	____	____	−3	−2	−1	0	+1	+2	+3
27. Major change in usual type and/or amount of recreation	____	____	−3	−2	−1	0	+1	+2	+3
28. Borrowing more than $10 000 (buying home, business, etc.)	____	____	−3	−2	−1	0	+1	+2	+3
29. Borrowing less than $10 000 (buying car, TV, getting school loan, etc.)	____	____	−3	−2	−1	0	+1	+2	+3
30. Being fired from job	____	____	−3	−2	−1	0	+1	+2	+3
31. *Male:* Wife/girlfriend having abortion *Female:* Having abortion	____	____	−3	−2	−1	0	+1	+2	+3
32. Major personal illness or injury	____	____	−3	−2	−1	0	+1	+2	+3
33. Major change in social activities—e.g., parties, movies, visiting (increased or decreased participation)	____	____	−3	−2	−1	0	+1	+2	+3
34. Major change in living conditions of family (building new home, remodeling, deterioration of home, neighborhood, etc.)	____	____	−3	−2	−1	0	+1	+2	+3
35. Divorce	____	____	−3	−2	−1	0	+1	+2	+3
36. Serious injury or illness of close friend	____	____	−3	−2	−1	0	+1	+2	+3
37. Retirement from work	____	____	−3	−2	−1	0	+1	+2	+3
38. Son or daughter leaving home (due to marriage, college, etc.)	____	____	−3	−2	−1	0	+1	+2	+3
39. Ending of formal schooling	____	____	−3	−2	−1	0	+1	+2	+3
40. Separation from spouse (due to work, travel, etc.)	____	____	−3	−2	−1	0	+1	+2	+3
41. Engagement	____	____	−3	−2	−1	0	+1	+2	+3
42. Breaking up with boyfriend/girlfriend	____	____	−3	−2	−1	0	+1	+2	+3
43. Leaving home for the first time	____	____	−3	−2	−1	0	+1	+2	+3
44. Reconciliation with boyfriend/girlfriend	____	____	−3	−2	−1	0	+1	+2	+3

Other recent experiences that have had an impact on your life. List and rate.

45. ______________________	____	____	−3	−2	−1	0	+1	+2	+3
46. ______________________	____	____	−3	−2	−1	0	+1	+2	+3
47. ______________________	____	____	−3	−2	−1	0	+1	+2	+3

Section II: For students only	0–6 months	7–12 months	Extremely negative	Moderately negative	Somewhat negative	No impact	Slightly positive	Moderately positive	Extremely positive
48. Beginning new school experience at a higher academic level (college, graduate school, professional school, etc.)	____	____	−3	−2	−1	0	+1	+2	+3
49. Changing to a new school at same academic level (undergraduate, graduate, etc.)	____	____	−3	−2	−1	0	+1	+2	+3
50. Academic probation	____	____	−3	−2	−1	0	+1	+2	+3
51. Being dismissed from dormitory or other residence	____	____	−3	−2	−1	0	+1	+2	+3
52. Failing an important exam	____	____	−3	−2	−1	0	+1	+2	+3
53. Changing a major	____	____	−3	−2	−1	0	+1	+2	+3
54. Failing a course	____	____	−3	−2	−1	0	+1	+2	+3
55. Dropping a course	____	____	−3	−2	−1	0	+1	+2	+3
56. Joining a fraternity/sorority	____	____	−3	−2	−1	0	+1	+2	+3

Scoring the Life Experience Survey

1. Add all the negative scores to arrive at your own distress score (negative stress).
2. Add all of the positive scores to arrive at a eustress score (positive stress).
3. It is possible to calculate scores for the last six months, or for the last year. The more recent the incident, the more likely it will be distressful.

Rating scale for life experiences and stress

	Sum of negative scores (distress)	Sum of positive scores (eustress)
May need counseling	14+	
Above average stress	9–13	
Average	6–9	9–10
Below average stress	<6	

Source: Sarason, I.G., Johnson, J.H., & Siegel, J.M. (1978). Assessing the impact of life changes: Development of the life experiences survey. *Journal of Consulting and Clinical Psychology, 46(5)*, 932-946. Copyright © 1978 by the American Psychological Association. Reprinted with permission. The use of APA information does not imply endorsement by APA.

ASSIGNMENT 13.2
WHAT IS YOUR BEHAVIOUR TYPE?

1. Which environments (social, work, school, family, and so on) tend to bring out type A behaviour in you? What is it about these environments that you believe elicits this behaviour?

2. Answer the questions above as they apply to type B behaviour.

3. Answer the questions above as they apply to type C behaviour.

4. Which personality traits do you think cause stress in your life?

5. Which personality traits do you think will positively assist you in a career in law enforcement? Why?

____

____

____

____

____

____

____

6. Which personality traits would you like to change? Why?

____

____

____

____

____

____

____

7. What coping strategies do you need to develop or enhance?

____

____

____

____

____

____

____

ASSIGNMENT 14.1 UNDERSTANDING SHIFT WORK BASED ON SLEEPING PATTERNS

1. Do you have problems falling asleep or staying asleep?

2. Have you ever suffered from jet lag? If so, what were the symptoms?

3. When you wake up, do you feel rested, refreshed, and able to feel alert throughout the day without a nap?

4. Have you lived in a household where someone was a shift worker? If so, how did it affect you?

5. Examine your sleeping environment.
   a. Is your bedroom a comfortable temperature? (Ideally around 18 °C.)
   b. Do you have a humidifier for the winter and an air conditioner for the summer? (Humidity levels that are too high or too low can affect your sleep.)
   c. Are your mattress and pillow in good condition, and are they comfortable?
   d. Is your bed partner disrupting your sleep?

   ____
   ____
   ____
   ____
   ____
   ____

6. List what you think might be the benefits and drawbacks of shift work.

   ____
   ____
   ____
   ____
   ____
   ____

If you have negative responses to most of these questions, you may be one of those people who has difficulty with sleep, which could lead to a sleep disorder or difficulty working shifts.

ASSIGNMENT 14.2 HOW WILL YOU COPE WITH SHIFT WORK?

1. What aspects of your life will you have to change to cope with shift work?

2. What changes in your house or other dwelling might make it a better place to sleep?

3. What nutritional concerns do you need to address to adjust to shift work?

4. What habits will you have to change to be able to sleep more effectively?

5. How do you think shift work will affect you socially? How can you moderate these effects?

6. How will you help your significant other and family members cope with your shift work?

7. What changes do you think you may have to make to ensure that you get the proper amount of fitness in?

ASSIGNMENT 16.1 PHYSICAL FITNESS LOG

As part of your physical fitness training goals, you should chart your progress throughout the two years. At the end of your first semester, you may have to change those goals that you have not been able to meet. Ultimately, it is your responsibility to know where you stand with your grades. Depending on the college, you will have certain standards to meet depending on which semester you are in. By charting your results, you will know where you stand and what areas you will have to address each semester. Your progress in each semester is ultimately your own responsibility.

STEP 1 Setting Specific Fitness Goals

Taking the goals that you developed in chapter 2, indicate five fitness goals that you need to address or achieve.

1. ______________________________
2. ______________________________
3. ______________________________
4. ______________________________
5. ______________________________

STEP 2 Setting Specific Goals for Test Protocols

Set specific goals in terms of time or numbers regarding test protocols. In the first semester, you may have to attempt a BFOR protocol before you can more accurately set a realistic goal for yourself. You may decide to do specific goal-setting charts for strength and endurance activities around weight training and plyometrics as well.

	Goal (in Terms of Time or Numbers)			
Test	**Semester __**	**Semester __**	**Semester __**	**Semester __**
PREP				
PARE				
COPAT				
Curl-ups				
Push-ups				
Sit and reach				
1.5-mile run				
Chin-ups				
100-m sprint				
Bench press				
Other tests				

STEP 3 Tracking Your Results

Use the log on the opposite page to keep track of your stats on how you are doing in class. After the first test, you might realize that you have set your goals too low or too high. If so, make sure that you adjust them accordingly so that you can be successful and/or continue to exceed the standards expected of you.

STEP 4 Assessing Your Goals

Take the time after four weeks to assess your progress. Some areas that you might consider addressing include:

- What I felt went well and why.
- What I felt did not go well and why.
- Strategies I will try in order to overcome future barriers.
- What I learned about myself and my progress in fitness.

PERSONAL FITNESS RESULTS PROGRESS CHECK FOR: ____________________

Canadian Fitness Standards	Result	SCORE	Result	SCORE	Result	SCORE	
Curl-ups							(/20)
Push-ups							(/20)
Sit and reach							(/10)
1.5-mile run							(/50)
(Maximum total = 100)	TOTAL =		TOTAL =		TOTAL =		

Strength and Endurance Tests	Result	SCORE	Result	SCORE	Result	SCORE	
Chin-ups							(/10)
Bench press							(/20)
Back assessment							(/10)
Max shuttle run							(/50)

BFOR Tests	Pursuit	SCORE	Shuttle	SCORE		Result	SCORE
PREP					PARE		
Pursuit (/30) / Shuttle (/20)					PARE		

NOTES

Glossary of Terms

1RM
one maximal repetition of weight

active living
a way of life in which individuals make meaningful and satisfying physical activities an integral part of daily living

amino acids
the fundamental constituents of proteins; amino acids can be divided into two types—complete (essential) and incomplete

aneurysm
a weak or thin area in a blood vessel that causes it to expand and fill with blood; aneurysms may occur as a result of a disease, an injury, or a congenital abnormality in the vessel

angina pectoris
severe chest pains associated with advanced cases of coronary heart disease

anorexia nervosa
an eating disorder in which individuals do not eat enough to maintain a healthy body weight

arteriosclerosis
a blanket term for a group of diseases characterized by a narrowing or hardening of the arteries

arteriovenous malformation
a malformation of the blood vessels of the brain, usually present at birth; an arteriovenous malformation can increase the risk of stroke

arthritis
a group of conditions in which there is a degeneration of the joint following trauma to the joint (as a result of an infection or aging)

atherosclerosis
a common type of arteriosclerosis; a slow, progressive disease in which arterial blockage results from fatty deposits collecting in the arteries

attitude
value added to one's beliefs

ballistic stretching
a stretching technique that promotes the stretch reflex but increases the risk of injury to muscles and tendons—it requires quick, well-coordinated action–reaction movements that stretch the muscles beyond their normal range of motion

basal metabolic rate (BMR)
the speed at which energy is used by the body

basal metabolism
the amount of energy a body at rest needs to maintain essential functions

belief
acceptance of an idea on the basis of knowledge and conviction

binge eating disorder (BED)
an eating disorder associated with obesity, where the person alternately eats obsessively and then diets and restricts eating; the disorder is diagnosed if the person does not follow the binge eating with compensatory behaviours such as vomiting, excessive exercise, or laxative abuse

blood cholesterol
the cholesterol produced by the liver

body composition
the proportion of lean tissue to fat in the body

body mass index (BMI) measurement
a method for assessing body composition, based on weight and height

Borg scale
a method for determining the intensity of exercise, used as an alternative to heart rate monitoring

bulimia nervosa
an eating disorder in which individuals have an intense fear of overweight and overfat that causes binge eating followed by self-induced vomiting

bursitis
inflammation of a bursa (a sac of fluid near a joint)

cardiac arrest
cessation of the heart's pumping action

cardiorespiratory endurance
heart and respiratory system endurance; the ability to perform prolonged large-muscle activities at moderate to high intensity

chronic time urgency
a constant state of stress due to putting pressure on yourself to do too much in too little time

circadian rhythm
the 24-hour cycle on which the human biological clock is based

concurrent training
training for either strength or power at the same time you train for endurance

coronary heart disease
a type of coronary artery disease in which fatty deposits block one or more coronary arteries (arteries supplying the heart)

critical incident
a situation faced by police and other emergency service personnel that causes them to experience unusually strong emotional reactions that have the potential to interfere with their ability to function at the scene (current stress) or later (residual stress)

DASH diet
a diet that follows *Canada's Food Guide* and the American Food Pyramid in order to reduce sodium, cholesterol, and fat in your diet

degenerative disc disease (DDD)
degeneration of the intervertebral disc

delayed-onset muscle soreness (DOMS)
soreness of muscles 12 hours or more after exercise

diabetes
a chronic disease in which your body cannot properly use glucose for energy

dietary cholesterol
the cholesterol in food

dietary fibre
food components that cannot be digested—found exclusively in plants; the two types of dietary fibre are insoluble and soluble

dynamic stretching
a stretching technique that involves performing movements within the full range of motion of the joint—it gradually increases reach and range of motion while the limbs are moving

exercise
a form of leisure-time physical activity that is planned, structured, and repetitive; its main objective is to improve or maintain physical fitness

exercising heart rate
your heart rate when your body is in motion during sustained exercise

extrinsic motivation
motivation to perform a task or goal based on external rewards

fartlek training
interval training of distances at intense levels followed by recovery periods at predetermined intervals

fatty acids
the fundamental constituents of fats; fatty acids can be divided into two types—saturated and unsaturated

female athlete triad
an eating disorder among female athletes defined by three conditions: disordered eating, amenorrhea, and osteoporosis

fibromyalgia
chronic disorder characterized by widespread musculoskeletal pain, fatigue, and multiple "tender points," particularly in the neck, spine, shoulders, and hips

five Cs
the five unique traits of the type C personality—control, commitment, challenge, choices in lifestyle, and connectedness

flexibility
the ability to move the joints freely through their full range of motion

frostbite
severe condition where both the skin and the underlying tissue (fat, muscle, and bone) are frozen

frostnip
a mild form of frostbite, where only the top layer of skin freezes

general adaptation
the process of preparing your muscles, joints, tendons, and ligaments for intense training by educating the neuromuscular component so that gains can be seen; characterized by higher repetitions, lower intensities, and short rest periods

general adaptation syndrome (GAS)
the body's reaction to stress

gestational diabetes
a temporary condition in which hormonal changes associated with pregnancy and the growth demands of the fetus increase insulin needs to two to three times the normal level; generally occurs after the 24th week of pregnancy and resolves after delivery

glucose
a simple form of sugar that acts as fuel for the body

health
the ability of an individual to function independently in a constantly changing environment

health benefits
improvements to physical, mental, and psychological health

health-related fitness
the aspects of fitness that are linked to a person's health

heat cramps
illness caused by a water and sodium deficiency; heat cramps feel like severe muscle pulls

heat exhaustion
illness caused by extreme body heat; excessive heat and dehydration can raise body temperature to 38–40 °C (100–104 °F)

heat stroke
illness caused by failure of the body's heat-regulating mechanism; may lead to permanent disability or death

high-density lipoprotein (HDL) cholesterol
the "good" cholesterol; it helps clean out undesirable LDL ("bad" cholesterol) deposits

high-intensity interval training (HIT)
a form of training to increase aerobic performance

hypertension
high blood pressure—the term *essential hypertension* is used for cases in which the cause is unknown

hypertrophy
the process characterized by high training volume with moderate training intensity in order to build muscle mass

hypothermia
condition occurring when the body's control mechanism can no longer maintain a normal body temperature, and the body's temperature drops to an abormally low level

impingement syndrome
squeezing of the rotator cuff (the group of muscles that surrounds the shoulder)

intentions
a determination to achieve an aim

interval training
training that is based on the concept that the body's energy systems can make both aerobic and anaerobic gains by training with relatively intense exercises followed by period of recovery

intervertebral discs
flexible, gelatinous, shock-absorbing pads that separate the vertebrae

intracerebral hemorrhage
bleeding in the brain resulting from the rupture of a blood vessel

intrinsic motivation
motivation to perform a task or goal based on enjoyment of doing the task itself

isokinetic action
one of the three common types of muscular action; isokinetic action occurs during exercises involving equipment that compensates for the varying amounts of force exerted by a muscle by maintaining a constant level of resistance

isometric action
one of the three common types of muscular action; isometric action occurs when muscle length remains constant, as is the case in certain exercises

isotonic action
one of the three common types of muscular action; isotonic action occurs when a muscle contracts in response to a constant force or load applied to it; there are two types of isotonic action—concentric and eccentric

kilocalorie (kcal)
a measure of the amount of energy in food; also referred to as a calorie; an individual's energy needs are the number of calories he or she must consume to maintain health based on age, sex, weight, height, and activity level

low-density lipoprotein (LDL) cholesterol
the "bad" cholesterol; it can build up in the arteries and cause health problems

maximal heart rate
your heart rate when your heart beats at maximal effort during a sustained aerobic activity

maximum aerobic capacity (VO_2 Max)
a measure of cardio fitness; estimated as the point at which oxygen uptake plateaus and does not increase with further increases in workload

mission statement
a concise statement of one's major values and goals, meant to give direction to the decisions one will make throughout the course of one's life

morbidity
number of ill people in a population, usually expressed as an annual rate

mortality
number of deaths in a population, usually expressed as an annual rate

muscular endurance
the ability of a muscle to sustain a prolonged contraction or to contract over and over again

muscular strength
the amount of force a muscle can produce with a single maximum effort

myocardial infarction
a heart attack

narcolepsy
a disorder that causes the malfunctioning of the brain, leading to one's falling asleep without warning

osteoporosis
a condition common in older people, in whom bones become increasingly soft and porous, thinner, and more brittle, making them susceptible to risk of fracture, particularly of the hip, spine, and wrist

overload principle
the principle that muscle mass can be built up only if the muscle is subjected to a greater than normal load

performance/skill-related fitness
the degree of fitness required to perform a particular job or sport

periodization
an organized approach to training that involves progressive cycling of various aspects of a training program during a specific period of time; overall training plan where an individual maximizes performances at peak times

personal goals
goals that reflect our personality—who we are, how we think, and how we look

physical activity
all leisure and non-leisure body movement that results in an expenditure of energy

physical fitness
a person's health and performance, specifically in the areas of cardiorespiratory fitness, body composition, muscular strength and endurance, and flexibility

plyometric training
a form of resistance training that works on developing strength and power

plyometrics
a method of training that enhances an individual's "explosive" reaction through rapid and powerful muscular contractions through stretch-shortening cycles; a concentric action immediately preceded by an eccentric action

post-traumatic stress disorder (PTSD)
disorder that changes the way the body responds to stress, probably as a result of chemical imbalances that increase the levels of stress hormones and alter the reaction of the nervous system

power training
the process where an athlete works to build overall body explosiveness and reactive ability by taking the strength gained in the strength phase and converting it to activity-specific power

principle of overload
refers to training and overloading our muscles that help us to adapt to more and more stress

principle of recovery
refers to the recuperation time or amount of rest required after a workout

principle of reversibility
refers to all the benefits of exercise that are lost if you stop training

principle of specificity
refers to the ability of the body to adapt to a particular type and amount of stress placed on it

procrastination
the postponement of unpleasant or burdensome tasks

professional goals
goals that reflect your career aspirations

proprioceptive neuromuscular facilitation (PNF)
a stretching technique that involves contracting and relaxing the muscles before stretching

psychosomatic symptoms
physical symptoms resulting from mental conflict

pyramid training
a system combining the light to heavy and heavy to light approaches for weight training

REM sleep
a stage of sleep that allows your body to recover from mental fatigue and helps to store memories and consolidate learning

repetition (rep)
one complete movement of an exercise

repetitive strain injury (RSI)
an injury that arises when soft tissue is subjected to repeated trauma (such as may be caused by typing or using a computer mouse) without the chance to recover from each trauma

resistance training
the most common form of weight training which incorporates exercises that result in gains to muscle mass and strength as well as the potential for improved flexibility and range of motion

resting heart rate
your heart rate when you are in a resting state such as sleep

restless legs syndrome (RLS)
a condition characterized by an overwhelming urge to move the legs when they are at rest

sciatica
pain anywhere along the sciatic nerve as the result of compression, inflammation, or irritation; generally, the pain travels from the back of the thigh to the back of the calf, and also may extend upwards, to the hip

self-efficacy
one's ability to take action and perform a specific behaviour

self-esteem
how one feels about oneself and one's characteristics

set
a group of repetitions

skinfold measurement
measurement of fat just below the skin surface at five points on the body to determine the percentage of body fat

sleep apnea
a breathing-related sleep disorder in which inappropriate brain signals do not tell the breathing muscles to initiate respiration

social involvement
the support of other people to assist you in achieving your goals

somatotype
body type—there are three somatotypes: ectomorphic, mesomorphic, and endomorphic

sprain
an injury to a ligament—a stretching or tearing

static stretching
a stretching technique that involves bringing a muscle to a maximum or near-maximum stretch by contracting the opposing muscle and holding the stretch for 20–30 seconds (without pain)

strain
an injury to a muscle or tendon—a twisting or pulling

stress
a "non-specific response of the body to any demands made upon it" (Dr. Hans Selye)

stressor
any physical, psychological, or environmental event or condition that initiates the stress response

stroke
paralysis and a sudden loss of consciousness caused by an interruption of blood flow to the brain; a thrombotic or thromboembolic stroke occurs when blood flow is interrupted by a blood clot that travels to the brain; a hemorrhagic stroke occurs when very high blood pressure causes a weakened blood vessel near the brain to break

subarachnoid hemorrhage
hemorrhage that occurs when a blood vessel on the surface of the brain bleeds into the space between the brain and the skull

superset training
a system involving performing two exercises in succession, without rest; often used to exercise opposing muscle groups and results in increased strength and muscle mass of the targeted muscle

grouptalk test
a method for determining the intensity of exercise, used as an alternative to heart rate monitoring; if a person is breathless and cannot carry on a conversation while exercising, he or she is working too hard

target heart rate (THR) zone
the zone that a person's heart rate must reach during exercise to improve or maintain aerobic fitness

tendinitis
inflammation of a tendon

trans fats
unsaturated fatty acids that have been hydrogenated to give them a longer shelf life; diets high in trans fats increase the risk of diseases like atherosclerosis and coronary heart disease

transient ischemic attack
a temporary interference with the blood supply to the brain

trisets
combining three exercises with little rest in between; can involve working the same muscle group from three different angles, working three different muscle groups, or working different areas of the same muscle from three different angles

type 1 diabetes
type of diabetes that occurs when the pancreas no longer produces insulin or produces very little

type 2 diabetes
type of diabetes that occurs when the pancreas cannot produce enough insulin or the body is unable to use the insulin effectively

values
the things that matter most to us and guide our daily behaviour, activities, and decisions

vertebrae
the bones of the spine (singular: vertebra)

vitality
an integrated approach to healthy living that shifts the focus away from rigid ideals, dieting, and overly prescriptive exercise toward acceptance of a range of body shapes and sizes and an emphasis on healthy eating, active living, and a positive self-image and body image

waist circumference (WC)
an indicator of health risk associated with abdominal fat

waist-to-hip ratio (WHR) measurement
a method for assessing body composition, based on the relationship between the girth of the waist and the girth of the hips

wellness
the ability of an individual to optimally function at his or her best

wind chill index (WCI)
measure representing how the temperature would feel on your skin if the wind were reduced to a walking pace of 4.8 km/h

Workplace Hazardous Materials Information System (WHMIS)
a system that familiarizes workers with safety information about potentially hazardous products in their workplace

Index

1RM, 99

active living, 6
agility, 58
amino acids, 148
aneurysm, 226
angina pectoris, 221
anorexia nervosa, 182
antioxidants, 144
arteriosclerosis, 219
arteriovenous malformation, 226
atherosclerosis, 219
arthritis, 252
attitude, 29
autogenic feedback, 286
 biofeedback, 288

back pain
 arthritis, and, 252
 cause, 243, 249
 injury treatment, 261
 nutritional considerations, 259
 prevention, 255-59
 repetitive strain injury (RSI), 253
 risk factors, 250
 sciatica, 255
balance, 58
ballistic stretching, 118
basal metabolic rate (BMR), 179
basal metabolism, 179
behaviour types, 282-83
belief, 29
beta-carotene, 144
binge eating disorder (BED), 184
biofeedback, 288
biological hazards, 328, 330
blood cholesterol, 147, 217
blood pressure, 231
body composition
 body mass index (BMI), 180
 defined, 57, 177
 eating disorders
  anorexia nervosa, 182
  binge eating disorder, 184
  bulimia nervosa, 183
  female athlete triad, 184
  warning signs, 183
 health risk classification, 180
 metabolism, 179
 misguided views, 175
 obesity, 179
 skinfold measurements, 181
 somatotypes, 178
 waist circumference (WC), 180
 waist-to-hip ratio (WHR) measurement, 182
body mass index (BMI), 180
Borg scale, 77, 79
breathing techniques, 103, 285
 hydrotherapy, 289
 hypnosis, 288
broken ribs, 318
bulimia nervosa, 183
bursitis, 316

caffeine, 160
calcium, 260
calories, 155
Canada's Food Guide, 136, 151, 152, 153, 303
carbohydrates
 function, 141
 glycemic index, and, 141
cardiac arrest, 221
cardiorespiratory endurance, 56
cardiorespiratory fitness
 assessment of, 74
 benefits of, 74
 importance, 73
 training program
  Borg scale, 77
  creation of, 79

cardiorespiratory fitness (cont.)
  training program (cont.)
    guidelines, 81
    heart rate monitoring, 77
    heart rates, 76
    shuttle run training, 83
    talk test, 78
    upper-limit training, 83
cardiovascular disease
  children, and, 218
  concern about, 214-17
  defined, 213
  heart
    anatomy of, 218
    function of, 218
  types of
    arteriosclerosis, 219
    coronary heart disease, 220-26
    hypertension, 229-32
    stroke, 226-29
change
  five stages of, 26
  nine processes of, 28
  process of, 25
  pros and cons, 33
chronic time urgency, 44
circadian rhythm, 300, 304
circuit training, 103
cholesterol, 147, 217
concurrent training, 64
coordination, 58
coronary heart disease, 220-26
critical incidents
  definition of, 275
  factors affected responses to, 276
  helping colleague cope, 279-81
  symptoms of stress arising out of, 277
  types of, 275
cruciferous vegetables, 144

DASH diet, 158, 229
degenerative disc disease (DDD), 246
dehydration, 325
delayed-onset muscle soreness (DOMS), 312-13
diabetes
  children, and, 197
  complications from, 197
  risk factors, 200
  shift work, and, 202
  symptoms of, 202
  types of, 196
diabetic dermopathy, 198
dietary cholesterol, 147
dietary fibre, 143
diets
  fasting, 158
  high-protein, 159
  low-carbohydrate, 159
  vegetarianism, 159
diminishing returns, 62
dislocated shoulder, 316
dynamic stretching, 118

EA Tracker, 165
eating disorders
  anorexia nervosa, 182
  binge eating disorder (BED), 184
  bulimia nervosa, 183
  female athlete triad, 184
  warning signs, 183
employee wellness initiatives, 166
endurance training, *see* strength and endurance training
energy drinks, 162
exercise, 4
exercising heart rate, 76
extension exercises, 256
extrinsic motivation, 26

fartlek training, 64
fats, 145
fatty acids, 145
female athlete triad, 184
fibre, 143
fibromyalgia, 252
fight-or-flight response, 270
first aid, *see* injuries
fitness
  active living, 6
  health-related, 5
  performance-related, 5
  vitality, 9
  wellness, relationship to, 4
FITT formula, 76
five Cs, 283
flexibility, 57, 115
flexion exercises, 256

food, *see also* nutrition
  function of, 137
  groups, 153
  labelling, 153
frostbite, 328
frostnip, 328

general adaptation, 94
general adaptation syndrome (GAS), 270
gestational diabetes, 197
glucose, 195
glycemic index, 141
goal setting
  change, process of, 25
  change, pros and cons, 33
  choice of, 31
  family relationships, 30
  mission statements, 33
  perseverance, 31
  personal goals, 30
  physical activity, 29
  professional goals, 30
  rewards, 32
  short- and long-term, 30
  understanding, 29

health
  benefits, 29
  defined, 9
  seven dimensions of, 10
heart
  anatomy of, 218
  function of, 218
heart rate
  monitoring, 77
  understanding, 76
heat cramps, 324
heat exhaustion, 324
heat stroke, 324
heavy to light training, 104
high-density lipoprotein (HDL) cholesterol, 148, 217
high-intensity interval training (HIT), 83
hydrotherapy, 289
hyperglycemia, 201
hypertension, 229
hypertrophy, 95, 99
hypnosis, 288
hypoglycemia, 201
hyponatremia, 162
hypothermia, 326

iliotibial band syndrome, 321
impingement syndrome, 316
injuries
  biological and chemical hazards, 328, 330
  cold-related injuries
    first aid, 327
    frostbite, 328
    frostnip, 328
    hypothermia, 326
    signs and symptoms, 327
  general treatments for, 311
  heat-related injuries
    dehydration, 325
    heat cramps, 324
    heat exhaustion, 324
    heat stroke, 324
    prevention, 325
  muscle soreness, 312-13
  RICE principle, 312
  sports-related injuries
    broken ribs, 318
    bursitis, 316
    dislocated shoulder, 316
    iliotibial band syndrome, 321
    impingement syndrome, 316
    knee ligament injuries, 322
    meniscus degeneration, 322-23
    Osgood-Schlatter disease, 320
    patello-femoral syndrome, 319
    plantar fasciitis, 320
    shin splints, 319
    sprain, 314
    strain, 314-15
    tendinitis, 315
insulin shock, 201
intentions, 29
Internet information, 163
interval training, 64
intervertebral disc, 245, 245
intracerebral hemorrhage, 226
intrinsic motivation, 27
isokinetic action, 96
isometric action, 97
isotonic action, 96

kilocalorie (kcal), 155
knee ligament injuries, 322

lifting techniques, 251
light to heavy training, 103
load, 103
Long Live Kids Program, 165
low-density lipoprotein (LDL) cholesterol, 147, 217
lower-fat food, 149

massage, 289
maximal heart rate, 76
maximum aerobic capacity (VO_2 max), 75
meditation, 285
meniscus degeneration, 322-23
metabolism, 179
minerals, 140
mission statements, 33
morbidity, 11
mortality, 11
muscle contraction, 118
muscle fibre, 93, 116, 151
muscle soreness, 312-13
muscular endurance, 57, 94
muscular strength, 57, 94
music, 288
myocardial infarction, 221

narcolepsy, 301
nutrition
back health, and, 259-60
basic nutrients
carbohydrates, 141
fibre, 143
minerals, 140, 260
proteins, 148
vitamins, 138
water, 138, 137
caloric value, nutrients, 155
Canada's Food Guide, 151
food groups, 153
portion size, 153-54
concerns, Canada, 136
content claims, 155
DASH diet, 158
diets
fasting, 158
high-protein, 159
low-carbohydrate, 159
vegetarianism, 159
food companies, nutritional education and, 164
food, function of, 137
food labels, 155
healthy weight, and, 136
Internet research, 163
performance-enhancing drinks
caffeine, 160
energy drinks, 162
hyponatremia, 162
sports drinks, 161
shift work, and, 303
sodium, role of, 157

obesity, 179
Ontario Police Fitness Award (OPFA) Standards
1.5-mile run, 353
curl-ups, 350
purpose, 338, 348
push-ups, 349
trunk forward flexion, 352
Osgood-Schlatter disease, 320-21
osteoporosis, 246-49
overload principle, 61, 94

PARE test
apprehension section, 345-47
faults and penalties, 347
purpose, 341
pursuit course, 343-45
screening, 342
torso bag carry, 348
Peel Regional Police Fitness Standards
100-yard sprint, 356
bench press, 353
chin-ups, 355
performance-enhancing substances, 100, 160
periodization, 63, 99
personal goals, 30
patello-femoral syndrome, 319
Physical Abilities Requirement Evaluation (PARE) test, *see* PARE test
physical activity
defined, 4
factors affecting participation, 29
health benefits of, 9

- physical benefits, 59
- psychological benefits, 60

physical fitness
- cardiorespiratory, *see* cardiorespiratory fitness
- defined, 5
- health-related fitness
  - body composition, 57
  - cardiorespiratory endurance, 56
  - flexibility, 57
  - muscular endurance, 57
  - muscular strength, 57
- performance-related fitness
  - agility, 58
  - balance, 58
  - coordination, 58
  - power, 59
  - reaction time, 58
  - speed, 58
- training, 56

physical fitness log, 356

Physical Readiness Evaluation for Police (PREP) test, *see* PREP test

physical training
- methods
  - concurrent, 64
  - fartlek, 64
  - interval, 64
  - periodization, 63
  - plyometric, 64
  - resistance, 64
- principles, 60
  - diminishing returns, 62
  - individuality, 62
  - progression, 62
  - progressive overload, 61
  - recovery, 63
  - reversibility, 62
  - specificity, 61
- program, guidelines for starting, 65

plantar fasciitis, 320

plyometric training, 64, 95, 104

police application process
- competencies, 15
- fitness testing, 17, 337-57
- local needs, police services, 17

portion size, 153

post-traumatic stress disorder (PTSD), 277

power, 59

power training, 95

PREP test
- aerobic fitness test, 340
- purpose, 338
- pursuit/restraint circuit, 339

principle of diminishing returns, 62

principle of overload, 61, 94

principle of progression, 62

principle of recovery, 63

principle of reversibility, 62

principle of specificity, 61

procrastination, 43

professional goals, 3

progression, 62

progressive muscle relaxation, 286

progressive overload, 61

proprioceptive neuromuscular facilitation (PNF), 119

protein, 148

protein supplements, 151

psychosomatic symptoms, 271

pyramid training, 104

reaction time, 58

recovery, 63

relaxation techniques
- autogenic feedback, 286
- biofeedback, 288
- breathing, 285
- hydrotherapy, 289
- hypnosis, 288
- massage, 289
- meditation, 285
- music, 288
- progressive muscle relaxation, 286
- shift work, and, 304
- T'ai Chi Ch'uan, 288
- visualization, 287
- yoga, 288

REM sleep, 299

repetitions, 95

repetitive strain injury (RSI), 253

resistance training, 64, 92

resting heart rate, 76

restless legs syndrome (RLS), 301

reversibility, 62

RICE principle, 312

saturated fats, 145
sciatica, 255
self-efficacy, 28
self-esteem, 27
set, 95
shift work
  coping strategies
    circadian rhythm, use of, 304
    eating nutritious food, 303
    light, role of, 303
    new friendships, development of, 305
    noise reduction, 305
    physical activity, 304
    power napping, 305
    relaxation techniques, 304
    sleeping effectively, 305
  diabetes, 202
  effects of
    physiological and psychological effects, 300
    sleep disorders, 301
    social effects, 302
  scheduling, 298
  sleep, importance of, 299
shin splints, 319
shuttle run, 83
skinfold measurements, 181
sleep apnea, 302
sleep disorders, 301
social involvement, 3
sodium, 157
somatotypes, 178
specificity, 61
speed, 58
spine, 244
sports drinks, 161
sprain, 314
static stretching, 119
strain, 314
strength and endurance training
  basics, 94
  frequency, 98
  goals, 102
  guidelines, 97
  hypertrophy in muscles, training and, 99
  importance of, 91
  muscle action, types of, 96
  muscle fibre, types of, 93
  performance-enhancing substances, 100
  periodization training, 99
  programs, 108
  variations on routines, 100
    breathing techniques, 103
    choice of system, 103
    correct form, importance of, 102
    load, determination of, 103
    plyometrics, 104
    program design, 105
    selecting and arranging exercises, 102
    trisets, 101
    warm-up, 102
stress
  additional, causes of, 281
  behaviour types, and
    type A, 282
    type B, 282
    type C, 282-83
  coping mechanisms, 283-84
  critical incidents
    definition of, 275
    factors affecting responses to, 276
    helping colleague cope, 279-81
    symptoms of stress arising out of, 277
    types of, 275
  definition of, 270
  effects of, 271
  relaxation techniques
    autogenic feedback, 286
    biofeedback, 288
    breathing, 285
    hydrotherapy, 289
    hypnosis, 288
    massage, 289
    meditation, 285
    music, 288
    progressive muscle relaxation, 286
    T'ai Chi Ch'uan, 288
    visualization, 287
    yoga, 288
  stress response, 270
  stressors
    daily life, 273
    law enforcement, 273
    workplace health and safety hazards, 274
  types of, 270
stressors
  daily life, 273

law enforcement, 273
workplace health and safety hazards, 274
stretching
benefits of, 116
exercises
Achilles stretch, 127
arm across body stretch, 123
back extension stretch, 124
biceps stretch, 120
calf stretch,127
chest stretch, 122
forward lunge, 126
front of shoulder and chest stretch, 122
groin stretch, 125, 126
hamstring stretch, 124, 127
head turn and tilt, 120
leg spinal twist, 125
lower-back stretch, 124
modified hurdle stretch, 125
quadriceps stretch, 126
shoulder stretch, 120
side stretch, 123
triceps stretch, 122
trunk stretch, 123
guidelines, 119
muscle contractions, types of, 118
muscle cooperation, and, 117
techniques
ballistic stretching, 118
dynamic stretching, 118
proprioceptive neuromuscular facilitation (PNF), 119
static stretching, 119
stroke, 226
stroke prevention, 228
subarachnoid hemorrhage, 226
superset training, 104

T'ai Chi Ch'uan, 288
talk test, 78
target heart rate (THR) zone, 77, 78
tendinitis, 316
time management
benefits of, 40
implementing activities, 42
delegation, 46
meetings, effective running, 46
organizing assignments, 45
procrastination, 43
prioritizing activities, 41
scheduling activities, 41
stages of, 40
trans fats, 145
transient ischemic attack, 226
trisets, 101
type 1 diabetes, 196
type 2 diabetes, 196

unsaturated fats, 147

values, 29
vegetarianism, 159
vehicles, sitting in, 258
vertebrae, 244
visualization, 287
vitality, 9
vitamins, 138, 139

waist circumference (WC), 180
waist-to-hip ratio (WHR) measurement, 182
warm-up, 102
water, 138
weight training, *see* strength and endurance training
wellness
defined, 9
relationship to fitness, 4
wellness/illness continuum, 12
wellness/illness continuum, 12
wellness profile, 3
wind chill index, 328
winter running, 80
Workplace Hazardous Materials Information System (WHMIS), 330

yoga, 288